Introduction to Meta-Analysis

Introduction to Meta-Analysis

Michael Borenstein
Biostat, Inc, New Jersey, USA.

Larry V. Hedges
Northwestern University, Evanston, USA.

Julian P.T. Higgins
MRC, Cambridge, UK.

Hannah R. Rothstein
Baruch College, New York, USA.

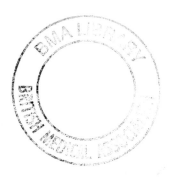

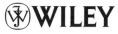

A John Wiley and Sons, Ltd., Publication

This edition first published 2009
© 2009 John Wiley & Sons, Ltd

Registered office
John Wiley & Sons Ltd, The Atrium, Southern Gate, Chichester, West Sussex, PO19 8SQ, United Kingdom

For details of our global editorial offices, for customer services and for information about how to apply for permission to reuse the copyright material in this book please see our website at www.wiley.com.

The right of the author to be identified as the author of this work has been asserted in accordance with the Copyright, Designs and Patents Act 1988.

Library of Congress Cataloguing-in-Publication Data

Introduction to meta-analysis / Michael Borenstein . . . [et al.].
       p.   ;   cm.
   Includes bibliographical references and index.
   ISBN 978-0-470-05724-7 (cloth)
   1. Meta-analysis.   I. Borenstein, Michael.
   [DNLM: 1. Meta-Analysis as Topic.   WA 950 I614 2009].
   R853.M48I58 2009
   610.72—dc22

                              2008043732

A catalogue record for this book is available from the British Library.

ISBN: 978-0-470-05724-7 (H/B)

Set in 10.5/13pt Times by Integra Software Services Pvt. Ltd, Pondicherry, India
Printed and bound by CPI Group (UK) Ltd, Croydon, CR0 4YY

8 2013

Contents

List of Tables

List of Figures

Acknowledgements

This book was funded by the following grants from the National Institutes of Health: *Combining data types in meta-analysis* (AG021360), *Publication bias in meta-analysis* (AG20052), *Software for meta-regression* (AG024771), From the National Institute on Aging, under the direction of Dr. Sidney Stahl; and *Forest plots for meta-analysis* (DA019280), from the National Institute on Drug Abuse, under the direction of Dr. Thomas Hilton.

These grants allowed us to convene a series of workshops on meta-analysis, and parts of this volume reflect ideas developed as part of these workshops. We would like to acknowledge and thank Doug Altman, Betsy Becker, Jesse Berlin, Michael Brannick, Harris Cooper, Kay Dickersin, Sue Duval, Roger Harbord, Despina Contopoulos-Ioannidis, John Ioannidis, Spyros Konstantopoulos, Mark Lipsey, Mike McDaniel, Ingram Olkin, Fred Oswald, Terri Pigott, Simcha Pollack, David Rindskopf, Stephen Senn, Will Shadish, Jonathan Sterne, Alex Sutton, Thomas Trikalinos, Jeff Valentine, Jack Vevea, Vish Viswesvaran, and David Wilson.

Steven Tarlow helped to edit this book and to ensure the accuracy of all formulas and examples.

As always, the people at Wiley made this endeavor a pleasure. We want to acknowledge and thank our editor Kathryn Sharples, and also Graham Woodward, Susan Barclay, Beth Dufour, Heather Kay, and Sunita Jayachandran.

Vivian Vargas and Shirley Rudolph at Biostat, and Patricia Ferguson at Northwestern University provided invaluable administrative assistance.

Preface

In his best-selling book *Baby and Child Care*, Dr. Benjamin Spock wrote 'I think it is preferable to accustom a baby to sleeping on his stomach from the beginning if he is willing'. This statement was included in most editions of the book, and in most of the 50 million copies sold from the 1950s into the 1990s. The advice was not unusual, in that many pediatricians made similar recommendations at the time.

During this same period, from the 1950s into the 1990s, more than 100,000 babies died of sudden infant death syndrome (SIDS), also called *crib death* in the United States and *cot death* in the United Kingdom, where a seemingly healthy baby goes to sleep and never wakes up.

In the early 1990s, researchers became aware that the risk of SIDS decreased by at least 50% when babies were put to sleep on their backs rather than face down. Governments in various countries launched educational initiatives such as the *Back to sleep* campaigns in the UK and the US, which led to an immediate and dramatic drop in the number of SIDS deaths.

While the loss of more than 100,000 children would be unspeakably sad in any event, the real tragedy lies in the fact that many of these deaths could have been prevented. Gilbert *et al.* (2005) write

> 'Advice to put infants to sleep on the front for nearly half a century was contrary to evidence available from 1970 that this was likely to be harmful. Systematic review of preventable risk factors for SIDS from 1970 would have led to earlier recognition of the risks of sleeping on the front and might have prevented over 10,000 infant deaths in the UK and at least 50,000 in the Europe, the USA and Australasia.'

AN ETHICAL IMPERATIVE

This example is one of several cited by Sir Iain Chalmers in a talk entitled *The scandalous failure of scientists to cumulate scientifically* (Chalmers, 2006). The theme of this talk was that we live in a world where the utility of almost any intervention will be tested repeatedly, and that rather than looking at any study in isolation, we need to look at the body of evidence. While not all systematic reviews carry the urgency of SIDS, the logic of looking at the body of evidence, rather than trying to understand studies in isolation, is always compelling.

Meta-analysis refers to the statistical synthesis of results from a series of studies. While the statistical procedures used in a meta-analysis can be applied to any set of data, the synthesis will be meaningful only if the studies have been collected systematically. This could be in the context of a systematic review, the process of systematically locating, appraising, and then synthesizing data from a large number of sources. Or, it could be in the context of synthesizing data from a select group of studies, such as those conducted by a pharmaceutical company to assess the efficacy of a new drug.

If a treatment effect (or effect size) is consistent across the series of studies, these procedures enable us to report that the effect is robust across the kinds of populations sampled, and also to estimate the magnitude of the effect more precisely than we could with any of the studies alone. If the treatment effect varies across the series of studies, these procedures enable us to report on the range of effects, and may enable us to identify factors associated with the magnitude of the effect size.

FROM NARRATIVE REVIEWS TO SYSTEMATIC REVIEWS

Prior to the 1990s, the task of combining data from multiple studies had been primarily the purview of the narrative review. An expert in a given field would read the studies that addressed a question, summarize the findings, and then arrive at a conclusion – for example, that the treatment in question was, or was not, effective. However, this approach suffers from some important limitations.

One limitation is the subjectivity inherent in this approach, coupled with the lack of transparency. For example, different reviewers might use different criteria for deciding which studies to include in the review. Once a set of studies has been selected, one reviewer might give more credence to larger studies, while another gives more credence to 'quality' studies and yet another assigns a comparable weight to all studies. One reviewer may require a substantial body of evidence before concluding that a treatment is effective, while another uses a lower threshold. In fact, there are examples in the literature where two narrative reviews come to opposite conclusions, with one reporting that a treatment is effective while the other reports that it is not. As a rule, the narrative reviewer will not articulate (and may not even be fully aware of) the decision-making process used to synthesize the data and arrive at a conclusion.

A second limitation of narrative reviews is that they become *less useful as more information becomes available*. The thought process required for a synthesis requires the reviewer to capture the finding reported in each study, to assign an appropriate *weight* to that finding, and then to synthesize these findings across all studies in the synthesis. While a reviewer may be able to synthesize data from a few studies in their head, the process becomes difficult and eventually untenable as the number of studies increases. This is true even when the treatment effect (or effect size) is consistent from study to study. Often, however, the treatment effect will vary as a function of study-level covariates, such as the patient population, the dose of medication, the outcome variable, and other factors. In these cases, a proper synthesis requires that the researcher be able to understand how the treatment effect varies as a function of these variables, and the narrative review is poorly equipped to address these kinds of issues.

THE SYSTEMATIC REVIEW AND META-ANALYSIS

For these reasons, beginning in the mid 1980s and taking root in the 1990s, researchers in many fields have been moving away from the narrative review, and adopting systematic reviews and meta-analysis.

For systematic reviews, a clear set of rules is used to search for studies, and then to determine which studies will be included in or excluded from the analysis. Since there is an element of subjectivity in setting these criteria, as well as in the conclusions drawn from the meta-analysis, we cannot say that the systematic review is entirely objective. However, because all of the decisions are specified clearly, the mechanisms are transparent.

A key element in most systematic reviews is the statistical synthesis of the data, or the meta-analysis. Unlike the narrative review, where reviewers implicitly assign some level of importance to each study, in meta-analysis the weights assigned to each study are based on mathematical criteria that are specified in advance. While the reviewers and readers may still differ on the substantive meaning of the results (as they might for a primary study), the statistical analysis provides a transparent, objective, and replicable framework for this discussion.

The formulas used in meta-analysis are extensions of formulas used in primary studies, and are used to address similar kinds of questions to those addressed in primary studies. In primary studies we would typically report a mean and standard deviation for the subjects. If appropriate, we might also use analysis of variance or multiple regression to determine if (and how) subject scores were related to various factors. Similarly, in a meta-analysis, we might report a mean and standard deviation for the treatment effect. And, if appropriate, we would also use procedures analogous to analysis of variance or multiple regression to assess the relationship between the effect and study-level covariates.

Meta-analyses are conducted for a variety of reasons, not only to synthesize evidence on the effects of interventions or to support evidence-based policy or practice. The purpose of the meta-analysis, or more generally, the purpose of any research synthesis has implications for *when* it should be performed, what model should be used to analyze the data, what sensitivity analyses should be undertaken, and how the results should be interpreted. Losing sight of the fact that meta-analysis is a tool with multiple applications causes confusion and leads to pointless discussions about *what is the right way to perform a research synthesis*, when there is no single right way. It all depends on the purpose of the synthesis, and the data that are available. Much of this book will expand on this idea.

META-ANALYSIS IS USED IN MANY FIELDS OF RESEARCH

In medicine, systematic reviews and meta-analysis form the core of a movement to ensure that medical treatments are based on the best available empirical data. For example, The Cochrane Collaboration has published the results of over 3700 meta-analyses (as of January 2009) which synthesize data on treatments in all areas of health care including headaches, cancer, allergies, cardiovascular disease, pain pre-vention, and depression. The reviews look at interventions relevant to neo-natal care, childbirth, infant and childhood diseases, as well as diseases common in adolescents, adults, and the elderly. The kinds of interventions assessed include surgery, drugs, acupuncture, and social interventions. BMJ publishes a series of journals on Evidence Based Medicine, built on the results from systematic reviews. Systematic reviews and meta-analyses are also used to examine the performance of diagnostic tests, and of epidemiological associations between exposure and disease prevalence, among other topics.

Pharmaceutical companies usually conduct a series of studies to assess the efficacy of a drug. They use meta-analysis to synthesize the data from these studies, yielding a more powerful test (and more precise estimate) of the drug's effect. Additionally, the meta-analysis provides a framework for evaluating the series of studies as a whole, rather than looking at each in isolation. These analyses play a role in internal research, in submissions to governmental agencies, and in market-ing. Meta-analyses are also used to synthesize data on adverse events, since these events are typically rare and we need to accumulate information over a series of studies to properly assess the risk of these events.

In the field of education, meta-analysis has been applied to topics as diverse as the comparison of distance education with traditional classroom learning, assess-ment of the impact of schooling on developing economies, and the relationship between teacher credentials and student achievement. Results of these and similar meta-analyses have influenced practice and policy in various locations around the world.

In psychology, meta-analysis has been applied to basic science as well as in support of evidence-based practice. It has been used to assess personality change over the life span, to assess the influence of media violence on aggressive behavior, and to examine gender differences in mathematics ability, leadership, and nonverbal communication. Meta-analyses of psychological interventions have been use to compare and select treatments for psychological problems, including obsessive-compulsive disorder, impulsivity disorder, bulimia nervosa, depression, phobias, and panic disorder.

In the field of criminology, government agencies have funded meta-analyses to examine the relative effectiveness of various programs in reducing criminal beha-vior. These include initiatives to prevent delinquency, reduce recidivism, assess the effectiveness of different strategies for police patrols, and for the use of special courts to deal with drug-related crimes.

In business, meta-analyses of the predictive validity of tests that are used as part of the hiring process, have led to changes in the types of tests that are used to select employees in many organizations. Meta-analytic results have also been used to guide practices for the reduction of absenteeism, turnover, and counterproductive behavior, and to assess the effectiveness of programs used to train employees.

In the field of ecology, meta-analyses are being used to identify the environmental impact of wind farms, biotic resistance to exotic plant invasion, the effects of changes in the marine food chain, plant reactions to global climate change, the effectiveness of conservation management interventions, and to guide conservation efforts.

META-ANALYSIS AS PART OF THE RESEARCH PROCESS

Systematic reviews and meta-analyses are used to synthesize the available evidence for a given question to inform policy, as in the examples cited above from medicine, social science, business, ecology, and other fields. While this is probably the most common use of the methodology, meta-analysis can also play an important role in other parts of the research process.

Systematic reviews and meta-analyses can play a role in designing new research. As a first step, they can help determine whether the planned study is necessary. It may be possible to find the required information by synthesizing data from prior studies, and in this case, the research should not be performed. Iain Chalmers (2007) made this point in an article entitled *The lethal consequences of failing to make use of all relevant evidence about the effects of medical treatments: the need for systematic reviews.*

In the event that the new study *is needed*, the meta-analysis may be useful in helping to design that study. For example, the meta-analysis may show that in the prior studies one outcome index had proven to be more sensitive than others, or that a specific mode of administration had proven to be more effective than others, and should be used in the planned study as well.

For these reasons, various government agencies, including institutes of health in various countries, have been encouraging (or requiring) researchers to conduct a meta-analysis of existing research prior to undertaking new funded studies.

The systematic review can also play a role in the publication of any new primary study. In the introductory section of the publication, a systematic review can help to place the new study in context by describing what we knew before, and what we hoped to learn from the new study. In the discussion section of the publication, a systematic review allows us to address not only the information provided by the new study, but the body of evidence as enhanced by the new study. Iain Chalmers and Michael Clarke (1998) see this approach as a way to avoid studies being reported without context, which they refer to as 'Islands in Search of Continents'. Systematic reviews would provide this context in a more rigorous and transparent manner than the narrative reviews that are typically used for this purpose.

THE INTENDED AUDIENCE FOR THIS BOOK

Since meta-analysis is a relatively new field, many people, including those who actually use meta-analysis in their work, have not had the opportunity to learn about it systematically. We hope that this volume will provide a framework that allows them to understand the logic of meta-analysis, as well as how to apply and interpret meta-analytic procedures properly.

This book is aimed at researchers, clinicians, and statisticians. Our approach is primarily conceptual. The reader will be able to skip the formulas and still understand, for example, the differences between fixed-effect and random-effects analysis, and the mechanisms used to assess the dispersion in effects from study to study. However, for those with a statistical orientation, we include all the relevant formulas, along with worked examples. Additionally, the spreadsheets and data files can be downloaded from the web at www.Meta-Analysis.com.

This book can be used as the basis for a course in meta-analysis. Supplementary materials and exercises are posted on the book's web site.

This volume is intended for readers from various substantive fields, including medicine, epidemiology, social science, business, ecology, and others. While we have included examples from many of these disciplines, the more important message is that meta-analytic methods that may have developed in any one of these fields have application to all of them.

Since our goal in using these examples is to explain the meta-analysis itself rather than to address the substantive issues, we provide only the information needed for this purpose. For example, we may present an analysis showing that a treatment reduces pain, while ignoring other analyses that show the same treatment increases the risk of adverse events. Therefore, any reader interested in the substantive issues addressed in an example should not rely on this book for that purpose.

AN OUTLINE OF THIS BOOK'S CONTENTS

Part 1 is an introduction to meta-analysis. We present a completed meta-analysis to serve as an example, and highlight the elements of this analysis – the effect size for each study, the summary effect, the dispersion of effects across studies, and so on. Our intent is to show where each element fits into the analysis, and thus provide the reader with a context as they move on to the subsequent parts of the book where each of the elements is explored in detail.

Part 2 introduces the effect sizes, such as the standardized mean difference or the risk ratio, that are computed for each study, and that serve as the unit of currency in the meta-analysis. We also discuss factors that determine the variance of an effect size and show how to compute the variance for each study, since this affects the weight assigned to that study in the meta-analysis.

Part 3 discusses the two computational models used in the vast majority of meta-analyses, the fixed-effect model and the random-effects model. We discuss the conceptual and practical differences between the two, and show how to compute a summary effect using either one.

Part 4 focuses on the issue of dispersion in effect sizes, the fact that the effect size varies from one study to the next. We discuss methods to quantify the heterogeneity, to test it, to incorporate it in the weighting scheme, and to understand it in a substantive as well as a statistical context. Then, we discuss methods to explain the heterogeneity. These include subgroup analyses to compare the effect in different subgroups of studies (analogous to analysis of variance in primary studies), and meta-regression (analogous to multiple regression).

Part 5 shows how to work with complex data structures. These include studies that report an effect size for two or more independent subgroups, for two or more outcomes or time-points, and for two or more comparison groups (such as two treatments being compared with the same control).

Part 6 is used to address three separate issues. One chapter discusses the procedure called vote counting, common in narrative reviews, and explains the problems with this approach. One chapter discusses statistical power for a meta-analysis. We show how meta-analysis often (but not always) yields a more powerful test of the null than do any of the included studies. Another chapter addresses the question of publication bias. We explain what this is, and discuss methods that have been developed to assess its potential impact.

Part 7 focuses on the issue of why we work with effect sizes in a meta-analysis. In one chapter we explain why we work with effect sizes rather than p-values. In another we explain why we compute an effect size for each study, rather than summing data over all studies and then computing an effect size for the summed data. The final chapter in this part shows how the use of inverse-variance weights can be extended to other applications including Bayesian meta-analysis and analyses based on individual participant data.

Part 8 includes chapters on methods that are sometimes used in meta-analysis but that fall outside the central narrative of this volume. These include meta-analyses based on p-values, alternate approaches (such as the Mantel-Haenszel method) for assigning study weights, and options sometimes used in psychometric meta-analyses.

Part 9 is dedicated to a series of general issues related to meta-analysis. We address the question of when it makes sense to perform a meta-analysis. This Part is also the location for a series of chapters on separate issues such as reporting the results of a meta-analysis, and the proper use of cumulative meta-analysis. Finally, we discuss some of the criticisms of meta-analysis and try to put them in context.

Part 10 is a discussion of resources for meta-analysis and systematic reviews. This includes an overview of several computer programs for meta-analysis. It also includes a discussion of organizations that promote the use of systematic reviews and meta-analyses in specific fields, and a list of useful web sites.

WHAT THIS BOOK DOES NOT COVER

Other elements of a systematic review

This book deals only with meta-analysis, the statistical formulas and methods used to synthesize data from a set of studies. A meta-analysis can be applied to any data, but if the goal of the analysis is to provide a synthesis of a body of data from various sources, then it is usually imperative that the data be compiled as part of a systematic review.

A systematic review incorporates many components, such as specification of the question to be addressed, determination of methods to be used for searching the literature and for including or excluding studies, specification of mechanisms to appraise the validity of the included studies, specification of methods to be used for performing the statistical analysis, and a mechanism for disseminating the results.

If the entire review is performed properly, so that the search strategy matches the research question, and yields a reasonably complete and unbiased collection of the relevant studies, then (providing that the included studies are themselves valid) the meta-analysis will also be addressing the intended question. On the other hand, if the search strategy is flawed in concept or execution, or if the studies are providing biased results, then problems exist in the review that the meta-analysis cannot correct.

In Part 10 we include an annotated listing of suggested readings for the other components in the systematic review, but these components are not otherwise addressed in this volume.

Other meta-analytic methods

In this volume we focus primarily on meta-analyses of effect sizes. That is, analyses where each study yields an estimate of some statistic (a standardized mean difference, a risk ratio, a prevalence, and so on) and our goal is to assess the dispersion in these effects and (if appropriate) compute a summary effect. The vast majority of meta-analyses performed use this approach. We deal only briefly (see Part 8) with other approaches, such as meta-analyses that combine p-values rather than effect sizes. We do not address meta-analysis of diagnostic tests.

Further Reading

Chalmers, I. (2007). The lethal consequences of failing to make use of all relevant evidence about the effects of medical treatments: the need for systematic reviews. In P. Rothwell(ed.), *Treating Individuals*, ed. London: Lancet: 37–58.

Chalmers, I., Hedges, L.V. & Cooper, H. (2002). A brief history of research synthesis. *Evaluation in the Health Professions*. 25(1): 12–37.

Clarke, M, Hopewell, S. & Chalmers, I. (2007). Reports of clinical trials should begin and end with up-to-date systematic reviews of other relevant evidence: a status report. *Journal of the Royal Society of Medicine*. 100: 187–190.

Hunt, M. (1999). *How Science Takes Stock: The Story of Meta-analysis*. New York: Russell Sage Foundation.

Sutton, A.J. & Higgins, J.P.T. (2008). Recent developments in meta-analysis. *Statistics in Medicine* 27: 625–650.

Web Site

The web site for this book is www.Meta-Analysis.com.
There, you will find easy access to

- All of the datasets used in this book
- All computations from this book as Excel spreadsheets
- Additional formulas for computing effect sizes
- Any corrections to this book
- Links to other meta-analysis sites
- A free trial of Comprehensive Meta Analysis

For those planning to use this book as a text, there are also worked examples and exercises.

Please send any questions or comments to MichaelB@Meta-Analysis.com

PART 1

Introduction

CHAPTER 1

How a Meta-Analysis Works

Introduction
Individual studies
The summary effect
Heterogeneity of effect sizes

INTRODUCTION

Figure 1.1 illustrates a meta-analysis that shows the impact of high dose versus standard dose of statins in preventing death and myocardial infarction (MI). This analysis is adapted from one reported by Cannon *et al.* and published in the *Journal of the American College of Cardiology* (2006).

Our goal in presenting this here is to introduce the various elements in a meta-analysis (the effect size for each study, the weight assigned to each effect size, the estimate of the summary effect, and so on) and show where each fits into the larger scheme. In the chapters that follow, each of these elements will be explored in detail.

INDIVIDUAL STUDIES

The first four rows on this plot represent the four studies. For each, the study name is shown at left, followed by the effect size, the relative weight assigned to the study for computing the summary effect, and the *p*-value. The effect size and weight are also shown schematically.

Effect size

The effect size, a value which reflects the magnitude of the treatment effect or (more generally) the strength of a relationship between two variables, is the unit of currency in a meta-analysis. We compute the effect size for each study, and then

Introduction to Meta-Analysis   M. Borenstein, L. V. Hedges, J. P. T. Higgins, H. R. Rothstein
© 2009, John Wiley & Sons, Ltd

Impact of Statin Dose
On Death and Myocardial Infarction

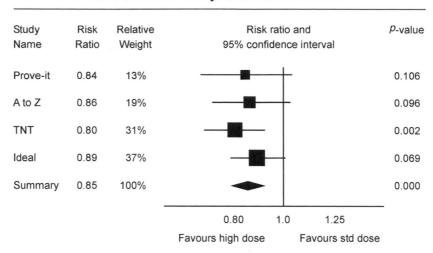

Study Name	Risk Ratio	Relative Weight	Risk ratio and 95% confidence interval				P-value
Prove-it	0.84	13%					0.106
A to Z	0.86	19%					0.096
TNT	0.80	31%					0.002
Ideal	0.89	37%					0.069
Summary	0.85	100%					0.000
			0.80	1.0	1.25		
			Favours high dose		Favours std dose		

Figure 1.1 High-dose versus standard-dose of statins (adapted from Cannon *et al.*, 2006).

work with the effect sizes to assess the consistency of the effect across studies and to compute a summary effect.

The effect size could represent the impact of an intervention, such as the impact of medical treatment on risk of infection, the impact of a teaching method on test scores, or the impact of a new protocol on the number of salmon successfully returning upstream. The effect size is not limited to the impact of interventions, but could represent *any relationship* between two variables, such as the difference in test scores for males versus females, the difference in cancer rates for persons exposed or not exposed to second-hand smoke, or the difference in cardiac events for persons with two distinct personality types. In fact, what we generally call an *effect size* could refer simply to the estimate of a single value, such as the prevalence of Lyme disease.

In this example the effect size is the risk ratio. A risk ratio of 1.0 would mean that the risk of death or MI was the same in both groups, while a risk ratio less than 1.0 would mean that the risk was lower in the high-dose group, and a risk ratio greater than 1.0 would mean that the risk was lower in the standard-dose group.

The effect size for each study is represented by a square, with the location of the square representing both the direction and magnitude of the effect. Here, the effect size for each study falls to the left of center (indicating a benefit for the high-dose group). The effect is strongest (most distant from the center) in the *TNT* study and weakest in the *Ideal* study.

Note. For measures of effect size based on ratios (as in this example) a ratio of 1.0 represents no difference between groups. For measures of effect based on differences (such as mean difference), a difference of 0.0 represents no difference between groups.

Precision

In the schematic, the effect size for each study is bounded by a confidence interval, reflecting the precision with which the effect size has been estimated in that study. The confidence interval for the last study (*Ideal*) is noticeably narrower than that for the first study (*Prove-it*), reflecting the fact that the *Ideal* study has greater precision. The meaning of precision and the factors that affect precision are discussed in Chapter 8.

Study weights

The solid squares that are used to depict each of the studies vary in size, with the size of each square reflecting the weight that is assigned to the corresponding study when we compute the summary effect. The *TNT* and *Ideal* studies are assigned relatively high weights, while somewhat less weight is assigned to the *A to Z* study and still less to the *Prove-it* study.

As one would expect, there is a relationship between a study's precision and that study's weight in the analysis. Studies with relatively good precision (*TNT* and *Ideal*) are assigned more weight while studies with relatively poor precision (*Prove-it*) are assigned less weight. Since precision is driven primarily by sample size, we can think of the studies as being weighted by sample size.

However, while precision is one of the elements used to assign weights, there are often other elements as well. In Part 3 we discuss different assumptions that one can make about the distribution of effect sizes across studies, and how these affect the weight assigned to each study.

p-values

For each study we show the *p*-value for a test of the null. There is a necessary correspondence between the *p*-value and the confidence interval, such that the *p*-value will fall under 0.05 if and only if the 95% confidence interval does not include the null value. Therefore, by scanning the confidence intervals we can easily identify the statistically significant studies. The role of *p*-values in the analysis, as well as the relationship between *p*-values and effect size, is discussed in Chapter 32.

In this example, for three of the four studies the confidence interval crosses the null, and the *p*-value is greater than 0.05. In one (the *TNT* study) the confidence interval does not cross the null, and the *p*-value falls under 0.05.

THE SUMMARY EFFECT

One goal of the synthesis is usually to compute a summary effect. Typically we report the effect size itself, as well as a measure of precision and a *p*-value.

Effect size

On the plot the summary effect is shown on the bottom line. In this example the summary risk ratio is 0.85, indicating that the risk of death (or MI) was 15% lower for patients assigned to the high dose than for patients assigned to standard dose.

The summary effect is nothing more than the weighted mean of the individual effects. However, the mechanism used to assign the weights (and therefore the meaning of the summary effect) depends on our assumptions about the distribution of effect sizes from which the studies were sampled. Under the fixed-effect model, we assume that all studies in the analysis share the same true effect size, and the summary effect is our estimate of this common effect size. Under the random-effects model, we assume that the true effect size varies from study to study, and the summary effect is our estimate of the mean of the distribution of effect sizes. This is discussed in Part 3.

Precision

The summary effect is represented by a diamond. The location of the diamond represents the effect size while its width reflects the precision of the estimate. In this example the diamond is centered at 0.85, and extends from 0.79 to 0.92, meaning that the actual impact of the high dose (as compared to the standard) likely falls somewhere in that range.

The precision addresses the accuracy of the summary effect as an estimate of the true effect. However, as discussed in Part 3 the exact meaning of the precision depends on the statistical model.

p-value

The *p*-value for the summary effect is 0.00003. This *p*-value reflects both the magnitude of the summary effect size and also the volume of information on which the estimate is based. Note that the *p*-value for the summary effect is substantially more compelling than that of any single study. Indeed, only one of the four studies had a *p*-value under 0.05. The relationship between *p*-values and effect sizes is discussed in Chapter 32.

HETEROGENEITY OF EFFECT SIZES

In this example the treatment effect is consistent across all studies (by a criterion explained in Chapter 16), but such is not always the case. A key theme in this volume is the importance of assessing the dispersion of effect sizes from study to study, and then taking this into account when interpreting the data. If the effect size is consistent, then we will usually focus on the summary effect, and note that this effect is robust across the domain of studies included in the analysis. If the effect size varies modestly, then we might still report the summary effect but note that the true effect in any given study could be somewhat lower or higher than this value. If the effect varies substantially from one study to the next, our attention will shift from the summary effect to the dispersion itself.

Because the dispersion in observed effects is partly spurious (it includes both real difference in effects and also random error), before trying to interpret the variation in effects we need to determine what part (if any) of the observed variation is real. In Part 4 we show how to partition the observed variance into the part due to error and the part that represents variation in true effect sizes, and then how to use this information in various ways.

In this example our goal was to estimate the summary effect in a single population. In some cases, however, we will want to compare the effect size for one subgroup of studies versus another (say, for studies that used an elderly population versus those that used a relatively young population). In other cases we may want to assess the impact of putative moderators (or covariates) on the effect size (say, comparing the effect size in studies that used doses of 10, 20, 40, 80, 160 mg.). These kinds of analyses are also discussed in Part 4.

SUMMARY POINTS

- To perform a meta-analysis we compute an effect size and variance for each study, and then compute a weighted mean of these effect sizes.
- To compute the weighted mean we generally assign more weight to the more precise studies, but the rules for assigning weights depend on our assumptions about the distribution of true effects.

CHAPTER 2

Why Perform a Meta-Analysis

INTRODUCTION

Why perform a meta-analysis? What are the advantages of using statistical methods to synthesize data rather than taking the results that had been reported for each study and then having these collated and synthesized by an expert?

In this chapter we start at the point where we have already selected the studies to be included in the review, and are planning the synthesis itself. We do not address the differences between systematic reviews and narrative reviews in the process of locating and selecting studies. These differences can be critically important, but (as always) our focus is on the data analysis rather than the full process of the review.

The goal of a synthesis is to understand the results of any study in the context of all the other studies. First, we need to know whether or not the effect size is consistent across the body of data. If it *is* consistent, then we want to estimate the effect size as accurately as possible and to report that it is robust across the kinds of studies included in the synthesis. On the other hand, if it varies substantially from study to study, we want to quantify the extent of the variance and consider the implications.

Meta-analysis is able to address these issues whereas the narrative review is not. We start with an example to show how meta-analysis and narrative review would approach the same question, and then use this example to highlight the key differences between the two.

Introduction to Meta-Analysis   M. Borenstein, L. V. Hedges, J. P. T. Higgins, H. R. Rothstein
© 2009, John Wiley & Sons, Ltd

THE STREPTOKINASE META-ANALYSIS

During the time period beginning in 1959 and ending in 1988 (a span of nearly 30 years) there were a total of 33 randomized trials performed to assess the ability of streptokinase to prevent death following a heart attack. Streptokinase, a so-called *clot buster* which is administered intravenously, was hypothesized to dissolve the clot causing the heart attack, and thus increase the likelihood of survival. The trials all followed similar protocols, with patients assigned at random to either treatment or placebo. The outcome, whether or not the patient died, was the same in all the studies.

The trials varied substantially in size. The median sample size was slightly over 100 but there was one trial with a sample size in the range of 20 patients, and two large scale trials which enrolled some 12,000 and 17,000 patients, respectively. Of the 33 studies, six were statistically significant while the other 27 were not, leading to the perception that the studies yielded conflicting results.

In 1992 Lau *et al.* published a meta-analysis that synthesized the results from the 33 studies. The presentation that follows is based on the Lau paper (though we use a risk ratio where Lau used an odds ratio).

The forest plot (Figure 2.1) provides context for the analysis. An effect size to the left of center indicates that treated patients were more likely to survive, while an

Study name	Statistics for each study				Sample size	Year	Risk ratio and 95% CI
	Risk ratio	Lower limit	Upper limit	p-Value	Total		
Fletcher	0.229	0.030	1.750	0.155	23	1959	
Dewar	0.571	0.196	1.665	0.305	42	1963	
European 1	1.349	0.743	2.451	0.325	167	1969	
European 2	0.703	0.534	0.925	0.012	730	1971	
Heikinheimo	1.223	0.669	2.237	0.513	426	1971	
Italian	1.011	0.551	1.853	0.973	321	1971	
Australian 1	0.779	0.478	1.268	0.315	517	1973	
Franfurt 2	0.457	0.252	0.828	0.010	206	1973	
NHLBI SMIT	2.377	0.649	8.709	0.191	107	1974	
Frank	0.964	0.332	2.801	0.946	108	1975	
Valere	1.048	0.481	2.282	0.907	91	1975	
Klein	2.571	0.339	19.481	0.361	23	1976	
UK-Collab	0.922	0.609	1.394	0.699	595	1976	
Austrian	0.608	0.417	0.886	0.010	728	1977	
Australian 2	0.702	0.443	1.110	0.130	230	1977	
Lasierra	0.282	0.034	2.340	0.241	24	1977	
N Ger Collab	1.161	0.840	1.604	0.366	483	1977	
Witchitz	0.813	0.263	2.506	0.718	58	1977	
European 3	0.612	0.356	1.050	0.075	315	1979	
ISAM	0.880	0.619	1.250	0.476	1741	1986	
GISSI-1	0.827	0.749	0.914	0.000	11712	1986	
Olson	0.429	0.041	4.439	0.477	52	1986	
Baroffio	0.079	0.005	1.350	0.080	59	1986	
Schreiber	0.333	0.038	2.925	0.322	38	1986	
Cribier	1.095	0.073	16.427	0.948	44	1986	
Sainsous	0.500	0.132	1.887	0.306	98	1986	
Durand	0.621	0.151	2.555	0.510	64	1987	
White	0.174	0.040	0.761	0.020	219	1987	
Bassand	0.604	0.188	1.944	0.398	107	1987	
Vlay	0.462	0.048	4.461	0.504	25	1988	
Kennedy	0.654	0.322	1.331	0.241	368	1988	
ISIS-2	0.769	0.704	0.839	0.000	17187	1988	
Wisenberg	0.244	0.051	1.164	0.077	66	1988	
	0.794	0.724	0.870	0.000			

Figure 2.1 Impact of streptokinase on mortality (adapted from Lau *et al.*, 1992).

effect size to the right of center indicates that control patients were more likely to survive.

The plot serves to highlight the following points.

- The effect sizes are reasonably consistent from study to study. Most fall in the range of 0.50 to 0.90, which suggests that it would be appropriate to compute a summary effect size.
- The summary effect is a risk ratio of 0.79 with a 95% confidence interval of 0.72 to 0.87 (that is, a 21% decrease in risk of death, with 95% confidence interval of 13% to 28%). The p-value for the summary effect is 0.0000008.
- The confidence interval that bounds each effect size indicates the precision in that study. If the interval excludes 1.0, the p-value is less than 0.05 and the study is statistically significant. Six of the studies were statistically significant while 27 were not.

In sum, the treatment reduces the risk of death by some 21%. And, this effect was reasonably consistent across all studies in the analysis.

Over the course of this volume we explain the statistical procedures that led to these conclusions. Our goal in the present chapter is simply to explain that meta-analysis does offer these mechanisms, whereas the narrative review does not. The key differences are as follows.

STATISTICAL SIGNIFICANCE

One of the first questions asked of a study is the statistical significance of the results. The narrative review has no mechanism for synthesizing the p-values from the different studies, and must deal with them as discrete pieces of data. In this example six of the studies were statistically significant while the other 27 were not, which led some to conclude that there was evidence against an effect, or that the results were inconsistent (see vote counting in Chapter 28). By contrast, the meta-analysis allows us to combine the effects and evaluate the statistical significance of the summary effect. The p-value for the summary effect is $p = 0.0000008$.

While one might assume that 27 studies failed to reach statistical significance because they reported small effects, it is clear from the forest plot that this is not the case. In fact, the treatment effect in many of these studies was actually *larger* than the treatment effect in the six studies that *were* statistically significant. Rather, the reason that 82% of the studies were not statistically significant is that these studies had small sample sizes and low statistical power. In fact, as discussed in Chapter 29, most had power of less than 20%. By contrast, power for the meta-analysis exceeded 99.9% (see Chapter 29).

As in this example, if the goal of a synthesis is to test the null hypothesis, then meta-analysis provides a mathematically rigorous mechanism for this purpose. However, meta-analysis also allows us to move beyond the question of statistical significance, and address questions that are more interesting and also more relevant.

CLINICAL IMPORTANCE OF THE EFFECT

Since the point of departure for a narrative review is usually the p-values reported by the various studies, the review will often focus on the question of whether or not the body of evidence allows us to reject the null hypothesis. There is no good mechanism for discussing the magnitude of the effect. By contrast, the meta-analytic approaches discussed in this volume allow us to compute an estimate of the effect size for each study, and these effect sizes fall at the core of the analysis.

This is important because the effect size is what we care about. If a clinician or patient needs to make a decision about whether or not to employ a treatment, they want to know if the treatment reduces the risk of death by 5% or 10% or 20%, and this is the information carried by the effect size. Similarly, if we are thinking of implementing an intervention to increase the test scores of students, or to reduce the number of incarcerations among at-risk juveniles, or to increase the survival time for patients with pancreatic cancer, the question we ask is about the magnitude of the effect. The p-value can tell us only that the effect is not zero, and to report simply that the effect is not zero is to miss the point.

CONSISTENCY OF EFFECTS

When we are working with a collection of studies, it is critically important to ask whether or not the effect size is consistent across studies. The implications are quite different for a drug that consistently reduces the risk of death by 20%, as compared with a drug that reduces the risk of death by 20% on average, but that increases the risk by 20% in some populations while reducing it by 60% in others.

The narrative review has no good mechanism for assessing the consistency of effects. The narrative review starts with p-values, and because the p-value is driven by the size of a study as well as the effect in that study, the fact that one study reported a p-value of 0.001 and another reported a p-value of 0.50 does not mean that the effect was larger in the former. The p-value of 0.001 *could* reflect a large effect size but it could also reflect a moderate or small effect in a large study (see the GISSI-1 study in Figure 2.1, for example). The p-value of 0.50 *could* reflect a small (or nil) effect size but could also reflect a large effect in a small study (see the Fletcher study, for example).

This point is often missed in narrative reviews. Often, researchers interpret a nonsignificant result to mean that there is no effect. If some studies are statistically significant while others are not, the reviewers see the results as conflicting. This problem runs through many fields of research. To borrow a phrase from Cary Grant's character in *Arsenic and Old Lace*, we might say that it practically gallops.

Schmidt (1996) outlines the impact of this practice on research and policy. Suppose an idea is proposed that will improve test scores for African-American children. A number of studies are performed to test the intervention. The effect size is positive and consistent across studies but power is around 50%, and only around 50% of the studies yield statistically significant results. Researchers report that the evidence is 'conflicting' and launch a series of studies to determine why the intervention had a positive effect in some studies but not others (Is it the teacher's attitude? Is it the students' socioeconomic status?), entirely missing the point that the effect was actually consistent from one study to the next. No pattern can be found (since none exists). Eventually, researchers decide that the issue cannot be understood. A promising idea is lost, and a perception builds that research is not to be trusted. A similar point is made by Meehl (1978, 1990).

Rossi (1997) gives an example from the field of memory research that shows what can happen to a field of research when reviewers work with discrete p-values. The issue of whether or not researchers could demonstrate the spontaneous recovery of previously extinguished associations had a bearing on a number of important learning theories, and some 40 studies on the topic were published between 1948 and 1969. Evidence of the effect (that is, statistically significant findings) was obtained in only about half the studies, which led most texts and reviews to conclude that the effect was ephemeral and 'the issue was not so much resolved as it was abandoned' (p. 179). Later, Rossi returned to these studies and found that the average effect size (d) was 0.39. If we assume that this is the population effect size, the mean power for these studies would have been slightly under 50%. On this basis we would expect about half the studies to yield a significant effect, which is exactly what happened.

Even worse, when the significant study was performed in one type of sample and the nonsignificant study was performed in another type of sample, researchers would sometimes interpret this difference as meaning that the effect existed in one population but not the other. Abelson (1997) notes that if a treatment effect yields a p-value of 0.07 for wombats and 0.05 for dingbats we are likely to see a discussion explaining why the treatment is effective only in the latter group— completely missing the point that the treatment effect may have been virtually identical in the two. The treatment effect may have even been *larger* for the wombats if the sample size was smaller.

By contrast, meta-analysis completely changes the landscape. First, we work with effect sizes (not p-values) to determine whether or not the effect size is consistent across studies. Additionally, we apply methods based on statistical theory to allow that some (or all) of the observed dispersion is due to random sampling variation rather than differences in the true effect sizes. Then, we apply formulas to partition the variance into random error versus real variance, to quantify the true differences among studies, and to consider the implications of this variance. In the Schmidt and the Rossi examples, a meta-analysis might have found that the effect size was consistent across studies, and that all of the observed variation in effects could be attributed to random sampling error.

SUMMARY POINTS

- Since the narrative review is based on discrete reports from a series of studies, it provides no real mechanism for synthesizing the data. To borrow a phrase from Abelson, it involves *doing arithmetic with words*. And, when the words are based on p-values *the words are the wrong words*.
- By contrast, in a meta-analysis we introduce two fundamental changes. First, we work directly with the effect size from each study rather than the p-value. Second, we include all of the effects in a single statistical synthesis. This is critically important for the goal of computing (and testing) a summary effect. Meta-analysis also allows us to assess the dispersion of effects, and distinguish between real dispersion and spurious dispersion.

PART 2

Effect Size and Precision

CHAPTER 3

Overview

Treatment effects and effect sizes
Parameters and estimates
Outline of effect size computations

TREATMENT EFFECTS AND EFFECT SIZES

The terms *treatment effects* and *effect sizes* are used in different ways by different people. Meta-analyses in medicine often refer to the effect size as a *treatment effect*, and this term is sometimes assumed to refer to odds ratios, risk ratios, or risk differences, which are common in meta-analyses that deal with medical interventions. Similarly, meta-analyses in the social sciences often refer to the effect size simply as an *effect size* and this term is sometimes assumed to refer to standardized mean differences or to correlations, which are common in social science meta-analyses.

In fact, though, both the terms *effect size* and *treatment effect* can refer to any of these indices, and the distinction between these terms lies not in the index itself but rather in the nature of the study. The term *effect size* is appropriate when the index is used to quantify the relationship between two variables or a difference between two groups. By contrast, the term *treatment effect* is appropriate only for an index used to quantify the impact of a deliberate intervention. Thus, the difference between males and females could be called an *effect size* only, while the difference between treated and control groups could be called either an *effect size* or a *treatment effect*.

While most meta-analyses focus on relationships between variables, some have the goal of estimating a mean or risk or rate in a single population. For example, a meta-analysis might be used to combine several estimates for the prevalence of Lyme disease in Wabash or the mean SAT score for students in Utah. In these cases the index is clearly not a treatment effect, and is also not an effect size, since *effect* implies a relationship. Rather, the parameter being estimated could be called simply a *single group summary*.

Introduction to Meta-Analysis   M. Borenstein, L. V. Hedges, J. P. T. Higgins, H. R. Rothstein
© 2009, John Wiley & Sons, Ltd

Note, however, that the classification of an index as an *effect size* and/or a *treatment effect* (or simply a *single group summary*) has no bearing on the computations. In the meta-analysis itself we have simply a series of values and their variances, and the same mathematical formulas apply. In this volume we generally use the term *effect size*, but we use it in a generic sense, to include also treatment effects, single group summaries, or even a generic statistic.

How to choose an effect size

Three major considerations should drive the choice of an effect size index. The first is that the effect sizes from the different studies should be comparable to one another in the sense that they measure (at least approximately) the same thing. That is, the effect size should not depend on aspects of study design that may vary from study to study (such as sample size or whether covariates are used). The second is that estimates of the effect size should be computable from the information that is likely to be reported in published research reports. That is, it should not require the re-analysis of the raw data (unless these are known to be available). The third is that the effect size should have good technical properties. For example, its sampling distribution should be known so that variances and confidence intervals can be computed.

Additionally, the effect size should be substantively interpretable. This means that researchers in the substantive area of the work represented in the synthesis should find the effect size meaningful. If the effect size is not inherently meaningful, it is usually possible to transform the effect size to another metric for presentation. For example, the analyses may be performed using the log risk ratio but then transformed to a risk ratio (or even to illustrative risks) for presentation.

In practice, the kind of data used in the primary studies will usually lead to a pool of two or three effect sizes that meet the criteria outlined above, which makes the process of selecting an effect size relatively straightforward. If the summary data reported by the primary study are based on means and standard deviations in two groups, the appropriate effect size will usually be either the raw difference in means, the standardized difference in means, or the response ratio. If the summary data are based on a binary outcome such as events and non-events in two groups the appropriate effect size will usually be the risk ratio, the odds ratio, or the risk difference. If the primary study reports a correlation between two variables, then the correlation coefficient itself may serve as the effect size.

PARAMETERS AND ESTIMATES

Throughout this volume we make the distinction between an underlying effect size parameter (denoted by the Greek letter θ) and the sample estimate of that parameter (denoted by Y).

If a study had an infinitely large sample size then it would yield an effect size Y that was identical to the population parameter θ. In fact, though, sample sizes are finite and so the effect size estimate Y always differs from θ by some amount. The value of Y will vary from sample to sample, and the distribution of these values is the sampling distribution of Y. Statistical theory allows us to estimate the sampling distribution of effect size estimates, and hence their standard errors.

OUTLINE OF EFFECT SIZE COMPUTATIONS

Table 3.1 provides an outline of the computational formulas that follow.

These are some of the more common effect sizes and study designs. A more extensive array of formulas is offered in Borenstein *et al.* (2009).

Table 3.1 Roadmap of formulas in subsequent chapters.

Effect sizes based on means (Chapter 4)
    Raw (unstandardized) mean difference (D)
        Based on studies with independent groups
        Based on studies with matched groups or pre-post designs
    Standardized mean difference (d or g)
        Based on studies with independent groups
        Based on studies with matched groups or pre-post designs
    Response ratios (R)
        Based on studies with independent groups
Effect sizes based on binary data (Chapter 5)
    Risk ratio (RR)
        Based on studies with independent groups
    Odds ratio (OR)
        Based on studies with independent groups
    Risk difference (RD)
        Based on studies with independent groups
Effect sizes based on correlational data (Chapter 6)
    Correlation (r)
        Based on studies with one group

CHAPTER 4

Effect Sizes Based on Means

Introduction
Raw (unstandardized) mean difference D
Standardized mean difference, d and g
Response ratios

INTRODUCTION

When the studies report means and standard deviations, the preferred effect size is usually the raw mean difference, the standardized mean difference, or the response ratio. These effect sizes are discussed in this chapter.

RAW (UNSTANDARDIZED) MEAN DIFFERENCE D

When the outcome is reported on a meaningful scale *and* all studies in the analysis use the same scale, the meta-analysis can be performed directly on the raw difference in means (henceforth, we will use the more common term, *raw mean difference*). The primary advantage of the raw mean difference is that it is intuitively meaningful, either inherently (for example, blood pressure, which is measured on a known scale) or because of widespread use (for example, a national achievement test for students, where all relevant parties are familiar with the scale).

Consider a study that reports means for two groups (Treated and Control) and suppose we wish to compare the means of these two groups. Let μ_1 and μ_2 be the true (population) means of the two groups. The population mean difference is defined as

$$\Delta = \mu_1 - \mu_2. \qquad (4.1)$$

In the two sections that follow we show how to compute an estimate D of this parameter and its variance from studies that used two independent groups and from studies that used paired groups or matched designs.

Introduction to Meta-Analysis   M. Borenstein, L. V. Hedges, J. P. T. Higgins, H. R. Rothstein
© 2009, John Wiley & Sons, Ltd

Computing D from studies that use independent groups

We can estimate the mean difference Δ from a study that used two independent groups as follows. Let $\bar{X}_1$ and $\bar{X}_2$ be the sample means of the two independent groups. The sample estimate of Δ is just the difference in sample means, namely

$$D = \bar{X}_1 - \bar{X}_2. \tag{4.2}$$

Note that uppercase D is used for the *raw* mean difference, whereas lowercase d will be used for the *standardized* mean difference (below).

Let S_1 and S_2 be the sample standard deviations of the two groups, and n_1 and n_2 be the sample sizes in the two groups. If we assume that the two population standard deviations are the same (as is assumed to be the case in most parametric data analysis techniques), so that $\sigma_1 = \sigma_2 = \sigma$, then the variance of D is

$$V_D = \frac{n_1 + n_2}{n_1 n_2} S_{pooled}^2, \tag{4.3}$$

where

$$S_{pooled} = \sqrt{\frac{(n_1 - 1)S_1^2 + (n_2 - 1)S_2^2}{n_1 + n_2 - 2}}. \tag{4.4}$$

If we don't assume that the two population standard deviations are the same, then the variance of D is

$$V_D = \frac{S_1^2}{n_1} + \frac{S_2^2}{n_2}. \tag{4.5}$$

In either case, the standard error of D is then the square root of V,

$$SE_D = \sqrt{V_D}. \tag{4.6}$$

For example, suppose that a study has sample means $\bar{X}_1 = 103.00$, $\bar{X}_2 = 100.00$, sample standard deviations $S_1 = 5.5$, $S_2 = 4.5$, and sample sizes $n_1 = n_2 = 50$. The raw mean difference D is

$$D = 103.00 - 100.00 = 3.00.$$

If we assume that $\sigma_1 = \sigma_2$ then the pooled standard deviation within groups is

$$S_{pooled} = \sqrt{\frac{(50 - 1) \times 5.5^2 + (50 - 1) \times 4.5^2}{50 + 50 - 2}} = 5.0249.$$

The variance and standard error of D are given by

$$V_D = \frac{50 + 50}{50 \times 50} \times 5.0249^2 = 1.0100,$$

and

$$SE_D = \sqrt{1.0100} = 1.0050.$$

If we do not assume that $\sigma_1 = \sigma_2$ then the variance and standard error of D are given by

$$V_D = \frac{5.5^2}{50} + \frac{4.5^2}{50} = 1.0100$$

and

$$SE_D = \sqrt{1.0100} = 1.0050.$$

In this example formulas (4.3) and (4.5) yield the same result, but this will be true only if the sample size and/or the estimate of the variances is the same in the two groups.

Computing *D* from studies that use matched groups or pre-post scores

The previous formulas are appropriate for studies that use two independent groups. Another study design is the use of matched groups, where pairs of participants are matched in some way (for example, siblings, or patients at the same stage of disease), with the two members of each pair then being assigned to different groups. The unit of analysis is the pair, and the advantage of this design is that each pair serves as its own control, reducing the error term and increasing the statistical power. The magnitude of the impact depends on the correlation between (for example) siblings, with a higher correlation yielding a lower variance (and increased precision).

The sample estimate of $\varDelta$ is just the sample mean difference, D. If we have the difference score for each pair, which gives us the mean difference $\overline{X}_{diff}$ and the standard deviation of these differences (S_{diff}), then

$$D = \overline{X}_{diff}, \tag{4.7}$$

$$V_D = \frac{S_{diff}^2}{n}, \tag{4.8}$$

where n is the number of pairs, and

$$SE_D = \sqrt{V_D}. \tag{4.9}$$

For example, if the mean difference is 5.00 with standard deviation of the difference of 10.00 and n of 50 pairs, then

$$D = 5.0000,$$

$$V_D = \frac{10.00^2}{50} = 2.0000, \tag{4.10}$$

and

$$SE_D = \sqrt{2.00} = 1.4142. \tag{4.11}$$

Alternatively, if we have the mean and standard deviation for each set of scores (for example, siblings A and B), the difference is

$$D = \overline{X}_1 - \overline{X}_2. \tag{4.12}$$

The variance is again given by

$$V_D = \frac{S^2_{diff}}{n}, \tag{4.13}$$

where n is the number of pairs, and the standard error is given by

$$SE_D = \sqrt{V_D}. \tag{4.14}$$

However, in this case we need to compute the standard deviation of the difference scores from the standard deviation of each sibling's scores. This is given by

$$S_{diff} = \sqrt{S_1^2 + S_2^2 - 2 \times r \times S_1 \times S_2} \tag{4.15}$$

where r is the correlation between 'siblings' in matched pairs. If $S_1 = S_2$, then (4.15) simplifies to

$$S_{diff} = \sqrt{2 \times S^2_{pooled}(1 - r)}. \tag{4.16}$$

In either case, as r moves toward 1.0 the standard error of the paired difference will decrease, and when $r = 0$ the standard error of the difference is the same as it would be for a study with two independent groups, each of size n.

For example, suppose the means for siblings A and B are 105.00 and 100.00, with standard deviations 10 and 10, the correlation between the two sets of scores is 0.50, and the number of pairs is 50. Then

$$D = 105.00 - 100.00 = 5.0000,$$

$$V_D = \frac{10.00^2}{50} = 2.0000,$$

and

$$SE_D = \sqrt{2.00} = 1.4142.$$

In the calculation of V_D, the S_{diff} is computed using

$$S_{diff} = \sqrt{10^2 + 10^2 - 2 \times 0.50 \times 10 \times 10} = 10.0000$$

or

$$S_{diff} = \sqrt{2 \times 10^2(1 - 0.50)} = 10.0000.$$

The formulas for matched designs apply to pre-post designs as well. The pre and post means correspond to the means in the matched groups, n is the number of subjects, and r is the correlation between pre-scores and post-scores.

Calculation of effect size estimates from information that is reported

When a researcher has access to a full set of summary data such as the mean, standard deviation, and sample size for each group, the computation of the effect size and its variance is relatively straightforward. In practice, however, the researcher will often be working with only partial data. For example, a paper may publish only the *p*-value, means and sample sizes from a test of significance, leaving it to the meta-analyst to back-compute the effect size and variance. For information on computing effect sizes from partial information, see Borenstein *et al.* (2009).

Including different study designs in the same analysis

Sometimes a systematic review will include studies that used independent groups and also studies that used matched groups. From a statistical perspective the effect size (*D*) has the same meaning regardless of the study design. Therefore, we can compute the effect size and variance from each study using the appropriate formula, and then include all studies in the same analysis. While there is no technical barrier to using different study designs in the same analysis, there may be a concern that studies which used different designs might differ in substantive ways as well (see Chapter 40).

For all study designs (whether using independent or paired groups) the direction of the effect ($\bar{X}_1 - \bar{X}_2$ or $\bar{X}_2 - \bar{X}_1$) is arbitrary, except that the researcher must decide on a convention and then apply this consistently. For example, if a positive difference will indicate that the treated group did better than the control group, then this convention must apply for studies that used independent designs and for studies that used pre-post designs. In some cases it might be necessary to reverse the computed sign of the effect size to ensure that the convention is followed.

STANDARDIZED MEAN DIFFERENCE, *d* AND *g*

As noted, the raw mean difference is a useful index when the measure is meaningful, either inherently or because of widespread use. By contrast, when the measure is less well known (for example, a proprietary scale with limited distribution), the use of a raw mean difference has less to recommend it. In any event, the raw mean difference is an option only if all the studies in the meta-analysis use the same scale. If different studies use different instruments (such as different psychological or educational tests) to assess the outcome, then the scale of measurement will differ from study to study and it would not be meaningful to combine raw mean differences.

In such cases we can divide the mean difference in each study by that study's standard deviation to create an index (the standardized mean difference) that would be comparable across studies. This is the same approach suggested by Cohen (1969, 1987) in connection with describing the magnitude of effects in statistical power analysis.

The standardized mean difference can be considered as being comparable across studies based on either of two arguments (Hedges and Olkin, 1985). If the outcome measures in all studies are linear transformations of each other, the standardized mean difference can be seen as the mean difference that would have been obtained if all data were transformed to a scale where the standard deviation within-groups was equal to 1.0.

The other argument for comparability of standardized mean differences is the fact that the standardized mean difference is a measure of overlap between distributions. In this telling, the standardized mean difference reflects the difference between the distributions in the two groups (and how each represents a distinct cluster of scores) even if they do not measure exactly the same outcome (see Cohen, 1987, Grissom and Kim, 2005).

Consider a study that uses two independent groups, and suppose we wish to compare the means of these two groups. Let μ_1 and σ_1 be the true (population) mean and standard deviation of the first group and let μ_2 and σ_2 be the true (population) mean and standard deviation of the other group. If the two population standard deviations are the same (as is assumed in most parametric data analysis techniques), so that $\sigma_1 = \sigma_2 = \sigma$, then the standardized mean difference parameter or population standardized mean difference is defined as

$$\delta = \frac{\mu_1 - \mu_2}{\sigma}. \tag{4.17}$$

In the sections that follow, we show how to estimate δ from studies that used independent groups, and from studies that used pre-post or matched group designs. It is also possible to estimate δ from studies that used other designs (including clustered designs) but these are not addressed here (see resources at the end of this Part). We make the common assumption that $\sigma_1^2 = \sigma_2^2$, which allows us to pool the estimates of the standard deviation, and do not address the case where these are assumed to differ from each other.

Computing *d* and *g* from studies that use independent groups

We can estimate the standardized mean difference (δ) from studies that used two independent groups as

$$d = \frac{\overline{X}_1 - \overline{X}_2}{S_{within}}. \tag{4.18}$$

In the numerator, $\overline{X}_1$ and $\overline{X}_2$ are the sample means in the two groups. In the denominator S_{within} is the within-groups standard deviation, pooled across groups,

$$S_{within} = \sqrt{\frac{(n_1 - 1)S_1^2 + (n_2 - 1)S_2^2}{n_1 + n_2 - 2}} \tag{4.19}$$

where n_1 and n_2 are the sample sizes in the two groups, and S_1 and S_2 are the standard deviations in the two groups. The reason that we pool the two sample estimates of the standard deviation is that even if we assume that the underlying population standard deviations are the same (that is $\sigma_1 = \sigma_2 = \sigma$), it is unlikely that the sample estimates S_1 and S_2 will be identical. By pooling the two estimates of the standard deviation, we obtain a more accurate estimate of their common value.

The sample estimate of the standardized mean difference is often called Cohen's *d* in research synthesis. Some confusion about the terminology has resulted from the fact that the index δ, originally proposed by Cohen as a *population parameter* for describing the size of effects for statistical power analysis is also sometimes called *d*. In this volume we use the symbol δ to denote the effect size parameter and *d* for the sample estimate of that parameter.

The variance of *d* is given (to a very good approximation) by

$$V_d = \frac{n_1 + n_2}{n_1 n_2} + \frac{d^2}{2(n_1 + n_2)}. \tag{4.20}$$

In this equation the first term on the right of the equals sign reflects uncertainty in the estimate of the mean difference (the numerator in (4.18)), and the second reflects uncertainty in the estimate of S_{within} (the denominator in (4.18)).

The standard error of *d* is the square root of V_d,

$$SE_d = \sqrt{V_d}. \tag{4.21}$$

It turns out that *d* has a slight bias, tending to overestimate the absolute value of δ in small samples. This bias can be removed by a simple correction that yields an unbiased estimate of δ, with the unbiased estimate sometimes called Hedges' *g* (Hedges, 1981). To convert from *d* to Hedges' *g* we use a correction factor, which is called *J*. Hedges (1981) gives the exact formula for *J*, but in common practice researchers use an approximation,

$$J = 1 - \frac{3}{4df - 1}. \tag{4.22}$$

In this expression, *df* is the degrees of freedom used to estimate S_{within}, which for two independent groups is $n_1 + n_2 - 2$. This approximation always has error of less than 0.007 and less than 0.035 percent when $df \geq 10$ (Hedges, 1981). Then,

$$g = J \times d, \tag{4.23}$$

$$V_g = J^2 \times V_d, \tag{4.24}$$

and

$$SE_g = \sqrt{V_g}. \tag{4.25}$$

For example, suppose a study has sample means $\overline{X}_1 = 103$, $\overline{X}_2 = 100$, sample standard deviations $S_1 = 5.5$, $S_2 = 4.5$, and sample sizes $n_1 = n_2 = 50$. We would estimate the pooled-within-groups standard deviation as

$$S_{within} = \sqrt{\frac{(50-1) \times 5.5^2 + (50-1) \times 4.5^2}{50+50-2}} = 5.0249.$$

Then,

$$d = \frac{103-100}{5.0249} = 0.5970,$$

$$V_d = \frac{50+50}{50 \times 50} + \frac{0.5970^2}{2(50+50)} = 0.0418,$$

and

$$SE_d = \sqrt{0.0418} = 0.2044.$$

The correction factor (J), Hedges' g, its variance and standard error are given by

$$J = \left(1 - \frac{3}{4 \times 98 - 1}\right) = 0.9923,$$

$$g = 0.9923 \times 0.5970 = 0.5924,$$

$$v_g = 0.9923^2 \times 0.0418 = 0.0411,$$

and

$$SE_g = \sqrt{0.0411} = 0.2028.$$

The correction factor (J) is always less than 1.0, and so g will always be less than d in absolute value, and the variance of g will always be less than the variance of d. However, J will be very close to 1.0 unless df is very small (say, less than 10) and so (as in this example) the difference is usually trivial (Hedges, 1981).

Some slightly different expressions for the variance of d (and g) have been given by different authors and even the same authors at different times. For example, the denominator of the second term of the variance of d is given here as $2(n_1 + n_2)$. This expression is obtained by one method (assuming the n's become large with δ fixed). An alternate derivation (assuming n's become large with $\sqrt{n}\delta$ fixed) leads to a denominator in the second term that is slightly different, namely $2(n_1 + n_2 - 2)$. Unless n_1 and n_2 are very small, these expressions will be almost identical.

Similarly, the expression given here for the variance of g is J^2 times the variance of d, but many authors ignore the J^2 term because it is so close to unity in most cases. Again, while it is preferable to include this correction factor, the inclusion of this factor is likely to make little practical difference.

Computing d and g from studies that use pre-post scores or matched groups

We can estimate the standardized mean difference (δ) from studies that used matched groups or pre-post scores in one group. The formula for the sample estimate of d is

$$d = \frac{\overline{Y}_{diff}}{S_{within}} = \frac{\overline{Y}_1 - \overline{Y}_2}{S_{within}}. \tag{4.26}$$

This is the same formula as for independent groups (4.18). However, when we are working with independent groups the natural unit of deviation is the standard deviation within groups and so this value is typically reported (or easily imputed). By contrast, when we are working with matched groups, the natural unit of deviation is the standard deviation *of the difference scores*, and so *this* is the value that is likely to be reported. To compute d from the standard deviation of the differences we need to impute the standard deviation within groups, which would then serve as the denominator in (4.26).

Concretely, when working with a matched study, the standard deviation within groups can be imputed from the standard deviation of the difference, using

$$S_{within} = \frac{S_{diff}}{\sqrt{2(1-r)}}, \tag{4.27}$$

where r is the correlation between pairs of observations (e.g., the pretest-posttest correlation). Then we can apply (4.26) to compute d. The variance of d is given by

$$V_d = \left(\frac{1}{n} + \frac{d^2}{2n} \right) 2(1-r), \tag{4.28}$$

where n is the number of pairs. The standard error of d is just the square root of V_d,

$$SE_d = \sqrt{V_d}. \tag{4.29}$$

Since the correlation between pre- and post-scores is required to impute the standard deviation within groups from the standard deviation of the difference, we must assume that this correlation is known or can be estimated with high precision. Otherwise we may estimate the correlation from related studies, and possibly perform a sensitivity analysis using a range of plausible correlations.

To compute Hedges' g and associated statistics we would use formulas (4.22) through (4.25). The degrees of freedom for computing J is $n - 1$, where n is the number of pairs.

For example, suppose that a study has pre-test and post-test sample means $\overline{X}_1 = 103$, $\overline{X}_2 = 100$, sample standard deviation of the difference $S_{diff} = 5.5$, sample size $n = 50$, and a correlation between pre-test and post-test of $r = 0.7$. The standard deviation within groups is imputed from the standard deviation of the difference by

$$S_{within} = \frac{5.5}{\sqrt{2(1-0.7)}} = 7.1005.$$

Then d, its variance and standard error are computed as

$$d = \frac{103 - 100}{7.1000} = 0.4225,$$

$$v_d = \left(\frac{1}{50} + \frac{0.4225^2}{2 \times 50} \right) (2(1 - 0.7)) = 0.0131,$$

and

$$SE_d = \sqrt{0.0131} = 0.1143.$$

The correction factor J, Hedges' g, its variance and standard error are given by

$$J = \left(1 - \frac{3}{4 \times 49 - 1} \right) = 0.9846,$$

$$g = 0.9846 \times 0.4225 = 0.4160,$$

$$V_g = 0.9846^2 \times 0.0131 = 0.0127,$$

and

$$SE_g = \sqrt{0.0127} = 0.1126.$$

Including different study designs in the same analysis

As we noted earlier, a single systematic review can include studies that used independent groups and also studies that used matched groups. From a statistical perspective the effect size (d or g) has the same meaning regardless of the study design. Therefore, we can compute the effect size and variance from each study using the appropriate formula, and then include all studies in the same analysis. While there are no technical barriers to using studies with different designs in the same analysis, there may be a concern that these studies could differ in substantive ways as well (see Chapter 40).

For all study designs the direction of the effect ($\bar{X}_1 - \bar{X}_2$ or $\bar{X}_2 - \bar{X}_1$) is arbitrary, except that the researcher must decide on a convention and then apply this consistently. For example, if a positive difference indicates that the treated group did better than the control group, then this convention must apply for studies that used independent designs and for studies that used pre-post designs. It must also apply for all outcome measures. In some cases (for example, if some studies defined outcome as the number of correct answers while others defined outcome as the number of mistakes) it will be necessary to reverse the computed sign of the effect size to ensure that the convention is applied consistently.

RESPONSE RATIOS

In research domains where the outcome is measured on a physical scale (such as length, area, or mass) and is unlikely to be zero, the ratio of the means in the two groups might serve as the effect size index. In experimental ecology this effect size index is called the response ratio (Hedges, Gurevitch, & Curtis, 1999). It is important to recognize that the response ratio is only meaningful when the outcome

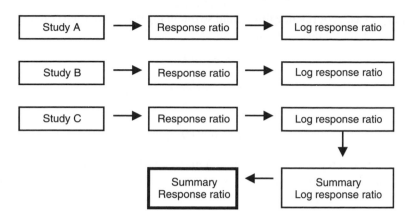

Figure 4.1 Response ratios are analyzed in log units.

is measured on a true ratio scale. The response ratio is not meaningful for studies (such as most social science studies) that measure outcomes such as test scores, attitude measures, or judgments, since these have no natural scale units and no natural zero points.

For response ratios, computations are carried out on a log scale (see the discussion under risk ratios, below, for an explanation). We compute the log response ratio and the standard error of the log response ratio, and use these numbers to perform all steps in the meta-analysis. Only then do we convert the results back into the original metric. This is shown schematically in Figure 4.1.

The response ratio is computed as

$$R = \frac{\overline{X}_1}{\overline{X}_2} \tag{4.30}$$

where $\overline{X}_1$ is the mean of group 1 and $\overline{X}_2$ is the mean of group 2. The log response ratio is computed as

$$lnR = \ln(R) = \ln\left(\frac{\overline{X}_1}{\overline{X}_2}\right) = \ln(\overline{X}_1) - \ln(\overline{X}_2). \tag{4.31}$$

The variance of the log response ratio is approximately

$$V_{lnR} = S^2_{pooled}\left(\frac{1}{n_1(\overline{X}_1)^2} + \frac{1}{n_2(\overline{X}_2)^2}\right), \tag{4.32}$$

where S_{pooled} is the pooled standard deviation. The approximate standard error is

$$SE_{\ln R} = \sqrt{V_{lnR}}. \tag{4.33}$$

Note that we do not compute a variance for the response ratio in its original metric. Rather, we use the *log* response ratio and its variance in the analysis to yield a summary effect, confidence limits, and so on, in log units. We then convert each of these values back to response ratios using

$$R = \exp(lnR), \tag{4.34}$$

$$LL_R = \exp(LL_{lnR}), \tag{4.35}$$

and

$$UL_R = \exp(UL_{lnR}), \tag{4.36}$$

where LL and UL represent the lower and upper limits, respectively.

For example, suppose that a study has two independent groups with means $\bar{X}_1 = 61.515$, $\bar{X}_2 = 51.015$, pooled within-group standard deviation 19.475, and sample size $n_1 = n_2 = 10$.

Then R, its variance and standard error are computed as

$$R = \frac{61.515}{51.015} = 1.2058,$$

$$lnR = \ln(1.2058) = 0.1871,$$

$$V_{lnR} = 19.475^2 \left(\frac{1}{10 \times (61.515)^2} + \frac{1}{10 \times (51.015)^2} \right) = 0.0246.$$

and

$$SE_{lnR} = \sqrt{0.0246} = 0.1581.$$

SUMMARY POINTS

- The raw mean difference (D) may be used as the effect size when the outcome scale is either inherently meaningful or well known due to widespread use. This effect size can only be used when all studies in the analysis used precisely the same scale.
- The standardized mean difference (d or g) transforms all effect sizes to a common metric, and thus enables us to include different outcome measures in the same synthesis. This effect size is often used in primary research as well as meta-analysis, and therefore will be intuitive to many researchers.
- The response ratio (R) is often used in ecology. This effect size is only meaningful when the outcome has a natural zero point, but when this condition holds, it provides a unique perspective on the effect size.
- It is possible to compute an effect size and variance from studies that used two independent groups, from studies that used matched groups (or pre-post designs) and from studies that used clustered groups. These effect sizes may then be included in the same meta-analysis.

CHAPTER 5

Effect Sizes Based on Binary Data (2 × 2 Tables)

INTRODUCTION

For data from a prospective study, such as a randomized trial, that was originally reported as the number of events and non-events in two groups (the classic 2 × 2 table), researchers typically compute a risk ratio, an odds ratio, and/or a risk difference. This data can be represented as cells A, B, C, and D, as shown in Table 5.1.

For example, assume a study with a sample size of 100 per group. Five patients died in the treated group, as compared with ten who died in the control group (see Table 5.2).

Table 5.1 Nomenclature for 2 × 2 table of outcome by treatment.

	Events	Non-Events	N
Treated	A	B	n_1
Control	C	D	n_2

Table 5.2 Fictional data for a 2 × 2 table.

	Dead	Alive	N
Treated	5	95	100
Control	10	90	100

Introduction to Meta-Analysis   M. Borenstein, L. V. Hedges, J. P. T. Higgins, H. R. Rothstein
© 2009, John Wiley & Sons, Ltd

From these data we might compute a risk ratio, an odds ratio, and/or a risk difference.

RISK RATIO

The risk ratio is simply the ratio of two *risks*. Here, the risk of death in the treated group is 5/100 and the risk of death in the control group is 10/100, so the ratio of the two risks is 0.50. This index has the advantage of being intuitive, in the sense that the meaning of a ratio is clear.

For risk ratios, computations are carried out on a log scale. We compute the log risk ratio, and the standard error of the log risk ratio, and will use these numbers to perform all steps in the meta-analysis. Only then will we convert the results back into the original metric. This is shown schematically in Figure 5.1.

The computational formula for the risk ratio is

$$RiskRatio = \frac{A/n_1}{C/n_2}. \tag{5.1}$$

The log risk ratio is then

$$LogRiskRatio = \ln(RiskRatio), \tag{5.2}$$

with approximate variance

$$V_{LogRiskRatio} = \frac{1}{A} - \frac{1}{n_1} + \frac{1}{C} - \frac{1}{n_2}, \tag{5.3}$$

and approximate standard error

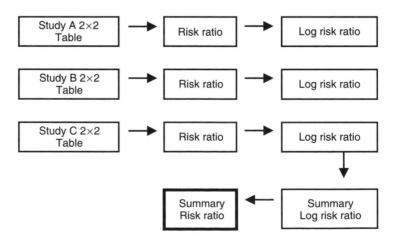

Figure 5.1 Risk ratios are analyzed in log units.

$$SE_{LogRiskRatio} = \sqrt{V_{LogRiskRatio}}. \tag{5.4}$$

Note that we do not compute a variance for the risk ratio in its original metric. Rather, we use the *log* risk ratio and its variance in the analysis to yield a summary effect, confidence limits, and so on, in log units. We then convert each of these values back to risk ratios using

$$RiskRatio = \exp(LogRiskRatio), \tag{5.5}$$

$$LL_{RiskRatio} = \exp(LL_{LogRiskRatio}), \tag{5.6}$$

and

$$UL_{RiskRatio} = \exp(UL_{LogRiskRatio}) \tag{5.7}$$

where *LL* and *UL* represent the lower and upper limits, respectively.

In the running example the risk ratio is

$$RiskRatio = \frac{5/100}{10/100} = 0.5000.$$

The log is

$$LogRiskRatio = \ln(0.5000) = -0.6932,$$

with variance

$$V_{LogRiskRatio} = \frac{1}{5} - \frac{1}{100} + \frac{1}{10} - \frac{1}{100} = 0.2800,$$

and standard error

$$SE_{LogRiskRatio} = \sqrt{0.280} = 0.5292.$$

Note 1. The log transformation is needed to maintain symmetry in the analysis. Assume that one study reports that the risk is twice as high in Group A while another reports that it is twice as high in Group B. Assuming equal weights, these studies should balance each other, with a combined effect showing equal risks (a risk ratio of 1.0). However, on the ratio scale these correspond to risk ratios of 0.50 and 2.00, which would yield a mean of 1.25. By working with log values we can avoid this problem. In log units the two estimates are -0.693 and $+0.693$, which yield a mean of 0.00. We convert this back to a risk ratio of 1.00, which is the correct value for this data.

Note 2. Although we defined the risk ratio in this example as

$$RiskRatio = \frac{5/100}{10/100} = 0.5000$$

(which gives the risk ratio of dying) we could alternatively have focused on the *risk* of staying alive, given by

$$RiskRatio = \frac{95/100}{90/100} = 1.0556.$$

The 'risk' of staying alive is *not* the inverse of the risk of dying (that is, 1.056 is not the inverse of 0.50), and therefore this should be considered a different measure of effect size.

ODDS RATIO

Where the risk ratio is the ratio of two *risks*, the odds ratio is the ratio of two *odds*. Here, the odds of death in the treated group would be 5/95, or 0.0526 (since probability of death in the treated group is 5/100 and the probability of life is 95/100), while the odds of death in the control group would be 10/90, or 0.1111. The ratio of the two odds would then be 0.0526/0.1111, or 0.4737.

Many people find this effect size measure less intuitive than the risk ratio, but the odds ratio has statistical properties that often make it the best choice for a meta-analysis. When the risk of the event is low, the odds ratio will be similar to the risk ratio.

For odds ratios, computations are carried out on a log scale (for the same reason as for risk ratios). We compute the log odds ratio, and the standard error of the log odds ratio, and will use these numbers to perform all steps in the meta-analysis. Only then will we convert the results back into the original metric. This is shown schematically in Figure 5.2.

The computational formula for the odds ratio is

$$OddsRatio = \frac{AD}{BC}. \tag{5.8}$$

The log odds ratio is then

$$LogOddsRatio = \ln(OddsRatio), \tag{5.9}$$

with approximate variance

$$V_{LogOddsRatio} = \frac{1}{A} + \frac{1}{B} + \frac{1}{C} + \frac{1}{D} \tag{5.10}$$

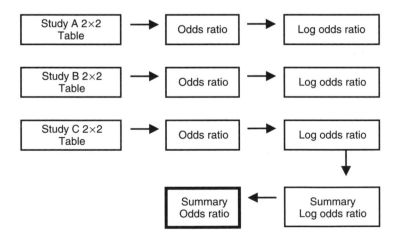

Figure 5.2 Odds ratios are analyzed in log units.

and approximate standard error

$$SE_{LogOddsRatio} = \sqrt{V_{LogOddsRatio}}. \tag{5.11}$$

Note that we do not compute a variance for the odds ratio. Rather, the log odds ratio and its variance are used in the analysis to yield a summary effect, confidence limits, and so on, in log units. We then convert each of these values back to odds ratios using

$$OddsRatio = \exp(LogOddsRatio), \tag{5.12}$$

$$LL_{OddsRatio} = \exp(LL_{LogOddsRatio}), \tag{5.13}$$

and

$$UL_{OddsRatio} = \exp(UL_{LogOddsRatio}), \tag{5.14}$$

where LL and UL represent the lower and upper limits, respectively.

In the running example

$$OddsRatio = \frac{5 \times 90}{95 \times 10} = 0.4737,$$

and

$$LogOddsRatio = \ln(0.4737) = -0.7472,$$

with variance

$$V_{LogOddsRatio} = \frac{1}{5} + \frac{1}{95} + \frac{1}{10} + \frac{1}{90} = 0.3216$$

and standard error

$$SE_{LogOddsRatio} = \sqrt{0.3216} = 0.5671.$$

Note. When working with the odds ratio or risk ratio we can place either the Treated group or the Control group in the numerator, as long we apply this consistently across all studies. If we put the Treated group in the denominator the log odds ratio would change signs (from -0.7472 to $+0.7472$) and the odds ratio would change to its inverse (from 0.4737 to 2.1110). The same thing happens to the odds ratio if we swap Dead and Alive within each group. However, this is *not* the case for the risk ratio.

RISK DIFFERENCE

The risk difference is the *difference* between two risks. Here, the risk in the treated group is 0.05 and the risk in the control group is 0.10, so the risk difference is -0.05.

Unlike the case for risk ratios and for odds ratios, computations for risk differences are carried out in raw units rather than log units.

The risk difference is defined as

$$RiskDiff = \left(\frac{A}{n_1}\right) - \left(\frac{C}{n_2}\right) \tag{5.15}$$

with approximate variance

$$V_{RiskDiff} = \frac{AB}{n_1^3} + \frac{CD}{n_2^3} \qquad (5.16)$$

and approximate standard error

$$SE_{RiskDiff} = \sqrt{V_{RiskDiff}}. \qquad (5.17)$$

In the running example

$$RiskDiff = \left(\frac{5}{100}\right) - \left(\frac{10}{100}\right) = -0.0500$$

with variance

$$V_{RiskDiff} = \frac{5 \times 95}{100^3} + \frac{10 \times 90}{100^3} = 0.0014$$

and standard error

$$SE_{RiskDiff} = \sqrt{0.00138} = 0.0371.$$

CHOOSING AN EFFECT SIZE INDEX

In selecting among the risk ratio, odds ratio, and risk difference the researcher needs to consider both substantive and technical factors.

The risk ratio and odds ratio are relative measures, and therefore tend to be relatively insensitive to differences in baseline events. By contrast, the risk difference is an absolute measure and as such is very sensitive to the baseline risk. If we wanted to test a compound and believed that it reduced the risk of an event by 20 % regardless of the baseline risk, then by using a ratio index we would expect to see the same effect size across studies even if the baseline risk varied from study to study. The risk difference, by contrast, would be higher in studies with a higher base rate.

At the same time, if we wanted to convey the clinical impact of the treatment, the risk difference might be the better measure. Suppose we perform a meta-analysis to assess the risk of adverse events for treated versus control groups. The risk is 1/1000 for treated patients versus 1/2000 for control patients, for a risk ratio of 2.00. At the same time, the risk difference is 0.0010 versus 0.0005 for a risk difference of 0.0005. These two numbers (2.00 and 0.0005) are both correct, but measure different things.

Because the ratios are less sensitive to baseline risk while the risk difference is sometimes more clinically meaningful, some suggest using the risk ratio (or odds ratio) to perform the meta-analysis and compute a summary risk (or odds) ratio. Then, they can use this to predict the risk difference for any given baseline risk.

SUMMARY POINTS

- We can compute the risk of an event (such as the risk of death) in each group (for example, treated versus control). The ratio of these risks then serves as an effect size (the risk ratio).
- We can compute the odds of an event (such as ratio of dying to living) in each group (for example, treated versus control). The ratio of these odds then serves as the odds ratio.
- We can compute the risk of an event (such as the risk of death) in each group (for example, treated versus control). The difference in these risks then serves as an effect size (the risk difference).
- To work with the risk ratio or odds ratio we transform all values to log values, perform the analyses, and then convert the results back to ratio values for presentation. To work with the risk difference we work with the raw values.

CHAPTER 6

Effect Sizes Based on Correlations

Introduction
Computing r
Other approaches

INTRODUCTION

For studies that report a correlation between two continuous variables, the correlation coefficient itself can serve as the effect size index. The correlation is an intuitive measure that, like δ, has been standardized to take account of different metrics in the original scales. The population parameter is denoted by ρ (the Greek letter rho).

COMPUTING r

The estimate of the correlation parameter ρ is simply the sample correlation coefficient, r. The variance of r is approximately

$$V_r = \frac{(1 - r^2)^2}{n - 1},$$ (6.1)

where n is the sample size.

Most meta-analysts do not perform syntheses on the correlation coefficient itself because the variance depends strongly on the correlation. Rather, the correlation is converted to the Fisher's z scale (not to be confused with the z-score used with significance tests), and all analyses are performed using the transformed values. The results, such as the summary effect and its confidence interval, would then be converted back to correlations for presentation. This is shown schematically in Figure 6.1, and is analogous to the procedure used with odds ratios or risk ratios where all analyses are performed using log transformed values, and then converted back to the original metric.

Introduction to Meta-Analysis   M. Borenstein, L. V. Hedges, J. P. T. Higgins, H. R. Rothstein
© 2009, John Wiley & Sons, Ltd

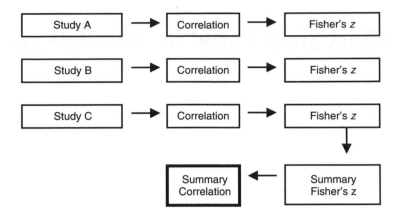

Figure 6.1 Correlations are analyzed in Fisher's z units.

The transformation from sample correlation r to Fisher's z is given by

$$z = 0.5 \times \ln\left(\frac{1+r}{1-r}\right). \tag{6.2}$$

The variance of z (to an excellent approximation) is

$$V_z = \frac{1}{n-3}, \tag{6.3}$$

and the standard error is

$$SE_z = \sqrt{V_z}. \tag{6.4}$$

When working with Fisher's z, we do not use the variance for the correlation. Rather, the Fisher's z score and its variance are used in the analysis, which yield a summary effect, confidence limits, and so on, in the Fisher's z metric. We then convert each of these values back to correlation units using

$$r = \frac{e^{2z} - 1}{e^{2z} + 1}. \tag{6.5}$$

For example, if a study reports a correlation of 0.50 with a sample size of 100, we would compute

$$z = 0.5 \times \ln\left(\frac{1+0.5}{1-0.5}\right) = 0.5493,$$

$$V_z = \frac{1}{100-3} = 0.0103,$$

and

$$SE_z = \sqrt{0.0103} = 0.1015.$$

To convert the Fisher's z value back to a correlation, we would use

$$r = \frac{e^{(2 \times 0.5493)} - 1}{e^{(2 \times 0.5493)} + 1} = 0.5000 \,.$$

OTHER APPROACHES

Hunter and Schmidt (2004) advocate an approach for working with correlations that differs in several ways from the one presented here. This approach is discussed in Chapter 38.

SUMMARY POINTS

- When studies report data as correlations, we usually use the correlation coefficient itself as the effect size. We transform the correlation using the Fisher's z transformation and perform the analysis using this index. Then, we convert the summary values back to correlations for presentation.

CHAPTER 7

Converting Among Effect Sizes

Introduction
Converting from the log odds ratio to d
Converting from d to the log odds ratio
Converting from r to d
Converting from d to r

INTRODUCTION

Earlier in this Part we discussed the case where different study designs were used to compute the same effect size. For example, studies that used independent groups and studies that used matched groups were both used to yield estimates of the standardized mean difference, g. There is no problem in combining these estimates in a meta-analysis since the effect size has the same meaning in all studies.

Consider, however, the case where some studies report a difference in means, which is used to compute a standardized mean difference. Others report a difference in proportions which is used to compute an odds ratio. And others report a correlation. All the studies address the same broad question, and we want to include them in one meta-analysis. Unlike the earlier case, we are now dealing with different indices, and we need to convert them to a common index before we can proceed.

The question of whether or not it is appropriate to combine effect sizes from studies that used different metrics must be considered on a case by case basis. The key issue is that it only makes sense to compute a summary effect from studies that we judge to be comparable in relevant ways. If we would be comfortable combining these studies if they had used the same metric, then the fact that they used different metrics should not be an impediment.

For example, suppose that several randomized controlled trials start with the same measure, on a continuous scale, but some report the outcome as a mean and others dichotomize the outcome and report it as success or failure. In this case, it may be highly appropriate to transform the standardized mean differences

Introduction to Meta-Analysis M. Borenstein, L. V. Hedges, J. P. T. Higgins, H. R. Rothstein
© 2009, John Wiley & Sons, Ltd

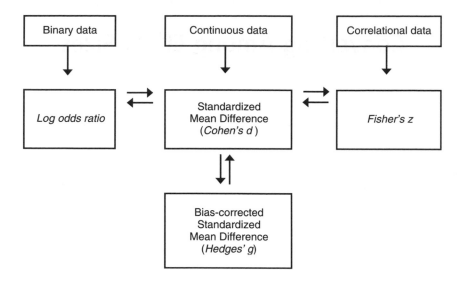

Figure 7.1 Converting among effect sizes.

and the odds ratios to a common metric and then combine them across studies. By contrast, observational studies that report correlations may be substantially different from observational studies that report odds ratios. In this case, even if there is no technical barrier to converting the effects to a common metric, it may be a bad idea from a substantive perspective.

In this chapter we present formulas for converting between an odds ratio and d, or between d and r. By combining formulas it is also possible to convert from an odds ratio, via d, to r (see Figure 7.1). In every case the formula for converting the effect size is accompanied by a formula to convert the variance.

When we convert between different measures we make certain assumptions about the nature of the underlying traits or effects. Even if these assumptions do not hold exactly, the decision to use these conversions is often better than the alternative, which is to simply omit the studies that happened to use an alternate metric. This would involve loss of information, and possibly the *systematic* loss of information, resulting in a biased sample of studies. A sensitivity analysis to compare the meta-analysis results with and without the converted studies would be important.

Figure 7.1 outlines the mechanism for incorporating multiple kinds of data in the same meta-analysis. First, each study is used to compute an effect size and variance of its *native* index, the log odds ratio for binary data, d for continuous data, and r for correlational data. Then, we convert all of these indices to a common index, which would be either the log odds ratio, d, or r. If the final index is d, we can move from there to Hedges' g. This common index and its variance are then used in the analysis.

CONVERTING FROM THE LOG ODDS RATIO TO d

We can convert from a log odds ratio ($LogOddsRatio$) to the standardized mean difference d using

$$d = LogOddsRatio \times \frac{\sqrt{3}}{\pi},\qquad(7.1)$$

where π is the mathematical constant (approximately 3.14159). The variance of d would then be

$$V_d = V_{LogOddsRatio} \times \frac{3}{\pi^2},\qquad(7.2)$$

where $V_{LogOddsRatio}$ is the variance of the log odds ratio. This method was originally proposed by Hasselblad and Hedges (1995) but variations have been proposed (see Sanchez-Meca, Marin-Martinez, & Chacon-Moscoso, 2003; Whitehead, 2002). It assumes that an underlying continuous trait exists and has a logistic distribution (which is similar to a normal distribution) in each group. In practice, it will be difficult to test this assumption.

For example, if the log odds ratio were $LogOddsRatio = 0.9069$ with a variance of $V_{LogOddsRatio} = 0.0676$, then

$$d = 0.9069 \times \frac{\sqrt{3}}{3.1416} = 0.5000$$

with variance

$$V_d = 0.0676 \times \frac{3}{3.1416^2} = 0.0205.$$

CONVERTING FROM d to the log odds ratio

We can convert from the standardized mean difference d to the log odds ratio ($LogOddsRatio$) using

$$LogOddsRatio = d \frac{\pi}{\sqrt{3}},\qquad(7.3)$$

where π is the mathematical constant (approximately 3.14159). The variance of $LogOddsRatio$ would then be

$$V_{LogOddsRatio} = V_d \frac{\pi^2}{3}.\qquad(7.4)$$

For example, if $d = 0.5000$ and $V_d = 0.0205$ then

$$LogOddsRatio = 0.5000 \times \frac{3.1416}{\sqrt{3}} = 0.9069,$$

and

$$V_{LogOddsRatio} = 0.0205 \times \frac{3.1416^2}{3} = 0.0676.$$

To employ this transformation we assume that the continuous data have the logistic distribution.

CONVERTING FROM *r* TO *d*

We convert from a correlation (*r*) to a standardized mean difference (*d*) using

$$d = \frac{2r}{\sqrt{1 - r^2}}. \tag{7.5}$$

The variance of *d* computed in this way (converted from *r*) is

$$V_d = \frac{4V_r}{(1 - r^2)^3}. \tag{7.6}$$

For example, if $r = 0.50$ and $V_r = 0.0058$, then

$$d = \frac{2 \times 0.50}{\sqrt{1 - 0.50^2}} = 1.1547$$

and the variance of *d* is

$$V_d = \frac{4 \times 0.0058}{\left(1 - 0.50^2\right)^3} = 0.0550.$$

In applying this conversion we assume that the continuous data used to compute *r* has a bivariate normal distribution and that the two groups are created by dichotomizing one of the two variables.

CONVERTING FROM *d* TO *r*

We can convert from a standardized mean difference (*d*) to a correlation (*r*) using

$$r = \frac{d}{\sqrt{d^2 + a}} \tag{7.7}$$

where *a* is a correction factor for cases where $n_1 \neq n_2$,

$$a = \frac{(n_1 + n_2)^2}{n_1 n_2}. \tag{7.8}$$

The correction factor (*a*) depends on the ratio of n_1 to n_2, rather than the absolute values of these numbers. Therefore, if n_1 and n_2 are not known precisely, use $n_1 = n_2$, which will yield $a = 4$. The variance of *r* computed in this way (converted from *d*) is

$$V_r = \frac{a^2 V_d}{\left(d^2 + a\right)^3}.$$ (7.9)

For example, if $n_1 = n_2$, $d = 1.1547$ and $v_d = 0.0550$, then

$$r = \frac{1.1547}{\sqrt{1.1547^2 + 4}} = 0.5000$$

and the variance of r converted from d will be

$$V_r = \frac{4^2 \times 0.0550}{\left(1.1547^2 + 4\right)^3} = 0.0058.$$

In applying this conversion assume that a continuous variable was dichotomized to create the treatment and control groups.

When we transform between Fisher's z and d we are making assumptions about the independent variable only. When we transform between the log odds ratio and d we are making assumptions about the dependent variable only. As such, the two sets of assumptions are independent of each other, and one has no implications for the validity of the other. Therefore, we can apply both sets of assumptions and transform from Fisher's z through d to the log odds ratio, as well as the reverse.

SUMMARY POINTS

- If all studies in the analysis are based on the same kind of data (means, binary, or correlational), the researcher should select an effect size based on that kind of data.
- When some studies use means, others use binary data, and others use correlational data, we can apply formulas to convert among effect sizes.
- Studies that used different measures may differ from each other in substantive ways, and we need to consider this possibility when deciding if it makes sense to include the various studies in the same analysis.

CHAPTER 8

Factors that Affect Precision

Introduction
Factors that affect precision
Sample size
Study design

INTRODUCTION

In the preceding chapter we showed how to compute the variance for specific effect sizes such as the standardized mean difference or a log risk ratio. Our goal in this chapter is to provide some context for those formulas.

We use the term precision as a general term to encompass three formal statistics, the variance, standard error, and confidence interval. These are all related to each other, so when we discuss the impact of a factor on precision, this translates into an impact on all three. In this chapter we outline the relationship between these three indices of precision. Then, we discuss two factors that affect precision and make some studies more precise than others.

Variance, standard error, and confidence intervals

The variance is a measure of the mean squared deviation from the mean effect. For an effect size Y (used generically), the variance would be denoted simply as

$$V_Y, \tag{8.1}$$

The computation of the variance is different for every effect size index (some formulas were presented in the preceding chapters).

The variance has properties that make it useful for some statistical computations, but because its metric is based on squared values it is not an intuitive index. A more accessible index is the standard error, which is on the same scale as the effect size

---

Introduction to Meta-Analysis   M. Borenstein, L. V. Hedges, J. P. T. Higgins, H. R. Rothstein
© 2009, John Wiley & Sons, Ltd

itself. If Y is the effect size and V_Y is the variance of Y, then the standard error of Y (SE_Y) is given by

$$SE_Y = \sqrt{V_Y}. \tag{8.2}$$

If we assume that the effect size is normally distributed then we can compute a 95% confidence interval using

$$LL_Y = \overline{Y} - 1.96 \times SE_Y \tag{8.3}$$

and

$$UL_Y = \overline{Y} + 1.96 \times SE_Y. \tag{8.4}$$

In these equations 1.96 is the Z-value corresponding to confidence limits of 95% (allowing for 2.5% error at either end of the distribution). We can also compute a test statistic Z as

$$Z_Y = \frac{\overline{Y}}{SE_Y}. \tag{8.5}$$

There is a perfect relationship between the p-value for Z and the confidence interval, such that the p-value will be less than 0.05 if and only if the confidence interval does not include the null value.

FACTORS THAT AFFECT PRECISION

Some of the factors that affect precision are unique to each effect size index, as explained in the preceding chapters. They are also unique to each study since each study has inherent factors, such as the homogeneity of the sample, which affect precision. Beyond these unique factors, however, are two factors that have an important and predictable impact on precision. One is the size of the sample, and the other is the study design (whether the study used paired groups, independent groups, or clustered groups). The impact of these two factors is explained here.

SAMPLE SIZE

A dominant factor in precision is the sample size, with larger samples yielding more precise estimates than smaller samples.

For example, consider the three studies in Table 8.1. These studies compared the means in two independent groups, and we computed the standardized mean

Table 8.1 Impact of sample size on variance.

Study	Design	N per Group	Standard Error	Variance
A	Independent	100	0.141	0.020
B	Independent	200	0.100	0.010
C	Independent	400	0.071	0.005

Impact of Sample Size on Variance

N per group	Standard Error	Variance	Standard difference in means (d) and 95% confidence interval
N = 100	0.141	0.020	
N = 200	0.100	0.010	
N = 400	0.071	0.005	

−0.50   −0.25   0.00   0.25   0.50

Figure 8.1 Impact of sample size on variance.

difference (d), which is 0.0 in this example. The sample sizes in the three studies (A, B, C) are 100, 200, and 400 per group, respectively, and the variances are 0.020, 0.010, and 0.005. In other words, as the sample size increases by a factor of 4 (compare studies A and C) the variance will decrease by a factor of 4 and the standard error will decrease by a factor of 2 (that is, by the square root of 4).

Note. In this example we assume that $d = 0.0$ which allows us to focus on the relationship between sample size and variance. When d is nonzero, d has an impact on the variance (though this impact is typically small).

The same information is presented graphically in Figure 8.1, where each study is represented by a box and bounded by a confidence interval. In this figure,

- The area of a box is proportional to the inverse of that study's variance.
- Any side on a box is proportional to the inverse of that study's standard error.
- The confidence interval for each box is proportional to that study's standard error.

Later, we will discuss how weights are assigned to each study in the meta-analysis. Under one scheme weights are inversely proportional to the variance, and study C would be assigned four times as much weight as study A.

STUDY DESIGN

In the preceding example (where we compared different sample sizes) we assumed that the studies used two independent groups. Here, we consider what happens if we use a comparable sample size but an alternate study design.

One alternate design is matched pairs, where each person in the treated group is matched with a similar person in the control group (say, a sibling, or a person at the same disease stage). This design allows us to work with differences within these pairs (rather than differences between groups) which can reduce the error term and thus increase the precision of the estimate. The impact on precision depends on the correlation between (for example) siblings, with a higher correlation yielding greater precision.

In Table 8.2 line D (*Independent*) shows the variance for a study with 100 subjects per group, and is identical to Study A in the prior table. The three lines

Table 8.2 Impact of study design on variance.

	Design	N per group	Intraclass Correlation	Correlation	Standard Error	Variance
A	Cluster	10 x 10	0.10		0.205	0.042
B	Cluster	10 x 10	0.05		0.175	0.031
C	Cluster	10 x 10	0.00		0.141	0.020
D	Independent	100			0.141	0.020
E	Paired	100 pairs		0.00	0.141	0.020
F	Paired	100 pairs		0.50	0.100	0.010
G	Paired	100 pairs		0.75	0.071	0.005

below this are based on paired (or matched groups) with the same sample size (100 pairs). If the pre-post correlation was 0.00 (line *E*) then the matching would have no impact and the variance would remain at 0.02, but if the correlation was 0.50 (line *F*) or 0.75 (line *G*), then the variance would drop to 0.01 or 0.005.

Another design is the clustered trial, where an entire cluster of participants is assigned to one condition or another. For example, the design might call for students within classrooms, where an entire classroom is assigned to a single condition. Just as the use of matched pairs served to *decrease* the error term, the use of clusters serves to *increase* the error term, and a study that used clustered groups would typically have a larger variance than one with two independent groups. In clustered trials the intraclass correlation reflects the difference between clusters. If the intraclass correlation was 0.0 (line *C*) then the clustering would have no impact and the variance would remain at 0.02, but if the intraclass correlation was 0.05 (line *B*) or 0.10 (line *A*) the variance would increase to 0.03 or 0.04 (assuming 10 clusters of 10 subjects per group).

Again, the same information is presented graphically in Figure 8.2 where the larger blocks (and narrower confidence intervals) represent studies with more precise estimates.

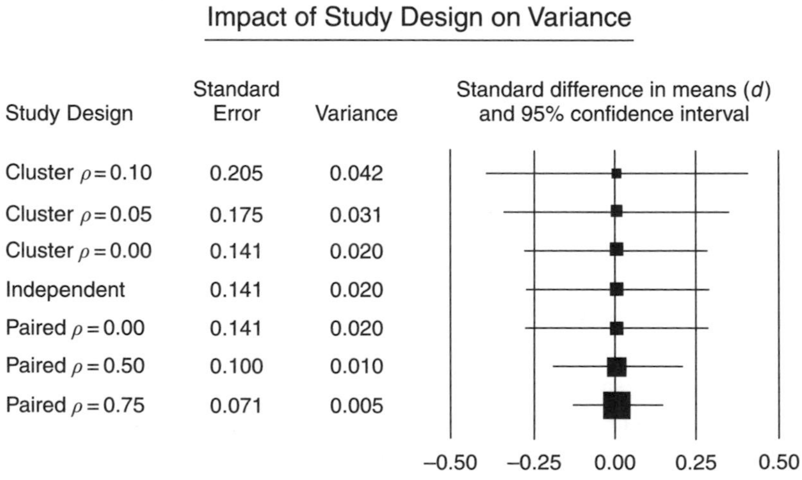

Impact of Study Design on Variance

Figure 8.2 Impact of study design on variance.

Concluding remarks

The information conveyed by precision is critically important in both primary studies and meta-analysis.

When we are working with individual studies the precision defines a range of likely values for the true effect. The precision, usually reported as a standard error or confidence interval, tells us how much confidence we can have in the effect size. To report that the effect size is 0.50 plus/minus 0.10 is very different than to report an effect size of 0.50 plus/minus 0.50.

As we turn our attention from the single study to the synthesis, our perspective shifts somewhat. A person performing a narrative review might look at a very precise study and decide to assign that study substantial weight in the analysis. This is formalized in the meta-analysis, with more weight being assigned to the more precise studies, as discussed in Part 4.

SUMMARY POINTS

- The precision with which we estimate an effect size can be expressed as a standard error or confidence interval (in the same metric as the effect size itself) or as a variance (in a squared metric).
- The precision is driven primarily by the sample size, with larger studies yielding more precise estimates of the effect size.
- Other factors affecting precision include the study design, with matched groups yielding more precise estimates (as compared with independent groups) and clustered groups yielding less precise estimates.
- In addition to these general factors, there are unique factors that affect the precision for each effect size index.
- Studies that yield more precise estimates of the effect size carry more information and are assigned more weight in the meta-analysis.

CHAPTER 9

Concluding Remarks

While many meta-analyses use one of the effect sizes presented above, other options exist. Researchers working in medicine sometimes use the hazard ratio (based on the time to event in two groups) or the rate ratio (based on events by time in two groups). Nor are we limited to indices that look at the impact of a treatment or the relationship between two variables. Some indices simply report the mean, risk, or rate in a single group. For example, we could perform a meta-analysis of studies that had estimated the prevalence of HIV infection in different countries.

As we move on to formulas for meta-analysis we will be using one or another effect size as an example in each chapter. However, it is important to understand that once we have computed an effect size and variance for each study, the formulas for computing a summary effect, for assessing heterogeneity, and so on, are the same regardless of whether the effect size is a raw difference in means, a standardized difference in means, a log risk ratio, or another index.

Further Reading

Borenstein, M., Hedges L.V., Higgins, J.P.T. & Rothstein, H. (2009). *Computing Effect Sizes for Meta-analysis*. Chichester, UK: John Wiley & Sons, Ltd.[*]

Cooper, H., Hedges, L.V. & Valentine, J. (2009). *The Handbook of Research Synthesis*, 2nd edn. New York: Russell Sage Foundation.

Deeks, J.J. (2002). Issues in the selection of a summary statistic for meta-analysis of clinical trials with binary outcomes. *Statistics in Medicine* 21: 1575–1600.

Glass, G., McGaw, B., & Smith, M. (1981). *Meta-analysis in Social Research*. Newbury Park, CA : Sage.

Hedges, L.V., Gurevitch, J., & Curtis, P. (1999). The meta-analysis of response ratios in experimental ecology. *Ecology* 80: 1150–1156.

Higgins, J.P.T. & Green, S. (eds) (2008). *Cochrane Handbook for Systematic Reviews of Interventions*. Chichester, UK: John Wiley & Sons, Ltd.

Lipsey, M., & Wilson, D. (2001). *Practical Meta-analysis*. Thousand Oaks, CA: Sage.

Rosenthal, R., Rosnow, R., & Rubin, D. (2000). *Contrasts and Effect Sizes in Behavioral Research: A Correlational Approach*. Cambridge, UK: Cambridge University Press.

Shadish, W. (2003). *Effect Size Calculator*. St. Paul, MN: Assessment Systems Corporation.

---

[*] Note. The first of these references (Borenstein *et al.*, 2009) is the companion volume to this text, dedicated entirely to the computation of effect sizes and their variance.

Concluding Remarks

Fixed-Effect Versus Random-Effects Models

CHAPTER 10

Overview

Introduction
Nomenclature

INTRODUCTION

Most meta-analyses are based on one of two statistical models, the fixed-effect model or the random-effects model.

Under the fixed-effect model we assume that there is one *true effect size* (hence the term *fixed effect*) which underlies all the studies in the analysis, and that all differences in observed effects are due to sampling error. While we follow the practice of calling this a fixed-effect model, a more descriptive term would be a *common-effect* model. In either case, we use the singular (*effect*) since there is only one true effect.

By contrast, under the random-effects model we allow that the true effect could vary from study to study. For example, the effect size might be higher (or lower) in studies where the participants are older, or more educated, or healthier than in others, or when a more intensive variant of an intervention is used, and so on. Because studies will differ in the mixes of participants and in the implementations of interventions, among other reasons, there may be *different effect sizes* underlying different studies. If it were possible to perform an infinite number of studies (based on the inclusion criteria for our analysis), the true effect sizes for these studies would be distributed about some mean. The effect sizes in the studies that actually *were performed* are assumed to represent a random sample of these effect sizes (hence the term *random effects*). Here, we use the plural (*effects*) since there is an array of true effects.

In the chapters that follow we discuss the two models and show how to compute a summary effect using each one. Because the computations for a summary effect are not always intuitive, it helps to keep in mind that the summary effect is nothing more than the mean of the effect sizes, with more weight assigned to the more precise studies. We need to consider what we mean by the *more precise* studies and

Introduction to Meta-Analysis   M. Borenstein, L. V. Hedges, J. P. T. Higgins, H. R. Rothstein
© 2009, John Wiley & Sons, Ltd

	True effect	Observed effect
Study	●	■
Combined	▼	◆

Figure 10.1 Symbols for true and observed effects.

how this translates into a study weight (this depends on the model), but not lose track of the fact that we are simply computing a weighted mean.

NOMENCLATURE

Throughout this Part we distinguish between a true effect size and an observed effect size. A study's *true effect size* is the effect size in the underlying population, and is the effect size that we would observe if the study had an infinitely large sample size (and therefore no sampling error). A study's *observed effect size* is the effect size that is actually observed.

In the schematics we use different symbols to distinguish between true effects and observed effects. For individual studies we use a circle for the former and a square for the latter (see Figure 10.1). For summary effects we use a triangle for the former and a diamond for the latter.

Worked examples

In meta-analysis the same formulas apply regardless of the effect size being used. To allow the reader to work with an effect size of their choosing, we have separated the formulas (which are presented in the following chapters) from the worked examples (which are presented in Chapter 14). There, we provide a worked example for the standardized mean difference, one for the odds ratio, and one for correlations.

The reader is encouraged to select one of the worked examples and follow the details of the computations while studying the formulas. The three datasets and all computations are available as Excel spreadsheets on the book's web site.

CHAPTER 11

Fixed-Effect Model

Introduction
The true effect size
Impact of sampling error
Performing a fixed-effect meta-analysis

INTRODUCTION

In this chapter we introduce the fixed-effect model. We discuss the assumptions of this model, and show how these are reflected in the formulas used to compute a summary effect, and in the meaning of the summary effect.

THE TRUE EFFECT SIZE

Under the fixed-effect model we assume that all studies in the meta-analysis share a common (true) effect size. Put another way, all factors that could influence the effect size are the same in all the studies, and therefore the true effect size is the same (hence the label *fixed*) in all the studies. We denote the true (unknown) effect size by theta (θ)

In Figure 11.1 the true overall effect size is 0.60 and this effect (represented by a triangle) is shown at the bottom. The true effect for each study is represented by a circle. Under the definition of a fixed-effect model the true effect size for each study must also be 0.60, and so these circles are aligned directly above the triangle.

IMPACT OF SAMPLING ERROR

Since all studies share the same true effect, it follows that the observed effect size varies from one study to the next only because of the random error inherent in each study. If each study had an infinite sample size the sampling error would be zero and the observed effect for each study would be the same as the true effect. If we were to plot the observed effects rather than the true effects, the observed effects would exactly coincide with the true effects.

Introduction to Meta-Analysis   M. Borenstein, L. V. Hedges, J. P. T. Higgins, H. R. Rothstein
© 2009, John Wiley & Sons, Ltd

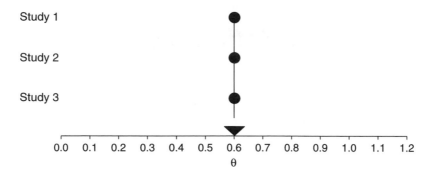

Figure 11.1 Fixed-effect model – true effects.

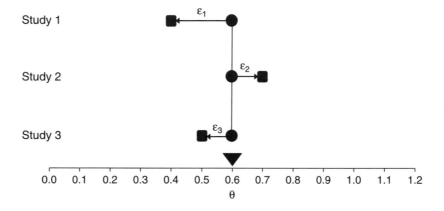

Figure 11.2 Fixed-effect model – true effects and sampling error.

In practice, of course, the sample size in each study is not infinite, and so there *is* sampling error and the effect observed in the study is not the same as the true effect. In Figure 11.2 the true effect for each study is still 0.60 (as depicted by the circles) but the observed effect (depicted by the squares) differs from one study to the next. In Study 1 the sampling error (ε_1) is -0.20, which yields an observed effect (Y_1) of

$$Y_1 = 0.60 - 0.20 = 0.40.$$

In Study 2 the sampling error (ε_2) is 0.10, which yields an observed effect (Y_2) of

$$Y_2 = 0.60 + 0.10 = 0.70.$$

In Study 3 the sampling error (ε_3) is -0.10, which yields an observed effect (Y_3) of

$$Y_3 = 0.60 - 0.10 = 0.50.$$

More generally, the observed effect Y_i for any study is given by the population mean plus the sampling error in that study. That is,

$$Y_i = \theta + \varepsilon_i. \tag{11.1}$$

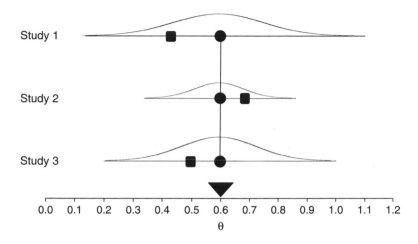

Figure 11.3 Fixed-effect model – distribution of sampling error.

While the error in any given study is random, we *can* estimate the sampling distribution of the errors. In Figure 11.3 we have placed a normal curve about the true effect size for each study, with the width of the curve being based on the variance in that study. In Study 1 the sample size was small, the variance large, and the observed effect is likely to fall anywhere in the relatively wide range of 0.20 to 1.00. By contrast, in Study 2 the sample size was relatively large, the variance is small, and the observed effect is likely to fall in the relatively narrow range of 0.40 to 0.80. (The width of the normal curve is based on the square root of the variance, or standard error).

PERFORMING A FIXED-EFFECT META-ANALYSIS

In an actual meta-analysis, of course, rather than starting with the population effect and making projections about the observed effects, we work backwards, starting with the observed effects and trying to estimate the population effect. In order to obtain the most precise estimate of the population effect (to minimize the variance) we compute a weighted mean, where the weight assigned to each study is the inverse of that study's variance. Concretely, the weight assigned to each study in a fixed-effect meta-analysis is

$$W_i = \frac{1}{V_{Y_i}},\qquad(11.2)$$

where V_{Y_i} is the within-study variance for study (i). The weighted mean (M) is then computed as

$$M = \frac{\sum_{i=1}^{k} W_i Y_i}{\sum_{i=1}^{k} W_i}, \tag{11.3}$$

that is, the sum of the products $W_i Y_i$ (effect size multiplied by weight) divided by the sum of the weights.

The variance of the summary effect is estimated as the reciprocal of the sum of the weights, or

$$V_M = \frac{1}{\sum_{i=1}^{k} W_i}, \tag{11.4}$$

and the estimated standard error of the summary effect is then the square root of the variance,

$$SE_M = \sqrt{V_M}. \tag{11.5}$$

Then, 95% lower and upper limits for the summary effect are estimated as

$$LL_M = M - 1.96 \times SE_M \tag{11.6}$$

and

$$UL_M = M + 1.96 \times SE_M. \tag{11.7}$$

Finally, a Z-value to test the null hypothesis that the common true effect θ is zero can be computed using

$$Z = \frac{M}{SE_M}. \tag{11.8}$$

For a one-tailed test the p-value is given by

$$p = 1 - \Phi(\pm|Z|), \tag{11.9}$$

where we choose '+' if the difference is in the expected direction and '−' otherwise, and for a two-tailed test by

$$p = 2\left[1 - \left(\Phi(|Z|)\right)\right], \tag{11.10}$$

where $\Phi(Z)$ is the standard normal cumulative distribution. This function is tabled in many introductory statistics books, and is implemented in Excel as the function =NORMSDIST(Z).

Illustrative example

We suggest that you turn to a worked example for the fixed-effect model before proceeding to the random-effects model. A worked example for the standardized mean difference (Hedges' g) is on page 87, a worked example for the odds ratio is on page 92, and a worked example for correlations is on page 97.

SUMMARY POINTS

- Under the fixed-effect model all studies in the analysis share a common true effect.
- The summary effect is our estimate of this common effect size, and the null hypothesis is that this common effect is zero (for a difference) or one (for a ratio).
- All observed dispersion reflects sampling error, and study weights are assigned with the goal of minimizing this within-study error.

CHAPTER 12

Random-Effects Model

Introduction
The true effect sizes
Impact of sampling error
Performing a random-effects meta-analysis

INTRODUCTION

In this chapter we introduce the random-effects model. We discuss the assumptions of this model, and show how these are reflected in the formulas used to compute a summary effect, and in the meaning of the summary effect.

THE TRUE EFFECT SIZES

The fixed-effect model, discussed above, starts with the assumption that the true effect size is the same in all studies. However, in many systematic reviews this assumption is implausible. When we decide to incorporate a group of studies in a meta-analysis, we assume that the studies have enough in common that it makes sense to synthesize the information, but there is generally no reason to assume that they are *identical* in the sense that the true effect size is *exactly the same* in all the studies.

For example, suppose that we are working with studies that compare the proportion of patients developing a disease in two groups (vaccinated versus placebo). If the treatment works we would expect the effect size (say, the risk ratio) to be *similar but not identical* across studies. The effect size might be higher (or lower) when the participants are older, or more educated, or healthier than others, or when a more intensive variant of an intervention is used, and so on. Because studies will differ in the mixes of participants and in the implementations of interventions, among other reasons, there may be *different effect sizes* underlying different studies.

Introduction to Meta-Analysis   M. Borenstein, L. V. Hedges, J. P. T. Higgins, H. R. Rothstein
© 2009, John Wiley & Sons, Ltd

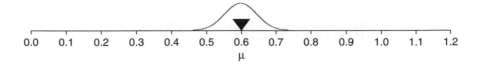

Figure 12.1 Random-effects model – distribution of true effects.

Or, suppose that we are working with studies that assess the impact of an educational intervention. The magnitude of the impact might vary depending on the other resources available to the children, the class size, the age, and other factors, which are likely to vary from study to study.

We might not have assessed these covariates in each study. Indeed, we might not even know what covariates actually are related to the size of the effect. Nevertheless, logic dictates that such factors do exist and will lead to variations in the magnitude of the effect.

One way to address this variation across studies is to perform a *random-effects* meta-analysis. In a random-effects meta-analysis we usually assume that the true effects are normally distributed. For example, in Figure 12.1 the mean of all true effect sizes is 0.60 but the individual effect sizes are distributed about this mean, as indicated by the normal curve. The width of the curve suggests that most of the true effects fall in the range of 0.50 to 0.70.

IMPACT OF SAMPLING ERROR

Suppose that our meta-analysis includes three studies drawn from the distribution of studies depicted by the normal curve, and that the true effects (denoted θ_1, θ_2, and θ_3) in these studies happen to be 0.50, 0.55 and 0.65 (see Figure 12.2).

If each study had an infinite sample size the sampling error would be zero and the observed effect for each study would be the same as the true effect for that study.

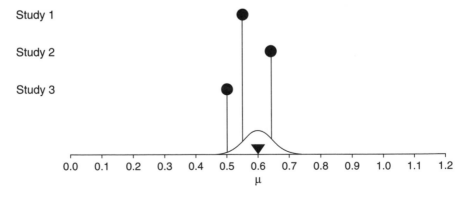

Figure 12.2 Random-effects model – true effects.

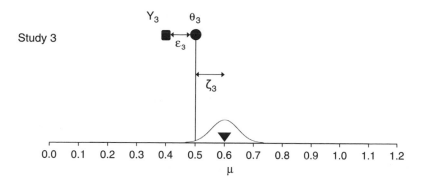

Figure 12.3 Random-effects model – true and observed effect in one study.

If we were to plot the observed effects rather than the true effects, the observed effects would exactly coincide with the true effects.

Of course, the sample size in any study is not infinite and therefore the sampling error is not zero. If the true effect size for a study is θ_i, then the observed effect for that study will be less than or greater than θ_i because of sampling error. For example, consider Study 3 in Figure 12.2. This study is the subject of Figure 12.3, where we consider the factors that control the observed effect. The true effect for Study 3 is 0.50 but the sampling error for this study is –0.10, and the observed effect for this study is 0.40.

This figure also highlights the fact that the distance between the overall mean and the observed effect in any given study consists of two distinct parts: true variation in effect sizes (ζ_i) and sampling error (ε_i). In Study 3 the total distance from μ to Y_3 is –0.20. The distance from μ to θ_3 (0.60 to 0.50) reflects the fact that the true effect size actually varies from one study to the next, while the distance from θ_3 to Y_3 (0.5 to 0.4) is sampling error.

More generally, the observed effect Y_i for any study is given by the grand mean, the deviation of the study's true effect from the grand mean, and the deviation of the study's observed effect from the study's true effect. That is,

$$Y_i = \mu + \zeta_i + \varepsilon_i. \tag{12.1}$$

Therefore, to predict how far the observed effect Y_i is likely to fall from μ in any given study we need to consider both the variance of ζ_i and the variance of ε_i.

The distance from μ (the triangle) to each θ_i (the circles) depends on the standard deviation of the distribution of the true effects across studies, called τ (tau) (or τ^2 for its variance). The same value of τ^2 applies to all studies in the meta-analysis, and in Figure 12.4 is represented by the normal curve at the bottom, which extends roughly from 0.50 to 0.70.

The distance from θ_i to Y_i depends on the sampling distribution of the sample effects about θ_i. This depends on the variance of the observed effect size from each study, V_{Y_i}, and so will vary from one study to the next. In Figure 12.4 the curve for Study 1 is relatively wide while the curve for Study 2 is relatively narrow.

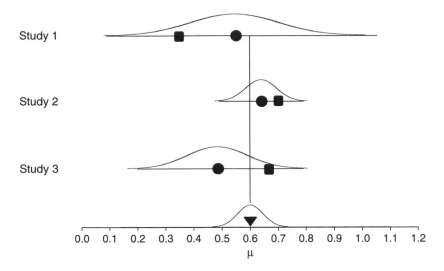

Figure 12.4 Random-effects model – between-study and within-study variance.

PERFORMING A RANDOM-EFFECTS META-ANALYSIS

In an actual meta-analysis, of course, rather than start with the population effect and make projections about the observed effects, we start with the observed effects and try to estimate the population effect. In other words our goal is to use the collection of Y_i to estimate the overall mean, μ. In order to obtain the most precise estimate of the overall mean (to minimize the variance) we compute a weighted mean, where the weight assigned to each study is the inverse of that study's variance.

To compute a study's variance under the random-effects model, we need to know both the within-study variance and τ^2, since the study's total variance is the sum of these two values. Formulas for computing the within-study variance were presented in Part 3. A method for estimating the between-studies variance is given here so that we can proceed with the worked example, but a full discussion of this method is deferred to Part 4, where we shall pursue the issue of heterogeneity in some detail.

Estimating tau-squared

The parameter τ^2 (tau-squared) is the between-studies variance (the variance of the effect size parameters across the population of studies). In other words, if we somehow knew the *true* effect size for each study, and computed the variance of these effect sizes (across an infinite number of studies), this variance would be τ^2. One method for estimating τ^2 is the method of moments (or the DerSimonian and Laird) method, as follows. We compute

$$T^2 = \frac{Q - df}{C} \ ,$$

(12.2)

where

$$Q = \sum_{i=1}^{k} W_i Y_i^2 - \frac{\left(\sum_{i=1}^{k} W_i Y_i \right)^2}{\sum_{i=1}^{k} W_i},$$ (12.3)

$$df = k - 1,$$ (12.4)

where k is the number of studies, and

$$C = \sum W_i - \frac{\sum W_i^2}{\sum W_i}.$$ (12.5)

Estimating the mean effect size

In the fixed-effect analysis each study was weighted by the inverse of its variance. In the random-effects analysis, too, each study will be weighted by the inverse of its variance. The difference is that the variance now includes the original (within-studies) variance plus the estimate of the between-studies variance, T^2. In keeping with the book's convention, we use τ^2 to refer to the parameter and T^2 to refer to the sample estimate of that parameter.

To highlight the parallel between the formulas here (random effects) and those in the previous chapter (fixed effect) we use the same notations but add an asterisk (*) to represent the random-effects version. Under the random-effects model the weight assigned to each study is

$$W_i^* = \frac{1}{V_{Y_i}^*},$$ (12.6)

where $V_{Y_i}^*$ is the within-study variance for study i plus the between-studies variance, T^2. That is,

$$V_{Y_i}^* = V_{Y_i} + T^2.$$

The weighted mean, M^*, is then computed as

$$M^* = \frac{\sum_{i=1}^{k} W_i^* Y_i}{\sum_{i=1}^{k} W_i^*},$$ (12.7)

that is, the sum of the products (effect size multiplied by weight) divided by the sum of the weights.

The variance of the summary effect is estimated as the reciprocal of the sum of the weights, or

$$V_{M^*} = \frac{1}{\sum\limits_{i=1}^{k} W_i^*},$$

(12.8)

and the estimated standard error of the summary effect is then the square root of the variance,

$$SE_{M^*} = \sqrt{V_{M^*}}.$$

(12.9)

The 95% lower and upper limits for the summary effect would be computed as

$$LL_{M^*} = M^* - 1.96 \times SE_{M^*},$$

(12.10)

and

$$UL_{M^*} = M^* + 1.96 \times SE_{M^*}.$$

(12.11)

Finally, a Z-value to test the null hypothesis that the mean effect μ is zero could be computed using

$$Z^* = \frac{M^*}{SE_{M^*}}.$$

(12.12)

For a one-tailed test the p-value is given by

$$p^* = 1 - \Phi(\pm|Z^*|),$$

(12.13)

where we choose '+' if the difference is in the expected direction or '−' otherwise, and for a two-tailed test by

$$p^* = 2[1 - (\Phi(|Z^*|))],$$

(12.14)

where $\Phi(Z^*)$ is the standard normal cumulative distribution. This function is tabled in many introductory statistics books, and is implemented in Excel as the function =NORMSDIST(Z*).

Illustrative example
As before, we suggest that you turn to one of the worked examples in the next chapter before proceeding with this discussion.

SUMMARY POINTS

- Under the random-effects model, the true effects in the studies are assumed to have been sampled from a distribution of true effects.
- The summary effect is our estimate of the mean of all relevant true effects, and the null hypothesis is that the mean of these effects is 0.0 (equivalent to a ratio of 1.0 for ratio measures).

- Since our goal is to estimate the mean of the distribution, we need to take account of two sources of variance. First, there is within-study error in estimating the effect in each study. Second (even if we knew the true mean for each of our studies), there is variation in the true effects across studies. Study weights are assigned with the goal of minimizing both sources of variance.

CHAPTER 13

Fixed-Effect Versus Random-Effects Models

INTRODUCTION

In Chapter 11 and Chapter 12 we introduced the fixed-effect and random-effects models. Here, we highlight the conceptual and practical differences between them.

Consider the forest plots in Figures 13.1 and 13.2. They include the same six studies, but the first uses a fixed-effect analysis and the second a random-effects analysis. These plots provide a context for the discussion that follows.

DEFINITION OF A SUMMARY EFFECT

Both plots show a summary effect on the bottom line, but the meaning of this summary effect is different in the two models. In the fixed-effect analysis we assume that the true effect size is the same in all studies, and the summary effect is our estimate of this common effect size. In the random-effects analysis we assume that the true effect size varies from one study to the next, and that the studies in our analysis represent a random sample of effect sizes that could

Introduction to Meta-Analysis   M. Borenstein, L. V. Hedges, J. P. T. Higgins, H. R. Rothstein
© 2009, John Wiley & Sons, Ltd

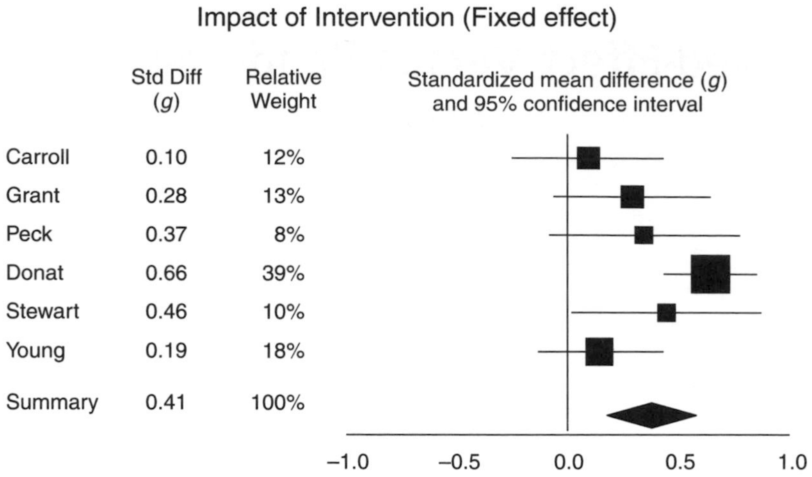

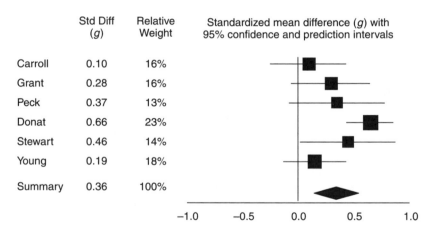

Figure 13.1 Fixed-effect model – forest plot showing relative weights.

Figure 13.2 Random-effects model – forest plot showing relative weights.

have been observed. The summary effect is our estimate of the mean of these effects.

ESTIMATING THE SUMMARY EFFECT

Under the fixed-effect model we assume that the true effect size for all studies is identical, and the only reason the effect size varies between studies is sampling error (error in estimating the effect size). Therefore, when assigning weights to the different studies we can largely ignore the information in the smaller studies since we have better information about the same effect size in the larger studies.

By contrast, under the random-effects model the goal is not to estimate one true effect, but to estimate the mean of a distribution of effects. Since each study provides information about a different effect size, we want to be sure that all these effect sizes are represented in the summary estimate. This means that we cannot discount a small study by giving it a very small weight (the way we would in a fixed-effect analysis). The estimate provided by that study may be imprecise, but it is information about an effect that no other study has estimated. By the same logic we cannot give too much weight to a very large study (the way we might in a fixed-effect analysis). Our goal is to estimate the mean effect in a range of studies, and we do not want that overall estimate to be overly influenced by any one of them.

In these graphs, the weight assigned to each study is reflected in the size of the box (specifically, the area) for that study. Under the fixed-effect model there is a wide range of weights (as reflected in the size of the boxes) whereas under the random-effects model the weights fall in a relatively narrow range. For example, compare the weight assigned to the largest study (Donat) with that assigned to the smallest study (Peck) under the two models. Under the fixed-effect model Donat is given about five times as much weight as Peck. Under the random-effects model Donat is given only 1.8 times as much weight as Peck.

EXTREME EFFECT SIZE IN A LARGE STUDY OR A SMALL STUDY

How will the selection of a model influence the overall effect size? In this example Donat is the largest study, and also happens to have the highest effect size. Under the fixed-effect model Donat was assigned a large share (39%) of the total weight and pulled the mean effect up to 0.41. By contrast, under the random-effects model Donat was assigned a relatively modest share of the weight (23%). It therefore had less pull on the mean, which was computed as 0.36.

Similarly, Carroll is one of the smaller studies and happens to have the smallest effect size. Under the fixed-effect model Carroll was assigned a relatively small proportion of the total weight (12%), and had little influence on the summary effect. By contrast, under the random-effects model Carroll carried a somewhat higher proportion of the total weight (16%) and was able to pull the weighted mean toward the left.

The operating premise, as illustrated in these examples, is that whenever τ^2 is nonzero, the relative weights assigned under random effects will be *more balanced* than those assigned under fixed effects. As we move from fixed effect to random effects, extreme studies will lose influence if they are large, and will gain influence if they are small.

CONFIDENCE INTERVAL

Under the fixed-effect model the only source of uncertainty is the within-study (sampling or estimation) error. Under the random-effects model there is this same source of uncertainty plus an additional source (between-studies variance). It follows that the variance, standard error, and confidence interval for the summary effect will always be larger (or wider) under the random-effects model than under the fixed-effect model (unless T^2 is zero, in which case the two models are the same). In this example, the standard error is 0.064 for the fixed-effect model, and 0.105 for the random-effects model.

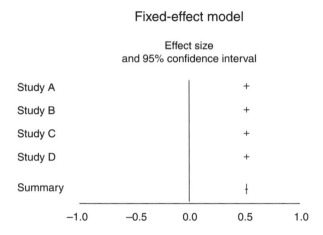

Figure 13.3 Very large studies under fixed-effect model.

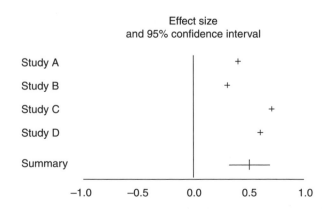

Figure 13.4 Very large studies under random-effects model.

Consider what would happen if we had five studies, and each study had an infinitely large sample size. Under either model the confidence interval for the effect size in each study would have a width approaching zero, since we know the effect size in that study with perfect precision. Under the fixed-effect model the summary effect would also have a confidence interval with a width of zero, since we know the common effect precisely (Figure 13.3). By contrast, under the random-effects model the width of the confidence interval would not approach zero (Figure 13.4). While we know the effect in each study precisely, these effects have been sampled from a universe of possible effect sizes, and provide only an estimate of the mean effect. Just as the error within a study will approach zero only as the sample size approaches infinity, so too the error of these studies as an estimate of the mean effect will approach zero only as the number of studies approaches infinity.

More generally, it is instructive to consider what factors influence the standard error of the summary effect under the two models. The following formulas are based on a meta-analysis of means from k one-group studies, but the conceptual argument applies to all meta-analyses. The within-study variance of each mean depends on the standard deviation (denoted σ) of participants' scores and the sample size of each study (n). For simplicity we assume that all of the studies have the same sample size and the same standard deviation (see Box 13.1 for details).

Under the fixed-effect model the standard error of the summary effect is given by

$$SE_M = \sqrt{\frac{\sigma^2}{k \times n}}. \qquad (13.1)$$

It follows that with a large enough sample size the standard error will approach zero, and this is true whether the sample size is concentrated on one or two studies, or dispersed across any number of studies.

Under the random-effects model the standard error of the summary effect is given by

$$SE_M = \sqrt{\frac{\sigma^2}{k \times n} + \frac{\tau^2}{k}}. \qquad (13.2)$$

The first term is identical to that for the fixed-effect model and, again, with a large enough sample size, this term will approach zero. By contrast, the second term (which reflects the between-studies variance) will only approach zero as the number of studies approaches infinity. These formulas do not apply exactly in practice, but the conceptual argument does. Namely, increasing the sample size within studies is not sufficient to reduce the standard error beyond a certain point (where that point is determined by τ^2 and k). If there is only a small number of studies, then the standard error could still be substantial even if the total n is in the tens of thousands or higher.

BOX 13.1   FACTORS THAT INFLUENCE THE STANDARD ERROR OF THE SUMMARY EFFECT.

To illustrate the concepts with some simple formulas, let us consider a meta-analysis of studies with the very simplest design, such that each study comprises a single sample of n observations with standard deviation σ. We combine estimates of the mean in a meta-analysis. The variance of each estimate is

$$V_{Y_i} = \frac{\sigma^2}{n}$$

so the (inverse-variance) weight in a fixed-effect meta-analysis is

$$W_i = \frac{1}{\sigma^2/n} = \frac{n}{\sigma^2}$$

and the variance of the summary effect under the fixed-effect model the standard error is given by

$$V_M = \frac{1}{\sum\limits_{i=1}^{k} W_i} = \frac{1}{k \times n/\sigma^2} = \frac{\sigma^2}{k \times n}.$$

Therefore under the fixed-effect model the (true) standard error of the summary mean is given by

$$SE_M = \sqrt{\frac{\sigma^2}{k \times n}}.$$

Under the random-effects model the weight awarded to each study is

$$W^*_i = \frac{1}{(\sigma^2/n) + \tau^2}$$

and the (true) standard error of the summary mean turns out to be

$$SE_{M^*} = \sqrt{\frac{\sigma^2}{k \times n} + \frac{\tau^2}{k}}.$$

THE NULL HYPOTHESIS

Often, after computing a summary effect, researchers perform a test of the null hypothesis. Under the fixed-effect model the null hypothesis being tested is that there is zero effect in *every study*. Under the random-effects model the null hypothesis being tested is that the *mean effect* is zero. Although some may treat these hypotheses as interchangeable, they are in fact different, and it is imperative to choose the test that is appropriate to the inference a researcher wishes to make.

WHICH MODEL SHOULD WE USE?

The selection of a computational model should be based on our expectation about whether or not the studies share a common effect size and on our goals in performing the analysis.

Fixed effect

It makes sense to use the fixed-effect model if two conditions are met. First, we believe that all the studies included in the analysis are functionally identical. Second, our goal is to compute the common effect size for the identified population, and not to generalize to other populations.

For example, suppose that a pharmaceutical company will use a thousand patients to compare a drug versus placebo. Because the staff can work with only 100 patients at a time, the company will run a series of ten trials with 100 patients in each. The studies arc identical in the sense that any variables which can have an impact on the outcome are the same across the ten studies. Specifically, the studies draw patients from a common pool, using the same researchers, dose, measure, and so on (we assume that there is no concern about practice effects for the researchers, nor for the different starting times of the various cohorts). All the studies are expected to share a common effect and so the first condition is met. The goal of the analysis is to see if the drug works in the population from which the patients were drawn (and not to extrapolate to other populations), and so the second condition is met, as well.

In this example the fixed-effect model is a plausible fit for the data and meets the goal of the researchers. It should be clear, however, that this situation is relatively rare. The vast majority of cases will more closely resemble those discussed immediately below.

Random effects

By contrast, when the researcher is accumulating data from a series of studies that had been performed by researchers operating independently, it would be unlikely that all the studies were functionally equivalent. Typically, the subjects or interventions in these studies would have differed in ways that would have impacted on the results, and therefore we should not assume a common effect size. Therefore, in these cases the random-effects model is more easily justified than the fixed-effect model.

Additionally, the goal of this analysis is usually to generalize to a range of scenarios. Therefore, if one did make the argument that all the studies used an identical, narrowly defined population, then it would not be possible to extrapolate from this population to others, and the utility of the analysis would be severely limited.

A caveat

There is one caveat to the above. If the number of studies is very small, then the estimate of the between-studies variance (τ^2) will have poor precision. While the random-effects model is still the appropriate model, we lack the information needed to apply it correctly. In this case the reviewer may choose among several options, each of them problematic.

One option is to report the separate effects and *not* report a summary effect. The hope is that the reader will understand that we cannot draw conclusions about the effect size and its confidence interval. The problem is that some readers will revert to vote counting (see Chapter 28) and possibly reach an erroneous conclusion.

Another option is to perform a fixed-effect analysis. This approach would yield a descriptive analysis of the included studies, but would not allow us to make inferences about a wider population. The problem with this approach is that (a) we do want to make inferences about a wider population and (b) readers will make these inferences even if they are not warranted.

A third option is to take a Bayesian approach, where the estimate of τ^2 is based on data from outside of the current set of studies. This is probably the best option, but the problem is that relatively few researchers have expertise in Bayesian meta-analysis. Additionally, some researchers have a philosophical objection to this approach.

For a more general discussion of this issue see *When does it make sense to perform a meta-analysis* in Chapter 40.

MODEL SHOULD NOT BE BASED ON THE TEST FOR HETEROGENEITY

In the next chapter we will introduce a test of the null hypothesis that the between-studies variance is zero. This test is based on the amount of between-studies variance observed, relative to the amount we would expect if the studies actually shared a common effect size.

Some have adopted the practice of starting with a fixed-effect model and then switching to a random-effects model if the test of homogeneity is statistically significant. This practice should be strongly discouraged because the decision to use the random-effects model should be based on our understanding of whether or not all studies share a common effect size, and not on the outcome of a statistical test (especially since the test for heterogeneity often suffers from low power).

If the study effect sizes are seen as having been sampled from a *distribution* of effect sizes, then the random-effects model, which reflects this idea, is the logical one to use. If the between-studies variance is substantial (and statistically significant) then the fixed-effect model is inappropriate. However, even if the between-studies variance does not meet the criterion for statistical significance (which may be due simply to low power) we should still take account of this variance when assigning weights. If T^2 turns out to be zero, then the random-effects analysis reduces to the fixed-effect analysis, and so there is no cost to using this model.

On the other hand, if one has elected to use the fixed-effect model *a priori* but the test of homogeneity is statistically significant, then it would be important to revisit the assumptions that led to the selection of a fixed-effect model.

CONCLUDING REMARKS

Our discussion of differences between the fixed-model and the random-effects model focused largely on the computation of a summary effect and the confidence intervals for the summary effect. We did not address the implications of the dispersion itself. Under the fixed-effect model we assume that all dispersion in observed effects is due to sampling error, but under the random-effects model we allow that some of that dispersion reflects real differences in effect size across studies. In the chapters that follow we discuss methods to quantify that dispersion and to consider its substantive implications.

Although throughout this book we define a fixed-effect meta-analysis as assuming that every study has a common true effect size, some have argued that the fixed-effect method is valid without making this assumption. The point estimate of the effect in a fixed-effect meta-analysis is simply a weighted average and does not strictly require the assumption that all studies estimate the same thing. For simplicity and clarity we adopt a definition of a fixed-effect meta-analysis that does assume homogeneity of effect.

SUMMARY POINTS

- A fixed-effect meta-analysis estimates a single effect that is assumed to be common to every study, while a random-effects meta-analysis estimates the mean of a distribution of effects.
- Study weights are more balanced under the random-effects model than under the fixed-effect model. Large studies are assigned less relative weight and small studies are assigned more relative weight as compared with the fixed-effect model.
- The standard error of the summary effect and (it follows) the confidence intervals for the summary effect are wider under the random-effects model than under the fixed-effect model.

- The selection of a model must be based solely on the question of which model fits the distribution of effect sizes, and takes account of the relevant source(s) of error. When studies are gathered from the published literature, the random-effects model is generally a more plausible match.
- The strategy of starting with a fixed-effect model and then moving to a random-effects model if the test for heterogeneity is significant is a mistake, and should be strongly discouraged.

Worked Examples (Part 1)

INTRODUCTION

In this chapter we present worked examples for continuous data (using the standardized mean difference), binary data (using the odds ratio) and correlational data (using the Fisher's z transformation).

All of the data sets and all computations are available as Excel spreadsheets on the book's website (www.Meta-Analysis.com).

WORKED EXAMPLE FOR CONTINUOUS DATA (PART 1)

In this example we start with the mean, standard deviation, and sample size, and will use the bias-corrected standardized mean difference (Hedges' g) as the effect size measure.

Summary data

The summary data for six studies are presented in Table 14.1.

Compute the effect size and its variance for each study

The first step is to compute the effect size (g) and variance for each study using the formulas in Chapter 4 (see (4.18) to (4.24)). For the first study (Carroll) we compute the pooled within-groups standard deviation

Introduction to Meta-Analysis   M. Borenstein, L. V. Hedges, J. P. T. Higgins, H. R. Rothstein
© 2009, John Wiley & Sons, Ltd

Table 14.1 Dataset 1 – Part A (basic data).

Study	Treated			Control		
	Mean	SD	n	Mean	SD	n
Carroll	94	22	60	92	20	60
Grant	98	21	65	92	22	65
Peck	98	28	40	88	26	40
Donat	94	19	200	82	17	200
Stewart	98	21	50	88	22	45
Young	96	21	85	92	22	85

Table 14.2 Dataset 1 – Part B (fixed-effect computations).

Study	Effect size	Variance Within	Weight	Calculated quantities		
	Y	V_Y	W	WY	WY^2	W^2
Carroll	0.095	0.033	30.352	2.869	0.271	921.214
Grant	0.277	0.031	32.568	9.033	2.505	1060.682
Peck	0.367	0.050	20.048	7.349	2.694	401.931
Donat	0.664	0.011	95.111	63.190	41.983	9046.013
Stewart	0.462	0.043	23.439	10.824	4.999	549.370
Young	0.185	0.023	42.698	7.906	1.464	1823.115
Sum			244.215	101.171	53.915	13802.325

Table 14.3 Dataset 1 – Part C (random-effects computations)

Study	Effect size Y	Variance Within V_Y	Variance Between T^2	Variance Total $V_Y + T^2$	Weight W^*	Calculated quantities W^*Y
Carroll	0.095	0.033	0.037	0.070	14.233	1.345
Grant	0.277	0.031	0.037	0.068	14.702	4.078
Peck	0.367	0.050	0.037	0.087	11.469	4.204
Donat	0.664	0.011	0.037	0.048	20.909	13.892
Stewart	0.462	0.043	0.037	0.080	12.504	5.774
Young	0.185	0.023	0.037	0.061	16.466	3.049
Sum					90.284	32.342

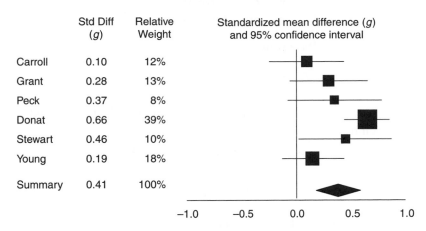

Figure 14.1 Forest plot of Dataset 1 – fixed-effect weights.

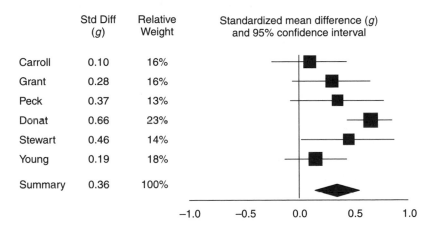

Figure 14.2 Forest plot of Dataset 1 – random-effects weights.

$$S_{within} = \sqrt{\frac{(60-1) \times 22^2 + (60-1) \times 20^2}{60 + 60 - 2}} = 21.0238.$$

Then we compute the standardized mean difference, d, and its variance as

$$d_1 = \frac{94 - 92}{21.0238} = 0.0951,$$

and
$$V_{d_1} = \frac{60 + 60}{60 \times 60} + \frac{0.0951^2}{2(60 + 60)} = 0.0334.$$

The correction factor (J) is estimated as
$$J = \left(1 - \frac{3}{4 \times 118 - 1}\right) = 0.9936.$$

Finally, the bias-corrected standardized mean difference, Hedges' g, and its variance are given by
$$g_1 = 0.9936 \times 0.0951 = 0.0945,$$

and
$$V_{g_1} = 0.9936^2 \times 0.0334 = 0.0329.$$

This procedure is repeated for all six studies.

Compute the summary effect using the fixed-effect model

The effect size and its variance are copied into Table 14.2 where they are assigned the generic labels Y and V_Y. We then compute the other values shown in the table. For Carroll,
$$W_1 = \frac{1}{0.0329} = 30.3515,$$

$$W_1 Y_1 = 30.3515 \times 0.0945 = 2.8690,$$

and so on for the other five studies. The sum of W is 244.215 and the sum of WY is 101.171. From these numbers we can compute the summary effect and related statistics, using formulas from Part 3 as follows (see (11.3) to (11.10)). In the computations that follow we use the generic M to represent Hedges' g.

$$M = \frac{101.171}{244.215} = 0.4143,$$

$$V_M = \frac{1}{244.215} = 0.0041,$$

$$SE_M = \sqrt{0.0041} = 0.0640,$$

$$LL_M = 0.4143 - 1.96 \times 0.0640 = 0.2889,$$

$$UL_M = 0.4143 + 1.96 \times 0.0640 = 0.5397,$$

and

$$Z = \frac{0.4143}{0.0640} = 6.4739.$$

For a one-tailed test the p-value is given by

$$p = 1 - \Phi(6.4739) < 0.0001,$$

and for a two-tailed test, by

$$p = 2[1 - \Phi(|6.4739|)] < 0.0001.$$

In words, using fixed-effect weights, the standardized mean difference (Hedges' g) is 0.41 with a 95% confidence interval of 0.29 to 0.54. The Z-value is 6.47, and the p-value is <0.0001 (one-tailed) or <0.0001 (two tailed). These results are illustrated in Figure 14.1.

Compute an estimate of τ^2

To estimate τ^2, the variance of the true standardized mean differences, we use the DerSimonian and Laird method (see (12.2) to (12.5)). Using sums from Table 14.2,

$$Q = 53.915 - \left(\frac{101.171^2}{244.215}\right) = 12.0033,$$

$$df = (6 - 1) = 5,$$

$$C - 244.215 \left(\frac{13802.325}{244.215}\right) = 187.698,$$

and

$$T^2 = \frac{12.0033 - 5}{187.698} = 0.0373.$$

Compute the summary effect using the random-effects model

To compute the summary effect using the random-effects model we use the same formulas as for the fixed effect, but the variance for each study is now the sum of the variance within studies plus the variance between studies (see (12.6) to (12.13)).
    For Carroll,

$$W_1^* = \frac{1}{(0.0329 + 0.0373)} = \frac{1}{(0.070)} = 14.2331,$$

and so on for the other studies as shown in Table 14.3. Note that the within-study variance is unique for each study, but there is only one value of τ^2, so this value (estimated as 0.037) is applied to all studies.

Then,

$$M^* = \frac{32.342}{90.284} = 0.3582, \tag{14.1}$$

$$V_{M^*} = \frac{1}{90.284} = 0.0111, \tag{14.2}$$

$$SE_{M^*} = \sqrt{0.0111} = 0.1052,$$

$$LL_{M^*} = 0.3582 - 1.96 \times 0.1052 = 0.1520,$$

$$UL_{M^*} = 0.3582 + 1.96 \times 0.1052 = 0.5645,$$

$$Z^* = \frac{0.3582}{0.1052} = 3.4038,$$

and, for a one-tailed test

$$p^* = 1 - \Phi(3.4038) = 0.0003$$

or, for a two-tailed test

$$p^* = 2[1 - \Phi(|3.4038|)] = 0.0007.$$

In words, using random-effect weights, the standardized mean difference (Hedges' g) is 0.36 with a 95% confidence interval of 0.15 to 0.56. The Z-value is 3.40, and the p-value is 0.0003 (one-tailed) or 0.0007 (two tailed). These results are illustrated in Figure 14.2.

WORKED EXAMPLE FOR BINARY DATA (PART 1)

In this example we start with the events and non-events in two independent groups and will use the odds ratio as the effect size measure.

Summary data

The summary data for six studies is presented in Table 14.4.

Compute the effect size and its variance for each study

For an odds ratio all computations are carried out using the log transformed values (see formulas (5.8) to (5.10)). For the first study (Saint) we compute the odds ratio, then the log odds ratio and its variance as

Table 14.4 Dataset 2 – Part A (basic data).

Study	Treated			Control		
	Events	Non-events	n	Events	Non-events	n
Saint	12	53	65	16	49	65
Kelly	8	32	40	10	30	40
Pilbeam	14	66	80	19	61	80
Lane	25	375	400	80	320	400
Wright	8	32	40	11	29	40
Day	16	49	65	18	47	65

Table 14.5 Dataset 2 – Part B (fixed-effect computations).

Study	Effect size	Variance Within	Weight	Calculated quantities		
	Y	V_Y	W	WY	WY^2	W^2
Saint	−0.366	0.185	5.402	−1.978	0.724	29.184
Kelly	−0.288	0.290	3.453	−0.993	0.286	11.925
Pilbeam	−0.384	0.156	6.427	−2.469	0.948	41.300
Lane	−1.322	0.058	17.155	−22.675	29.971	294.298
Wright	−0.417	0.282	3.551	−1.480	0.617	12.607
Day	−0.159	0.160	6.260	−0.998	0.159	39.190
Sum			42.248	−30.594	32.705	428.503

Table 14.6 Dataset 2 – Part C (random-effects computations).

Study	Effect size Y	Variance Within V_Y	Variance Between T^2	Variance Total $V_Y + T^2$	Weight W^*	Calculated quantities $W^* Y$
Saint	−0.366	0.185	0.173	0.358	2.793	−1.023
Kelly	−0.288	0.290	0.173	0.462	2.162	−0.622
Pilbeam	−0.384	0.156	0.173	0.329	3.044	−1.169
Lane	−1.322	0.058	0.173	0.231	4.325	−5.717
Wright	−0.417	0.282	0.173	0.455	2.200	−0.917
Day	−0.159	0.160	0.173	0.333	3.006	−0.479
Sum					17.531	−9.928

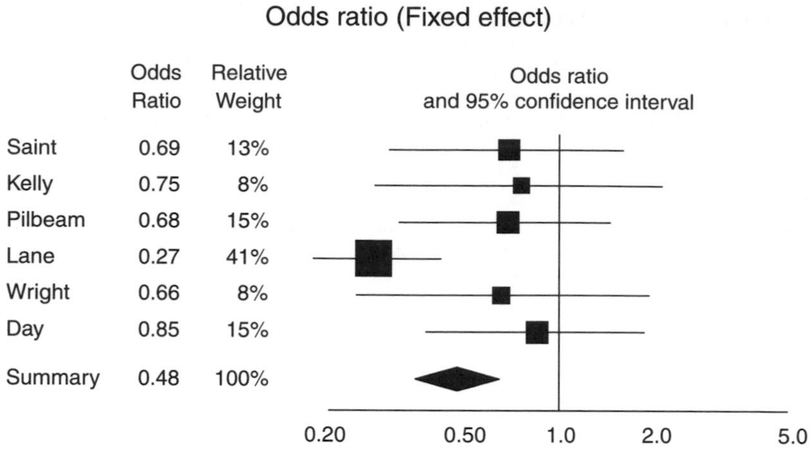

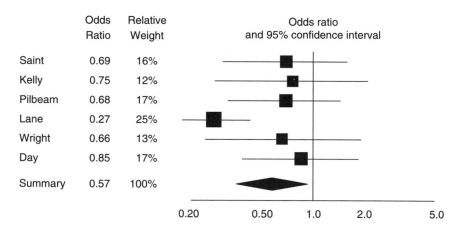

Figure 14.3 Forest plot of Dataset 2 – fixed-effect weights.

Figure 14.4 Forest plot of Dataset 2 – random-effects weights.

$$OddsRatio_1 = \frac{12 \times 49}{53 \times 16} = 0.6934,$$

$$LogOddsRatio_1 = \ln(0.6934) = -0.3662,$$

and

$$V_{LogOddsRatio_1} = \frac{1}{12} + \frac{1}{53} + \frac{1}{16} + \frac{1}{49} = 0.1851.$$

This procedure is repeated for all six studies.

Compute the summary effect using the fixed-effect model

The effect size and its variance (in log units) are copied into Table 14.5 where they are assigned the generic labels Y and V_Y.

For Saint

$$W_1 = \frac{1}{0.1851} = 5.4021,$$

$$W_1 Y_1 = 5.4021 \times (-0.3662) = -1.9780,$$

and so on for the other five studies.

The sum of W is 42.248 and the sum of WY is -30.594. From these numbers we can compute the summary effect and related statistics as follows (see (11.3) to (11.10)). In the computations that follow we use the generic M to represent the log odds ratio.

$$M = \frac{-30.594}{42.248} = -0.7241,$$

$$V_M = \frac{1}{42.248} = 0.0237,$$

$$SE_M = \sqrt{0.0237} = 0.1539,$$

$$LL_M = (-0.7241) - 1.96 \times 0.1539 = -1.0257,$$

$$UL_M = (-0.7241) + 1.96 \times 0.1539 = -0.4226,$$

and

$$Z = \frac{-0.7241}{0.1539} = -4.7068.$$

For a one-tailed test the p-value is given by

$$p = 1 - \Phi(-4.7068) < 0.0001,$$

and for a two-tailed test, by

$$p = 2[1 - \Phi(|-4.7068|)] < 0.0001.$$

We can convert the log odds ratio and confidence limits to the odds ratio scale using

$$OddsRatio = \exp(-0.7241) = 0.4847,$$

$$LL_{OddsRatio} = \exp(-1.0257) = 0.3586,$$

and

$$UL_{OddsRatio} = \exp(-0.4226) = 0.6553.$$

In words, using fixed-effect weights, the summary odd ratio is 0.48 with a 95% confidence interval of 0.36 to 0.66. The Z-value is -4.71, and the p-value is <0.0001 (one-tailed) or <0.0001 (two tailed). These results are illustrated in Figure 14.3.

Compute an estimate of τ^2

To estimate τ^2, the variance of the true log odds ratios, we use the DerSimonian and Laird method (see (12.2) to (12.5)). Using sums from Table 14.5,

$$Q = 32.705 - \left(\frac{-30.594^2}{42.248}\right) = 10.5512,$$

$$df = (6 - 1) = 5,$$

$$C = 42.248 - \left(\frac{428.503}{42.248}\right) = 32.1052,$$

and

$$T^2 = \frac{10.5512 - 5}{32.1052} = 0.1729.$$

These values are reported only on a log scale.

Compute the summary effect using the random-effects model

To compute the summary effect using the random-effects model, we use the same formulas as for the fixed effect, but the variance for each study is now the sum of the variance within studies plus the variance between studies (see (12.6) to (12.13)).
    For Saint,

$$W_1^* = \frac{1}{(0.1851 + 0.1729)} = \frac{1}{(0.3580)} = 2.7932,$$

and so on for the other studies as shown in Table 14.6. Note that the within-study variance is unique for each study, but there is only one value of τ^2, so this value (estimated as 0.173) is applied to all studies.
    Then,

$$M^* = \frac{-9.928}{17.531} = -0.5663, \tag{14.3}$$

$$V_{M^*} = \frac{1}{17.531} = 0.0570, \tag{14.4}$$

$$SE_{M^*} = \sqrt{0.0570} = 0.2388,$$

$$LL_{M^*} = (-0.5663) - 1.96 \times 0.2388 = -1.0344,$$

$$UL_{M^*} = (-0.5663) + 1.96 \times 0.2388 = -0.0982,$$

$$Z^* = \frac{-0.5663}{0.2388} = -2.3711,$$

and, for a one-tailed test

$$p^* = 1 - \Phi(-2.3711) = 0.0089$$

or, for a two-tailed test

$$p^* = 2[1 - \Phi(|-2.3711|)] = 0.0177.$$

We can convert the log odds ratio and confidence limits to the odds ratio scale using

$$OddsRatio^* = \exp(-0.5663) = 0.5676,$$

$$LL_{OddsRatio^*} = \exp(-1.0344) = 0.3554,$$

and

$$UL_{OddsRatio^*} = \exp(-0.0982) = 0.9065.$$

In words, using random-effects weights, the summary odds ratio is 0.57 with a 95% confidence interval of 0.36 to 0.91. The Z-value is -2.37, and the p-value is 0.0089 (one-tailed) or 0.0177 (two tailed). These results are illustrated in Figure 14.4.

WORKED EXAMPLE FOR CORRELATIONAL DATA (PART 1)

Summary data

In this example we start with the correlation and sample size in six studies, as shown in Table 14.7.

Compute the effect size and its variance for each study

For correlations, all computations are carried out using the Fisher's z transformed values (see formulas (6.2) to (6.3)). For the first study (Fonda) we compute the Fisher's z value and its variance as

$$z_1 = 0.5 \times \ln\left(\frac{1 + 0.50}{1 - 0.50}\right) = 0.5493,$$

and

$$V_1 = \frac{1}{40 - 3} = 0.0270.$$

This procedure is repeated for all six studies.

Table 14.7 Dataset 3 – Part A (basic data).

Study	Correlation	N
Fonda	0.50	40
Newman	0.60	90
Grant	0.40	25
Granger	0.20	400
Milland	0.70	60
Finch	0.45	50

Table 14.8 Dataset 3 – Part B (fixed-effect computations)

Study	Effect size	Variance Within	Weight	Calculated quantities		
	Y	V_Y	W	WY	WY^2	W^2
Fonda	0.5493	0.0270	37.000	20.324	11.164	1369.000
Newman	0.6931	0.0115	87.000	60.304	41.799	7569.000
Grant	0.4236	0.0455	22.000	9.320	3.949	484.000
Granger	0.2027	0.0025	397.000	80.485	16.317	157609.000
Milland	0.8673	0.0175	57.000	49.436	42.876	3249.000
Finch	0.4847	0.0213	47.000	22.781	11.042	2209.000
Sum			647.000	242.650	127.147	172489.000

Table 14.9 Dataset 3 – Part C (random-effects computations).

Study	Effect size Y	Variance Within V_Y	Variance Between T^2	Variance Total $V_Y + T^2$	Weight W^*	Calculated quantities W^*Y
Fonda	0.549	0.027	0.082	0.109	9.183	5.044
Newman	0.693	0.012	0.082	0.093	10.711	7.424
Grant	0.424	0.046	0.082	0.127	7.854	3.327
Granger	0.203	0.003	0.082	0.084	11.850	2.402
Milland	0.867	0.018	0.082	0.099	10.059	8.724
Finch	0.485	0.021	0.082	0.103	9.695	4.699
Sum					59.351	31.621

Correlation (Fixed effect)

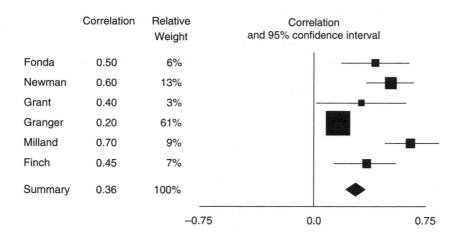

	Correlation	Relative Weight	Correlation and 95% confidence interval
Fonda	0.50	6%	
Newman	0.60	13%	
Grant	0.40	3%	
Granger	0.20	61%	
Milland	0.70	9%	
Finch	0.45	7%	
Summary	0.36	100%	

Figure 14.5 Forest plot of Dataset 3 – fixed-effect weights.

Correlation (Random effects)

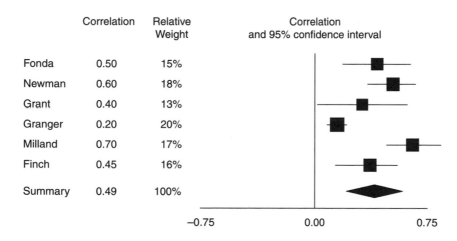

	Correlation	Relative Weight	Correlation and 95% confidence interval
Fonda	0.50	15%	
Newman	0.60	18%	
Grant	0.40	13%	
Granger	0.20	20%	
Milland	0.70	17%	
Finch	0.45	16%	
Summary	0.49	100%	

Figure 14.6 Forest plot of Dataset 3 – random-effects weights.

Compute the summary effect using the fixed-effect model

The effect size and its variance (in the Fisher's z metric) are copied into Table 14.8 where they are assigned the generic labels Y and V_Y.

For Fonda

$$W_1 = \frac{1}{0.0270} = 37.0000,$$

$$W_1 Y_1 = 37.000 \times (0.5493) = 20.3243,$$

and so on for the other five studies.

The sum of W is 647.000 and the sum of WY is 242.650. From these numbers we can compute the summary effect and related statistics as follows (see (11.3) to (11.10)). In the computations that follow we use the generic M to represent the Fisher's z score.

$$M = \frac{242.650}{647.000} = 0.3750,$$

$$V_M = \frac{1}{647.000} = 0.0015,$$

$$SE_M = \sqrt{0.0015} = 0.0393,$$

$$LL_M = 0.3750 - 1.96 \times 0.0393 = 0.2980,$$

$$UL_M = 0.3750 + 1.96 \times 0.0393 = 0.4521,$$

and

$$Z = \frac{0.3750}{0.0393} = 9.5396.$$

For a one-tailed test the p-value is given by

$$p = 1 - \Phi(9.5396) < 0.0001,$$

and for a two-tailed test, by

$$p = 2[1 - \Phi(|9.5396|)] < 0.0001.$$

We can convert the effect size and confidence limits from the Fisher's z metric to correlations using

$$r = \frac{e^{(2 \times 0.3750)} - 1}{e^{(2 \times 0.3750)} + 1} = 0.3584,$$

$$LL_r = \frac{e^{(2 \times 0.2980)} - 1}{e^{(2 \times 0.2980)} + 1} = 0.2895,$$

and

$$UL_r = \frac{e^{(2 \times 0.4521)} - 1}{e^{(2 \times 0.4521)} + 1} = 0.4236.$$

In words, using fixed-effect weights, the summary estimate of the correlation is 0.36 with a 95% confidence interval of 0.29 to 0.42. The Z-value is 9.54, and the p-value is <0.0001 (one-tailed) or <0.0001 (two tailed). These results are illustrated in Figure 14.5.

Compute an estimate of τ^2

To estimate τ^2, the variance of the true Fishers'z, we use the DerSimonian and Laird method (see (12.2) to (12.5)). Using sums from Table 14.8,

$$Q = 127.147 - \left(\frac{242.650^2}{647.000} \right) = 36.1437,$$

$$df = (6 - 1) = 5,$$

$$C = 647.000 - \left(\frac{172489.000}{647.000} \right) = 380.4019,$$

and

$$T^2 = \frac{36.1437 - 5}{380.4019} = 0.0819.$$

Compute the summary effect using the random-effects model

To compute the summary effect using the random-effects model, we use the same formulas as for the fixed effect, but the variance for each study is now the sum of the variance within studies plus the variance between studies (see (12.6) to (12.13)).
For Fonda,

$$W_1^* = \frac{1}{(0.0270 + 0.0819)} = \frac{1}{(0.1089)} = 9.1829,$$

and so on for the other studies as shown in Table 14.9. Note that the within-study variance is unique for each study, but there is only one value of τ^2, so this value (estimated as 0.0819) is applied to all studies.
Then,

$$M^* = \frac{31.621}{59.351} = 0.5328, \tag{14.5}$$

$$V_{M^*} = \frac{1}{59.351} = 0.0168, \tag{14.6}$$

$$SE_{M^*} = \sqrt{0.0168} = 0.1298,$$

$$LL_{M^*} = (0.5328) - 1.96 \times 0.1298 = 0.2784,$$

$$UL_{M^*} = (0.5328) + 1.96 \times 0.1298 = 0.7872,$$

and

$$Z^* = \frac{0.5328}{0.1298} = 4.1045.$$

Then, for a one-tailed test

$$p^* = 1 - \Phi(4.1045) < 0.0001,$$

or, for a two-tailed test

$$p^* = 2[1 - \Phi(|4.1045|)] < 0.0001.$$

We can convert the effect size and confidence limits from the Fisher's z metric to correlations using

$$r^* = \frac{e^{(2 \times 0.5328)} - 1}{e^{(2 \times 0.5328)} + 1} = 0.4875,$$

$$LL_{r^*} = \frac{e^{(2 \times 0.2784)} - 1}{e^{(2 \times 0.2784)} + 1} = 0.2714,$$

and

$$UL_{r^*} = \frac{e^{(2 \times 0.7872)} - 1}{e^{(2 \times 0.7872)} + 1} = 0.6568.$$

In words, using random-effects weights, the summary estimate of the correlation is 0.49 with a 95% confidence interval of 0.27 to 0.66. The Z-value is 4.10, and the p-value is <0.0001 (one-tailed) or <0.0001 (two tailed). These results are illustrated in Figure 14.6.

SUMMARY POINTS

- This chapter includes worked examples showing how to compute the summary effect using fixed-effect and random-effects models.
- For the standardized mean difference we work with the effect sizes directly.
- For ratios we work with the log transformed data.
- For correlations we work with the Fisher's z transformed data.
- These worked examples are available as Excel files on the book's web site.

PART 4

Heterogeneity

CHAPTER 15

Overview

Introduction
Nomenclature
Worked examples

INTRODUCTION

A central theme in this volume is that the goal of a synthesis is not simply to compute a summary effect, but rather to make sense of the pattern of effects. An intervention that consistently reduces the risk of criminal behavior by 40% across a range of studies is very different from one that reduces the risk by 40% *on average* with a risk reduction that ranges from 10% in some studies to 70% in others. If the effect size is consistent across studies we need to know that and to consider the implications, and if it varies we need to know that and consider the different implications.

The first chapter in this Part deals with the question of how to identify and quantify the heterogeneity in effect sizes. The problem we need to address is that the *observed* variation in the estimated effect sizes is partly spurious, in that it includes both true variation in effect sizes and also random error. We show how to isolate the true variance and then use it to create an array of measures that provide various perspectives on the dispersion. These are the Q statistic (a measure of weighted squared deviations), the results of a statistical test based on the Q statistic (p), the between-studies variance (T^2), the between-studies standard deviation (T), and the ratio of true heterogeneity to total observed variation (I^2). Then, we show how these measures can be used to address the following questions.

- Is there evidence of heterogeneity in true effect sizes?
- What is the variance of the true effects?
- What are the substantive implications of this heterogeneity?
- What proportion of the observed dispersion is real?

The other chapters in this Part address methods to explore the reasons for heterogeneity. In Chapter 19 we show how to compare the effect size in different

Introduction to Meta-Analysis   M. Borenstein, L. V. Hedges, J. P. T. Higgins, H. R. Rothstein
© 2009, John Wiley & Sons, Ltd

subgroups of studies (such as studies that used different populations, or studies that used different variants of the intervention), similar to analysis of variance in primary studies. In Chapter 20 we show how to assess the relationship between effect size and covariates (such as the dose of a drug or the mean age in the study sample), similar to multiple regression in primary studies. Finally, Chapter 21 includes a discussion of issues (and some important caveats) related to both techniques.

NOMENCLATURE

As we did in the previous part we distinguish between a true effect size and an observed effect size. A study's *true effect size* is the effect size in the underlying population, and is the effect size that we would observe if the study had an infinitely large sample size (and therefore no sampling error). A study's *observed effect size* is the effect size that is actually observed.

We use the terms *variation* and *dispersion* to refer to differences among values, sometimes true effects and sometimes observed effects, depending on the context. By contrast, we use *heterogeneity* to mean heterogeneity in true effects only.

We shall introduce several measures of heterogeneity, one of which is tau-squared, defined as the variance of the true effect sizes. We will use τ^2 to refer to the parameter (the population value) and T^2 to refer to our estimate of this parameter.

WORKED EXAMPLES

The discussion of formulas and concepts in Chapter 16 is followed by a section with worked examples using a series of effect sizes (standardized mean differences, odds ratios, and correlations). While reading the sections on formulas and concepts, it will be helpful to refer to one or more of the worked examples.

These examples are continuations of the three worked examples in Chapter 14, and are all available as Excel spreadsheets on the book's web site.

CHAPTER 16

Identifying and Quantifying Heterogeneity

Introduction
Isolating the variation in true effects
Computing Q
Estimating τ^2
The I^2 statistic
Comparing the measures of heterogeneity
Confidence intervals for τ^2
Confidence intervals (or uncertainty intervals) for I^2

INTRODUCTION

Under the random-effects model we allow that the true effect size may vary from study to study. In this chapter we discuss approaches to identify and then quantify this heterogeneity.

ISOLATING THE VARIATION IN TRUE EFFECTS

The mechanisms for describing the variation among scores in a primary study are well known. We can compute the standard deviation of the scores and discuss the proportion of subjects falling within a given range. We can compute the variance of the scores and discuss what proportion of variance can be explained by covariates.

Our goals are similar in a meta-analysis, in the sense that we want to describe the variation, using indices such as the standard deviation and variance. However, the process is more complicated for the following reason. When we speak about the *heterogeneity* in effect sizes we mean the variation in the *true* effect sizes. However, the variation that we actually observe is partly spurious, incorporating both (true) heterogeneity and also random error.

Introduction to Meta-Analysis   M. Borenstein, L. V. Hedges, J. P. T. Higgins, H. R. Rothstein
© 2009, John Wiley & Sons, Ltd

To understand the problem, suppose for a moment that all studies in the analysis shared the same *true* effect size, so that the (true) heterogeneity is zero. Under this assumption, we would not expect the observed effects to be identical to each other. Rather, because of within-study error, we would expect each to fall *within some range* of the common effect.

Now, assume that the true effect size *does* vary from one study to the next. In this case, the observed effects vary from one another for two reasons. One is the real heterogeneity in effect size, and the other is the within-study error. If we want to quantify the heterogeneity we need to partition the observed variation into these two components, and then focus on the former.

The mechanism that we use to extract the true between-studies variation from the observed variation is as follows.

1. We compute the total amount of study-to-study variation actually observed.
2. We estimate how much the observed effects would be expected to vary from each other if the true effect was actually the same in all studies.
3. The excess variation (if any) is assumed to reflect real differences in effect size (that is, the heterogeneity).

Consider the top row in Figure 16.1. The observed effects (and therefore variation in the observed effects) are identical in *A* and *B*. The difference between *A* and *B* is that the confidence intervals for each study in *A* are relatively wide, while the confidence intervals for each study in *B* are relatively narrow. The visual impression in *A* is that all studies could share a common effect, with the observed dispersion falling within the umbrella of the confidence intervals. By contrast, the confidence

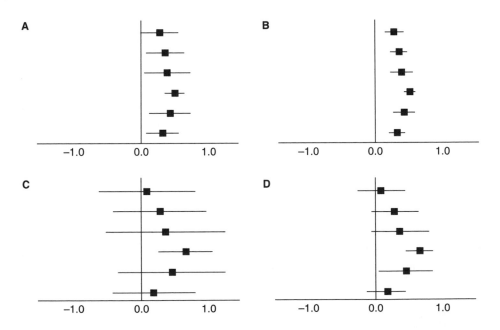

Figure 16.1 Dispersion across studies relative to error within studies.

intervals for the B studies are quite narrow, and cannot comfortably account for the observed dispersion.

Similarly, consider the bottom row in this plot. Again, the *observed* effects are identical in C and D, but C has wider confidence intervals around each study. In C, the effects can be fully explained by within-study error, while in D they cannot.

The difference between A and B (on the one hand) versus C and D (on the other) is that we have changed the *absolute value* (or the scale) of the dispersion. To move from A to C we multiplied both the within-study variance and the observed variance by 2.0 so that the scale has increased but the ratio (observed/within) is unchanged. The same holds true for B and D. While the effects are more widely dispersed in the second row than in the first, this is not relevant to the purpose of isolating the true dispersion. What matters is only the *ratio* of observed to expected dispersion, which is the same in A and C (and is the same in B and D).

It is this aspect of the dispersion – the one reflected in the difference of A versus B, and of C versus D that we want to capture for the purpose of isolating the true variation. In other words, we need a statistic that is sensitive to the *ratio* of the observed variation to the within-study error, rather than their absolute values. The statistic that we use for this purpose is Q.

COMPUTING Q

The first step in partitioning the variation is to compute Q, defined as

$$Q = \sum_{i=1}^{k} W_i (Y_i - M)^2, \tag{16.1}$$

where W_i is the study weight ($1/V_i$), Y_i is the study effect size, and M is the summary effect and k is the number of studies. In words, we compute the deviation of each effect size from the mean, square it, weight this by the inverse-variance for that study, and sum these values over all studies to yield the weighted sum of squares (*WSS*), or Q.

The same formula can be written as

$$Q = \sum_{i=1}^{k} \left(\frac{Y_i - M}{S_i} \right)^2 \tag{16.2}$$

to highlight the fact that Q is a standardized measure, which means that it is not affected by the metric of the effect size index. The analogy would be to the standardized mean difference d, where the mean difference is divided by the within-study standard deviation.

Finally, an equivalent formula, useful for computations, is

$$Q = \sum_{i=1}^{k} W_i Y_i^2 - \frac{\left(\sum_{i=1}^{k} W_i Y_i \right)^2}{\sum_{i=1}^{k} W_i}. \tag{16.3}$$

The expected value of Q based on within-study error

The next step is to determine the expected value of Q on the assumption that all studies share a common effect size, and (it follows) all the variation is due to sampling error within studies. Because Q is a standardized measure the expected value does not depend on the metric of effect size, but is simply the degrees of freedom (df),

$$df = k - 1, \tag{16.4}$$

where k is the number of studies.

The excess variation

Since Q is the observed WSS and df is the expected WSS (under the assumption that all studies share a common effect), the difference,

$$Q - df,$$

reflects the excess variation, the part that will be attributed to differences in the true effects from study to study.

Ratio of observed to expected variation

Earlier, we used Figure 16.1 to introduce the concept of excess variation, and showed that it needs to be based on the ratio of observed variance to the within-study variance. In Figure 16.2 we reproduce the same four plots but add the

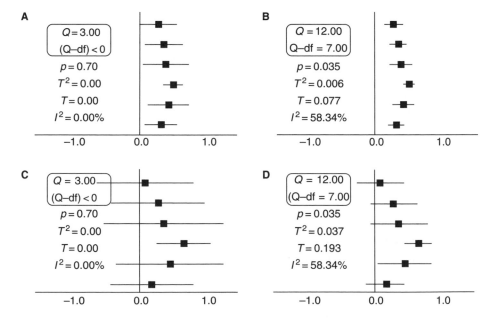

Figure 16.2 Q in relation to df as measure of dispersion.

Q statistic, which quantifies this concept. The plot also includes additional statistics, which will be explained below.

First, consider the top row. For plot A the observed value of Q is 3.00, versus an expected value (under the assumption of a common effect size) of 5.00 (that is, $k-1$). In this case the observed variation is less than we would expect based on within-study error (Q is less than the degrees of freedom). For plot B the observed value of Q is 12.00, versus an expected value of 5.00, so the observed variation is greater than we would expect based on within-study error (Q is greater than the degrees of freedom). This, of course, is consistent with the visual impression discussed earlier. We see the same thing in the second row, where for plot C the observed value of Q is 3.00, versus an expected value of 5.00, ($Q < df$) and for plot D the observed value of Q is 12.00, versus an expected value of 5.00, ($Q > df$).

Note that Q is the same (3.00) in A and C because these plots share the same ratio, despite the fact that the absolute range of effects is higher in C. Similarly, the value of Q is the same (12.00) in B and D because these plots share the same ratio, despite the fact that the absolute range of effects is higher in D.

At this point we have the values Q, which reflects the total dispersion (WSS) and $Q-df$, which reflects the excess dispersion. However, Q is not an intuitive measure. For one thing, Q is a sum (rather than a mean) and, as such, depends strongly on the number of studies. For another, Q is on a standardized scale, and for some purposes we will want to express the dispersion either as a ratio or on the same scale as the effect size itself.

Now that we have Q, however, we can use it to construct measures that do address specific needs, as outlined in Figure 16.3. To test the assumption of homogeneity we will work directly with Q, and take advantage of the fact that it is on a standardized

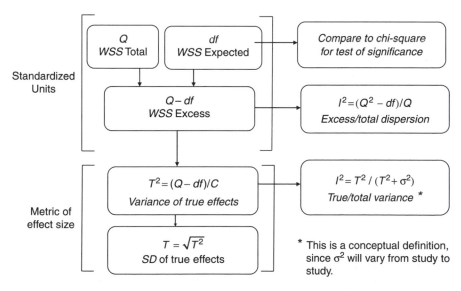

Figure 16.3 Flowchart showing how T^2 and I^2 are derived from Q and df.

scale and is sensitive to the number of studies. To estimate the variance (and standard deviation) of the true effects we will start with Q, remove the dependence on the number of studies, and return to the original metric. These estimates are called T^2 and T. Finally, to estimate what proportion of the observed variance reflects real differences among studies (rather than random error) we will start with Q, remove the dependence on the number of studies, and express the result as a ratio (called I^2).

Testing the assumption of homogeneity in effects

Researchers typically ask if the heterogeneity is statistically significant, and we can use Q (and df) to address this question. Formally, we pose the null hypothesis that all studies share a common effect size and then test this hypothesis. Under the null hypothesis Q will follow a central chi-squared distribution with degrees of freedom equal to $k-1$, so we can report a p-value for any observed value of Q. Typically, we set alpha at 0.10 or at 0.05, with a p-value less than alpha leading us to reject the null, and conclude that the studies do not share a common effect size.

This test of significance, like all tests of significance, is sensitive both to the magnitude of the effect (here, the excess dispersion) and the precision with which this effect is estimated (here, based on the number of studies).

The impact of the excess dispersion on the p-value is evident if we compare plots A versus B in Figure 16.4. These plots both have six studies, and as the excess dispersion increases (Q moves from 3.00 in A to 12.00 in B) the p-value moves from 0.70 to 0.035. Similarly, compare plots C and D, which both have twelve studies. As we move from C to D, Q moves from 6.62 to 27.12 and the p-value moves from 0.830 to 0.004.

The impact of the number of studies is evident if we compare plots A versus C. The two plots are essentially identical, except that A has six studies and C has twelve studies with the same estimated value of between-studies variation (prior to being truncated at zero). With the additional precision the p-value moves *away from zero*, from 0.70 (for A) to 0.83 (for C).

Similarly, the impact of the number of studies is evident if we compare plots B versus D. The two plots are essentially identical, except that (again) B has six studies and D has twelve studies with the same estimated value of between-studies variation ($T^2 = 0.037$). With the additional precision the p-value moves *towards zero*, from 0.035 (for B) to 0.004 (for D).

Note that the p-value for the left-hand columns moved toward 1.0 as we added studies, while the p-value for the left-hand columns moved toward 0.0 as we added studies. At left, since Q is less than df the additional evidence strengthens the case that the excess dispersion *is zero*, and moves the p-value towards 1.0. At right, since Q exceeds df, the additional evidence strengthens the case that the excess dispersion is *not* zero, and moves the p-value towards 0.0.

Concluding remarks about Q and its p-value

The test of the null hypothesis (that all studies share a common effect size) is subject to the same caveats as all tests of significance, as follows.

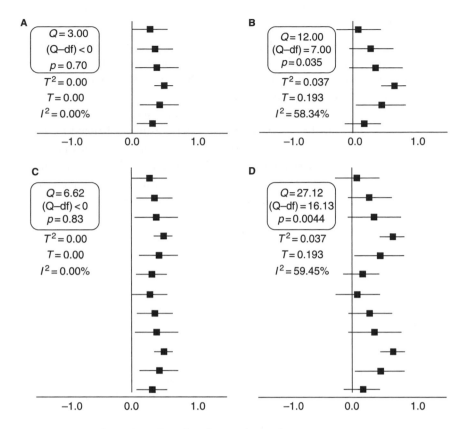

Figure 16.4 Impact of Q and number of studies on the p-value.

First, while a significant p-value provides evidence that the true effects vary, the converse is not true. A nonsignificant p-value should not be taken as evidence that the effect sizes are consistent, since the lack of significance may be due to low power. With a small number of studies and/or large within-study variance (small studies), even substantial between-studies dispersion might yield a nonsignificant p-value.

Second, the Q statistic and p-value address only the test of significance and should never be used as surrogates for the amount of true variance. A nonsignificant p-value *could* reflect a trivial amount of observed dispersion, but could also reflect a substantial amount of observed dispersion with imprecise studies. Similarly, a significant p-value *could* reflect a substantial amount of observed dispersion, but could also reflect a minor amount of observed dispersion with precise studies.

In sum, the purpose served by this test is to assess the viability of the null hypothesis, and not to estimate the magnitude of the true dispersion. There are several ways that we *can* describe the dispersion of true effect sizes, and we shall deal with each of these in the balance of this chapter.

ESTIMATING τ^2

The parameter tau-squared (τ^2) is defined as the variance of the true effect sizes. In other words, if we had an infinitely large sample of studies, each, itself, infinitely large (so that the estimate in each study was the true effect) and computed the variance of these effects, this variance would be τ^2.

Since we cannot observe the true effects we cannot compute this variance directly. Rather, we estimate it from the observed effects, with the estimate denoted T^2. To yield this estimate we start with the difference ($Q - df$) which represents the dispersion in true effects on a standardized scale. We divide by a quantity (C) which has the effect of putting the measure back into its original metric and also of making it an average, rather than a sum, of squared deviations. Concretely,

$$T^2 = \frac{Q - df}{C} \tag{16.5}$$

where

$$C = \sum W_i - \frac{\sum W_i^2}{\sum W_i}. \tag{16.6}$$

This means that T^2 is in the same metric (squared) as the effect size itself, and also reflects the absolute amount of variation in that scale.

While the actual variance of the true effects (τ^2) can never be less than zero, our estimate of this value (T^2) can be less than zero if, because of sampling error, the observed variance is less than we would expect based on within-study error – in other words, if $Q < df$. In this case, T^2 is simply set to zero.

If $Q > df$ then T^2 will be positive, and it will be based on two factors. The first is the amount of excess variation ($Q - df$), and the second is the metric of the effect size index.

The impact of the excess variation on our estimate of T^2 is evident if we compare plots A versus B in Figure 16.5. The within-study error is smaller in B. Therefore, while the observed variation is the same in both plots, a higher proportion of this variation is assumed to be real in B. As we move from A to B, Q moves from 12.00 to 48.01, and T^2 from 0.037 to 0.057.

The impact of the scale on our estimate of T^2 is evident if we compare plots C versus D in Figure 16.5. Q and df are the same in the two plots, which means that the same proportion of the observed variance will be attributed to between-studies variance. However, the absolute amount of the variance is larger in D, so this proportion translates into a larger estimate of τ^2. As we move from C to D, T^2 moves from 0.037 to 0.096.

Concluding remarks about T^2

As our estimate for the variance of the true effects, T^2 is used to assign weights under the random-effects model, where the weight assigned to each study is

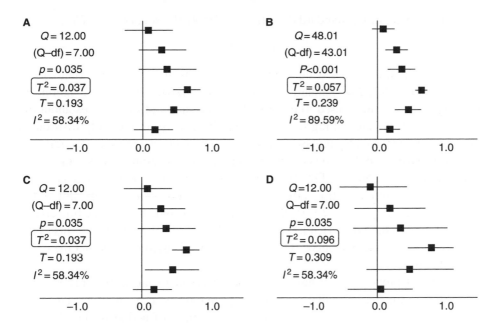

Figure 16.5 Impact of excess dispersion and absolute dispersion on T^2.

$$W_i^* = \frac{1}{V_{\bar{Y}_i}^*} = \frac{1}{V_{Y_i} + T^2}. \qquad (16.7)$$

In words, the total variance for a study (V_Y^*) is the sum of the within-study variance (V_Y) and the between-studies variance, (T^2).

This method of estimating the variance between studies is the most popular, and is known as the *method of moments* or the *DerSimonian and Laird method*. This method does not make any assumptions about the distribution of the random effects. It also has the advantage of being the easiest to compute and the easiest to explain, which makes it useful for a text. Alternatives exist, and some statisticians favor a restricted maximum likelihood (REML) method.

Interestingly, one of the authors of the key DerSimonian and Laird paper has since argued that the simple method we describe should no longer be used, since computational simplicity is no longer an important consideration. However, we believe that it is instructive to describe this simple method, and note that differences in results from one method to the other are likely to be small. Formulas to compute confidence intervals for T^2 are presented at the end of this chapter.

Tau

Above, we discussed the variance of the true effect sizes, where τ^2 refers to the actual variance and T^2 is our estimate of this parameter. Now, we turn to the standard deviation of the true effect sizes. Here, τ refers to the actual standard deviation and T is our estimate of this parameter.

T, the estimate of the standard deviation, is simply the square root of T^2,

$$T = \sqrt{T^2}. \tag{16.8}$$

Like T^2, T is on the same scale as the effect size itself, but T^2 (a variance) is a squared value, while T (a standard deviation) is not. Like the standard deviation in a primary study, T can be used to describe the distribution of effect sizes about the mean effect. If we are willing to assume that the effects are normally distributed (and we have a reasonably precise estimate of T), we can get a sense for the range of true effect sizes, and then consider the substantive implications of this range.

Figure 16.6 is identical to Figure 16.5 but this time we have added to each plot the expected distribution of true effects, based on T. For example, in plot A the summary effect is 0.41 and T is 0.193. We expect that some 95% of the true effects will fall in the range of 0.41 plus or minus 1.96 T, or 0.04 to 0.79, and this is the range reflected in the bell curve. The same approach is used to construct the curve for all the plots.

Recall that plots A and B have the same observed variance, but differ in the proportion of this variance that is attributed to real differences in effect size. In A, the bell curve is relatively narrow, and captures only a fraction of the observed

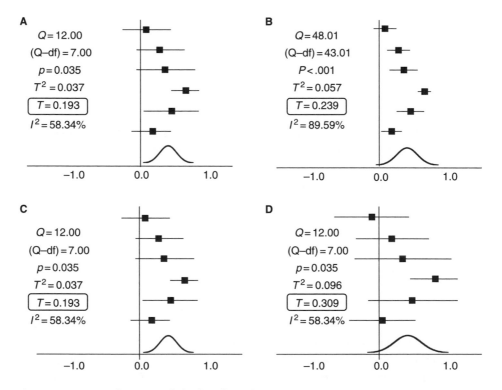

Figure 16.6 Impact of excess and absolute dispersion on T.

dispersion – the rest is assumed to reflect error. In B, the bell curve is relatively wide, and captures a larger fraction of the dispersion, since most of the dispersion is here assumed to be real.

Similarly, recall that in plots C and D the ratio of true to observed variance is the same, but the observed dispersion (the scale) is larger in D. The bell curve is wider in D than in C (because of the different scale), but in both cases a comparable proportion of the effects fall within the range of the curve (because the ratio is the same).

Concluding remarks about T

Our estimate T of the standard deviation of the true effects enables us to talk about the substantive importance of the dispersion. Suppose an intervention has a summary effect size of 0.50. If T is 0.10, then most of the effects (95 %) fall in the approximate range of 0.30 to 0.70. If T is 0.20 then most of the true effects fall in the approximate range of 0.10 to 0.90. If T is 0.30 then most of the true effects fall in the approximate range of -0.10 to $+1.10$. We still need to attach a value judgment to these ranges (what effect size is *harmful*, what effect size is *trivial*, what effect size is *useful*), but by having a sense of the distribution we have at least a starting point for these discussions.

In this example we assume that the effect size and T are estimated accurately. In practice, if we wanted to make predictions about the distribution of true effects we would need to take account of the error in estimating both of these values. Toward the end of this chapter we show how to compute confidence intervals for the value of T, and in Chapter 17 we show how to compute prediction intervals that take account of these sources of error.

THE I^2 STATISTIC

The utility of T^2 and T lies in the fact that they are absolute measures, which means that they quantify deviation on the same scale as the effect size index. In some cases, however, we would prefer to think about heterogeneity independent of scale and ask *What proportion of the observed variance reflects real differences in effect size?*

Higgins *et al.* (2003) proposed using a statistic, I^2, to reflect this proportion, that could serve as a kind of signal-to-noise ratio. It is computed as

$$I^2 = \left(\frac{Q - df}{Q} \right) \times 100\%, \qquad (16.9)$$

that is, the ratio of excess dispersion to total dispersion. The statistic I^2 can be viewed as a statistic of the form

$$I^2 = \left(\frac{Variance_{bet}}{Variance_{total}} \right) \times 100\% = \left(\frac{\tau^2}{\tau^2 + V_Y} \right) \times 100\%, \qquad (16.10)$$

that is, the ratio of true heterogeneity to total variance across the observed effect estimates. However, this is not a true definition of I^2 because in reality

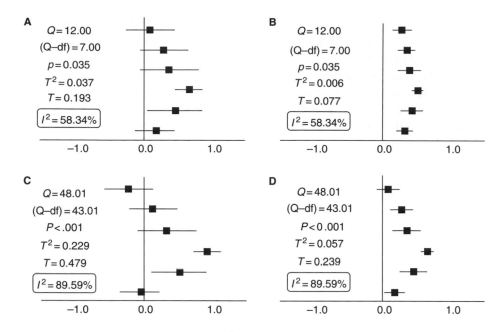

Figure 16.7 Impact of excess dispersion on I^2.

there is not a single V_Y, since the within-study variances vary from study to study. The I^2 statistic is a descriptive statistic and not an estimate of any underlying quantity.

To get a sense of the factors that control (and do not control) I^2, consider Figure 16.7. For any given df, I^2 moves in tandem with Q. As such, it is driven entirely by the ratio of observed dispersion to within-study dispersion. In the top row, both plots A and B have a Q value of 12.00 with 5 degrees of freedom. Therefore, they both have the same value of I^2, 58.34%. The fact that A has a wider scale than B (which yields a higher value of T^2) does not impact on I^2. Similarly, in the bottom row both plots C and D have a Q value of 48.01 with 5 degrees of freedom, and therefore both have the same I^2, 89.59%. Again, the fact that C has a wider scale than D does not impact on I^2.

I^2 reflects the extent of overlap of confidence intervals, which is not dependent on the actual location or spread of the true effects. As such it is convenient to view I^2 as a measure of *inconsistency* across the findings of the studies, and not as a measure of the real variation across the underlying true effects.

The scale of I^2 has a range of 0–100%, regardless of the scale used for the meta-analysis itself. It can be interpreted as a ratio, and has the additional advantage of being analogous to indices used in psychometrics (where reliability is the ratio of true to total variance) or regression (where R^2 is the proportion of the total variance that can be explained by the covariates). Importantly, I^2 is not directly affected by the number of studies in the analysis.

Concluding remarks about I^2

The I^2 index allows us to discuss the amount of variance on a *relative* scale. For example, if we are planning to speculate about reasons for the variation, we should first use I^2 to determine what proportion of the observed variance is real. If I^2 is near zero, then almost all the observed variance is spurious, which means that there is nothing to explain. By contrast, if I^2 is large, then it would make sense to speculate about reasons for the variance, and possibly to apply techniques such as subgroup analysis or meta-regression to try and explain it. Formulas to compute confidence intervals for I^2 are presented at the end of this chapter.

Higgins *et al.* (2003) provide some tentative benchmarks for I^2. They suggest that values on the order of 25%, 50%, and 75% might be considered as *low*, *moderate*, and *high*, respectively. Some context for the interpretation of I^2 is provided by a survey of meta-analyses of clinical trials in the Cochrane Database of Systematic Reviews, reported by Higgins *et al.* (2003). The value of I^2 was zero for about half of the meta-analyses, and was distributed evenly between 0% to 100% for the other half. It is likely that I^2 would be distributed differently in meta-analyses of other fields or other kinds of studies.

Note that the benchmarks (like the index itself) refer to the question of what *proportion* of the observed variation is real, and not to the variation on an absolute scale. An I^2 value near 100% means only that most of the observed variance is real, but does not imply that the effects are dispersed over a wide range (they could fall in a narrow range but be estimated precisely). Nor does a low value of I^2 imply that the effect are clustered in a narrow range (the observed effects could vary across a wide range, in studies with a lot of error). As such, I^2 is not meant to address the substantive implications of the dispersion.

COMPARING THE MEASURES OF HETEROGENEITY

We have described five ways of measuring heterogeneity, Q, p, T^2, T, and I^2. Table 16.1 shows the relationship among these measures. Since all the indices are based on Q (in relation to df), it follows that all will be low (or zero) if the total dispersion is low relative to the error within studies, and higher if the total dispersion is high, relative to the error within studies. However, the various measures of heterogeneity build on this core in different ways which makes each useful for a specific purpose.

Table 16.1 Factors affecting measures of dispersion.

	Range of possible values	Depends on number of studies	Depends on scale
Q	$0 \leq Q$	✓	
p	$0 \leq p \leq 1$	✓	
T^2	$0 \leq T^2$		✓
T	$0 \leq T$		✓
I^2	$0\% \leq I^2 < 100\%$		

Note that *the estimates* T^2 and T are based on the excess dispersion, but the population values (τ^2 and of τ) are defined solely by the variance of the true effects.

- The Q statistic and its *p*-value serve as a test of significance. The qualities that make these useful for this purpose are that they are sensitive to the number of studies and they are not sensitive to the metric of the effect size index.
- Our estimate of τ^2 serves as the between-studies variance in the analysis and our estimate of τ serves as the standard deviation of the true effects. The qualities that make these useful for this purpose are that they are sensitive to the metric of the effect size, and they are not sensitive to the number of studies.
- I^2 is the ratio of true heterogeneity to total variation in observed effects, a kind of signal to noise ratio. The qualities that make it useful for this purpose are that it is not sensitive to the metric of the effect size and it is not sensitive to the number of studies.

It is important to understand that T^2 and T (on the one hand) and I^2 (on the other) serve two entirely different functions. The statistics T^2 (and T) reflect the *amount* of true heterogeneity (the variance or the standard deviation) while I^2 reflects the proportion of observed dispersion that is due to this heterogeneity. In a sense, if we were to multiply the observed variance by I^2, we would get T^2 (this is meant as an illustration only, since the actual computation is more complicated). As such, the two tend to move in tandem, but have very different meanings.

I^2 reflects only the proportion of variance that is true, and says nothing about the absolute value of this variance. In Figure 16.8, plots A and B have the same value of I^2 (58.34%) but in A the true effects are clustered in a small range ($T^2 = 0.006$) while in B they are dispersed across a wider range ($T^2 = 0.037$).

Conversely, T^2 reflects only the absolute value of the true variance and says nothing about the proportion of observed variance that is true. In Figure 16.9, T^2 is the same in both plots, but in A it is a large part ($I^2 = 58.34\%$) of a small observed dispersion whereas in B it is a small part ($I^2 = 16.01\%$) of a large observed dispersion.

Note also that T^2 is tied to the effect size index while I^2 is not. For example, T^2 for a synthesis of risk ratios will be in the metric of log risk ratios while T^2 for a

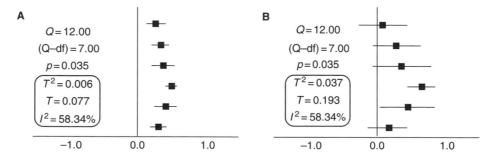

Figure 16.8 Factors affecting T^2 but not I^2.

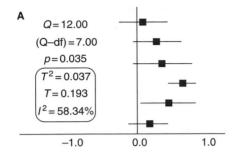
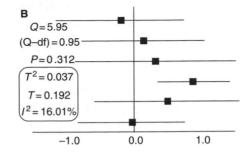

Figure 16.9 Factors affecting I^2 but not T^2.

synthesis of standardized mean differences will be in the metric of standardized mean differences. It would not be meaningful to compare the T^2 values for two syntheses unless they were in the same metric. By contrast, I^2 is on a ratio scale of 0% to 100%, and it is possible to compare this value from different syntheses.

In context

It is common for researchers who perform a meta-analysis to ask whether or not the effects are 'heterogeneous'. As we have tried to show in this chapter, to report that the data are, or are not, heterogeneous, is not terribly informative. We need to consider what is meant by 'heterogeneous' and then respond with the relevant statistics.

Researchers often focus their attention on the Q statistic and its p-value. A significant Q conjures up images of effects that are widely dispersed and a non-significant Q is taken as assurance that the effects are consistent. This use of Q is clearly incorrect for two reasons. First, the Q-statistic and its p-value only address the viability of the null hypothesis (*Is the true dispersion exactly zero*) and not the amount of excess dispersion. Second, Q is sensitive to *relative* variance (the kind tracked by I^2) and not absolute variance (the kind tracked by T^2 and T). These are two very different aspects of heterogeneity with very different implications (see below) and when a researcher reports Q alone, the consumer is not likely to make this distinction.

Researchers may also report T^2, since this is a key component in any random-effects meta-analysis. However, because T^2 is a variance (and reported in the squared metric), it is not an intuitive measure. The problem of interpretation is even worse when the index is on a log scale.

One way to think about the substantive implications of the dispersion is to think about the range of effects, and how the utility of the intervention (or the importance of the relationship) varies over this range. The index that addresses this issue is T. Just as we might report the mean and standard deviation in a primary study to describe the distribution of scores, we can report the summary effect and standard deviation (that is, T) in a meta-analysis to describe the distribution of true effects. For example, suppose that an effect size in the range of 0.0 to 0.20 would be considered *trivial*, 0.20 to 0.50 would be considered *moderate*, and 0.50 or above would be considered *high*. If the summary effect is 0.50 with a T of 0.10, most effects will fall in the range of 0.30 to 0.70, all in the moderate to high range. By contrast, if the summary effect is 0.50 with T of 0.20, some proportion of effects will fall in the trivial range. This approach works equally well when the index is on a log scale. Here, we compute the range of effects using this log scale, and then convert to the natural units for reporting. (Note that these intervals ignore uncertainty in the mean and in T. In Chapter 17 we describe a predictive interval that is more appropriate for this purpose).

Another way to think about the substantive implications of the dispersion is to ask what proportion of the observed variance is real. Faced with a forest plot of risk ratios (for example) that range from 0.50 to 4.0, a researcher may be tempted to look for covariates that can explain the mechanism responsible for this dispersion. Before embarking on this quest, it makes sense to ask how much (if any) of this dispersion is real. An I^2 near zero tells us that almost all of the dispersion will be attributed to random error, and any attempt to explain the variance is really an attempt to explain something that is (by definition) random. By contrast, as I^2 moves away from zero we know that some of the variance is real and can potentially be explained by subgroup analysis or meta-regression. These are the subjects of Chapters 19 to 21.

An informative presentation of heterogeneity indices requires both a measure of the magnitude and a measure of uncertainty. Magnitude may be represented by the degree of true variation on the scale of the effect measure (T^2) or the degree of inconsistency (I^2), or both. Uncertainty over whether apparent heterogeneity is genuine may be expressed using the p-value for Q or using confidence intervals for T^2 or I^2.

Note that uncertainty around T^2 or I^2 is often very large. If the studies themselves have poor precision (wide confidence intervals), this could mask the presence of real (possibly substantively important) heterogeneity, resulting in an estimate of zero for T^2 and I^2. Therefore, it would be a mistake to interpret a T^2 or I^2 of zero as meaning that the effect sizes are consistent unless this is justified by confidence intervals for T^2 and I^2 that exclude large values.

CONFIDENCE INTERVALS FOR τ^2

If we assume that the effect sizes are normally distributed, the standard error of T^2 may be estimated as follows.

First, compute

$$A = \left[df + 2\left(sw1 - \frac{sw2}{sw1} \right)\tau^2 + \left(sw2 - 2\left(\frac{sw3}{sw1} \right) + \frac{(sw2)^2}{(sw1)^2} \right)\tau^4 \right], \qquad (16.11)$$

where

$$sw1 = \sum_{i=1}^{k} w_i,$$

$$sw2 = \sum_{i=1}^{n} w_i^2,$$

and

$$sw3 = \sum_{i=1}^{n} w_i^3.$$

Then, the variance of T^2 is

$$V_{T^2} = 2 \times \left(\frac{A}{C^2} \right) \qquad (16.12)$$

and its standard error is given by

$$SE_{T^2} = \sqrt{V_{T^2}}. \qquad (16.13)$$

Because the distribution of T^2 is not well approximated by a normal distribution, computing the confidence interval as the estimate of τ^2 plus or minus two standard errors will not yield very accurate confidence intervals unless the number of studies is very large. There are several methods for obtaining a confidence interval for τ^2. A simple method is as follows.

First, if $Q > (df + 1)$, compute

$$B = 0.5 \times \frac{\ln(Q) - \ln(df)}{\sqrt{2Q} - \sqrt{2 \times df - 1}}, \qquad (16.14)$$

or if $Q \leq (df + 1)$, compute

$$B = \sqrt{\frac{1}{2 \times (df - 1) \times \left(1 - \left(\frac{1}{3 \times (df - 1)^2} \right) \right)}}. \qquad (16.15)$$

Then compute intermediate values

$$L = \mathrm{Exp}\left(0.5 \times \ln\left(\frac{Q}{df} \right) - 1.96 \times B \right) \qquad (16.16)$$

and

$$U = \mathrm{Exp}\left(0.5 \times \ln\left(\frac{Q}{df} \right) + 1.96 \times B \right). \qquad (16.17)$$

Finally, the 95% confidence intervals for τ^2 may then be obtained as

$$LL_{T^2} = \frac{df \times (L^2 - 1)}{C} \tag{16.18}$$

and

$$UL_{T^2} = \frac{df \times (U^2 - 1)}{C}. \tag{16.19}$$

Any value (T^2, lower limit or upper limit) that is computed as less than zero is set to zero. If the lower limit exceeds zero, then T^2 should be statistically significant. However, since T^2 is based on Q, and the sampling distribution of Q is better known, the preferred method would be to test Q for significance, and use this as the test for τ^2 being nonzero.

The 95% confidence interval for τ may be obtained by taking the square roots of the confidence limits for τ^2, namely

$$LL_T = \sqrt{LL_{T^2}}$$

and

$$UL_T = \sqrt{UL_{T^2}}.$$

CONFIDENCE INTERVALS (OR UNCERTAINTY INTERVALS) FOR I^2

There are several methods for obtaining an interval to convey uncertainty in I^2. Because I^2 does not estimate any underlying quantity, these intervals would be better described as uncertainty intervals rather than confidence intervals. However, we will continue to describe them as confidence intervals since the distinction is not practically important. A simple method to obtain confidence intervals is as follows.

First, if $Q > (df + 1)$, compute

$$B = 0.5 \times \frac{\ln(Q) - \ln(df)}{\sqrt{2Q} - \sqrt{2 \times df - 1}}, \tag{16.20}$$

or if $Q \leq (df + 1)$, compute

$$B = \sqrt{\frac{1}{2 \times (df - 1) \times \left(1 - \left(\frac{1}{3 \times (df - 1)^2}\right)\right)}}. \tag{16.21}$$

Then

$$L = \exp\left(0.5 \times \ln\left(\frac{Q}{df}\right) - 1.96 \times B\right) \tag{16.22}$$

and

$$U = \exp\left(0.5 \times \ln\left(\frac{Q}{df}\right) + 1.96 \times B\right). \tag{16.23}$$

The 95% confidence intervals may then be obtained as

$$LL_{I^2} = \left(\frac{L^2 - 1}{L^2}\right) \times 100\% \qquad (16.24)$$

and

$$UL_{I^2} = \left(\frac{U^2 - 1}{U^2}\right) \times 100\%. \qquad (16.25)$$

Any value (I^2, lower limit or upper limit) that is computed as less than zero is set to zero.

If the lower limit of I^2 exceeds zero, then I^2 should be statistically significant. However, since I^2 is based on Q, and the sampling distribution of Q is better known than the sampling distribution of I^2, the preferred method would be to test Q for significance, and use this as the test for I^2 being nonzero.

Worked examples for all of these computations are included in Chapter 18.

SUMMARY POINTS

- When we speak about dispersion in effect sizes from study to study we are usually concerned with the dispersion in true effect sizes, but the *observed* dispersion includes both true variance and random error.
- The mechanism used to isolate the true variance is to compare the observed dispersion with the amount we would expect to see if all studies shared a common effect size. The excess portion is assumed to reflect real differences among studies. This portion of the variance is then used to create several measures of heterogeneity.
- Q is the weighted sum of squares (*WSS*) on a standardized scale. As a standard score it can be compared with the expected *WSS* (on the assumption that all studies share a common effect) to yield a test of the null and also an estimate of the excess variance.
- T^2 is the variance of the true effects, on the same scale (squared) as the effects themselves. This value is used to assign study weights under the random-effects model.
- T is the standard deviation of the true effects, on the same scale as the effects themselves. We can use this to estimate the distribution of true effects, and consider the substantive implications of this distribution.
- I^2 is the proportion of observed dispersion that is real, rather than spurious. It is not dependent on the scale, and is expressed as a ratio with a range of 0% to 100%.

Prediction Intervals

INTRODUCTION

When we report the results of a meta-analysis we often focus on the summary effect size and its confidence interval. These give us an estimate of the mean effect size and its precision, *but they say nothing about how the true effects are distributed* about the summary effect.

In a fixed-effect analysis this is appropriate, since we assume that the true effect is the same in all studies. In a random-effects analysis, however, we need to consider not only the mean effect size, but also how the true effects are distributed about this mean. A mean effect size (say, a standardized mean difference) of 0.50 where all true effects are clustered in the range of 0.40 to 0.60 may have very different implications than the same mean effect where the true effects are scattered over the range of 0.00 to 1.00.

Our goal in this chapter is to show how we can use a prediction interval to describe the distribution of true effect sizes. We will review how the prediction interval is used in primary studies, and then show how the same mechanism can be used for meta-analysis.

PREDICTION INTERVALS IN PRIMARY STUDIES

Suppose we are interested in math scores for a population of children. We want to create a prediction interval, defined as the interval within which a new student's score would fall if that student were selected at random from this population.

The 80% prediction interval would include that score 80% of the time, the 95% interval would include that score 95% of the time, and so on. As such, the interval yields an intuitive picture of the distribution of scores.

If we somehow knew the population mean (μ) and standard deviation (σ), and were willing to assume that the scores are normally distributed, we could create a prediction interval, using

$$LL_{pred} = \mu - Z^\alpha \sqrt{\sigma^2} \qquad (17.1)$$

and

$$UL_{pred} = \mu + Z^\alpha \sqrt{\sigma^2}, \qquad (17.2)$$

where Z^α is the Z-value corresponding to the desired confidence level (for the 95 % interval, Z^α would be 1.96). For example, if μ is 0.50 and σ is 0.10, then the lower and upper limits of a 95% prediction interval are

$$LL_{pred} = 0.500 - 1.96 \times 0.100 = 0.3040$$

and

$$UL_{pred} = 0.500 + 1.96 \times 0.100 = 0.6960.$$

Formulas (17.1) and (17.2) are intuitive but are not useful in practice because they assume that we know both μ and σ exactly. When these values are estimated from the sample (as they almost always are) we instead use the formulas

$$LL_{pred} = \overline{X} - t_{df}^\alpha \sqrt{S^2 + \frac{S^2}{n}} \qquad (17.3)$$

and

$$UL_{pred} = \overline{X} + t_{df}^\alpha \sqrt{S^2 + \frac{S^2}{n}}, \qquad (17.4)$$

where $\overline{X}$ is the sample mean, t_{df}^α is the t-value corresponding to (for example if $\alpha = 0.05$) the 95% interval when there are df degrees of freedom, and S is the standard deviation of scores in the sample. These formulas have the same structure as (17.1) and (17.2) but to allow for error in the estimates of μ and σ they incorporate the following changes. First, we multiply by t rather than Z. Second, t is multiplied by a quantity that involves both the variance of the observations (the standard deviation squared, or S^2) and also the variance of the mean (the standard error squared, or S^2/n).

For example, if $X = 0.50$, $S = 0.10$ and $n = 30$, then

$$LL_{pred} = 0.5000 - 2.0452 \times \sqrt{0.1000^2 + \frac{0.1000^2}{30}} = 0.2921$$

and

$$UL_{pred} = 0.5000 + 2.0452 \times \sqrt{0.1000^2 + \frac{0.1000^2}{30}} = 0.7079,$$

where a t-value of 2.045 corresponds to the t-value for alpha of 0.05 with 29 df. In Excel, the function tinv(0.05,29) returns 2.0452.

Note that the prediction intervals based on the statistics (0.292 to 0.708) are wider than those based on the parameters (0.304 to 0.696).

PREDICTION INTERVALS IN META-ANALYSIS

We can follow a similar approach in meta-analysis. If we somehow knew the mean effect size (μ) and the standard deviation of true effect sizes (τ), and were willing to assume that the effect sizes are normally distributed, we could create a prediction interval using

$$LL_{pred} = \mu - Z^\alpha \sqrt{\tau^2} \tag{17.5}$$

and

$$UL_{pred} = \mu + Z^\alpha \sqrt{\tau^2}. \tag{17.6}$$

This is similar to (17.1) and (17.2) except that τ^2, the variance of the true effects in a meta-analysis, has replaced σ^2, the variance of the scores in a primary study.

Actually, we introduced this idea in Chapter 16 when we discussed the interpretation of T as an estimate of the standard deviation of true effect sizes. For example, if μ is 0.358 and τ^2 is 0.0373, then the 95% prediction interval is

$$LL_{pred} = 0.358 - 1.96 \times \sqrt{0.0373} = -0.0205$$

and

$$UL_{pred} = 0.358 + 1.96 \times \sqrt{0.0373} = 0.7365.$$

In a forest plot we would typically use a simple line (from -0.020 to 0.737) to represent the prediction interval, but in Figure 17.1 we use a bell curve to convey the idea that the true effect sizes are expected to be normally distributed within this range. Note that the bell curve has been truncated at either end (-0.020 and 0.737) so that it covers 95% of expected true effects.

Formulas (17.5) and (17.6) assume that we actually know the values of μ and τ, and make no allowance for error in these estimates. Higgins *et al.* propose the following formulas for computing a prediction interval when these values are estimated from the sample. The formulas are

$$LL_{pred} = M^* - t_{df}^\alpha \sqrt{T^2 + V_{M^*}} \tag{17.7}$$

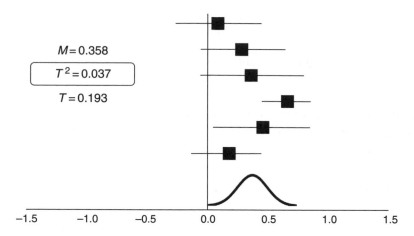

Figure 17.1 Prediction interval based on population parameters μ and τ^2.

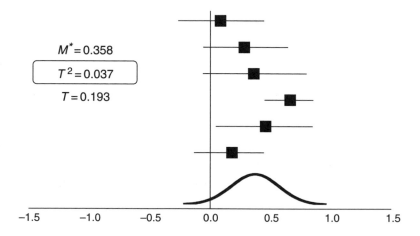

Figure 17.2 Prediction interval based on sample estimates M^* and T^2.

and

$$UL_{pred} = M^* + t_{df}^{\alpha} \sqrt{T^2 + V_{M^*}}, \tag{17.8}$$

where M^* is the mean effect size in the sample, T^2 is the sample estimate of the variance of true effect sizes, and V_{M^*} is the variance of M^*. The factor t is the t-value corresponding to (for example if $\alpha = 0.05$) the 95% interval when there are df degrees of freedom.

These formulas have the same structure as (17.5) and (17.6) but we multiply by the t-value (rather than the Z-value) and apply this factor to a quantity that involves both the variance of the *true effects* (T^2) and the variance of the *mean effect* (V_{M^*}). The degrees of freedom (df) is often taken as the number of studies minus 2 (that is, $k-2$).

For example, if $k = 6$, $M^* = 0.3582$, $T^2 = 0.0373$, and $V_{M*} = 0.0111$, then

$$LL_{pred} = 0.3582 - 2.7764 \times \sqrt{0.0373 + 0.0111} = -0.2525$$

and

$$UL_{pred} = 0.3582 + 2.7764 \times \sqrt{0.0373 + 0.0111} = 0.9690.$$

The value 2.7764 is the t-value corresponding to alpha of 0.05 with 4 df. In Excel, the function =TINV(0.05,4) returns 2.7764.

Figure 17.2 is identical to Figure 17.1 except that this time the prediction interval is based on the sample values M^* and T^2 rather than the population parameters μ and τ^2. Note that the bell curve is wider in Figure 17.2 (the 95% interval is -0.25 to $+0.97$) than in Figure 17.1 (where the interval was -0.02 to $+0.74$) which reflects the uncertainty in the estimates.

CONFIDENCE INTERVALS AND PREDICTION INTERVALS

Traditionally, the summary line in a forest plot uses a diamond to depict the mean effect size (the center of the diamond) and its confidence interval (the width of the diamond). Now, we want to add a visual indicator of the prediction interval, and we do so by adding a horizontal line to either end of the diamond, as in Figure 17.3.

The meta-analysis line in the plot now shows *two distinct items of information*. First, in 95% of cases the mean effect size falls inside the diamond. Second, in 95% of cases the true effect in a new study will fall inside the horizontal lines. It is important to understand that these two items address two distinct issues. The confidence interval quantifies *the accuracy of the mean*, while the prediction interval addresses the actual *dispersion of effect sizes*, and the two measures are not interchangeable.

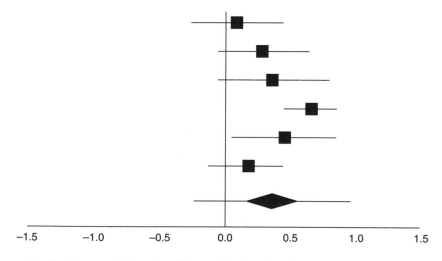

Figure 17.3 Simultaneous display of confidence interval and prediction interval.

As always, how we choose to interpret the effects depends on our goals. We may want to focus on the null effect. If the full diamond exceeds zero then we are 95% certain that the mean effect size exceeds zero. If the full prediction interval exceeds zero then the true effect in 95% of new studies will exceed zero.

Or, we may want to focus on a clinically important effect (say, a standardized mean difference of 0.20). If the full diamond exceeds 0.20 then we are 95% certain that the mean effect size exceeds 0.20. If the full prediction interval exceeds 0.20 then the true effect in 95 % of new studies will exceed 0.20.

COMPARING THE CONFIDENCE INTERVAL WITH THE PREDICTION INTERVAL

Earlier, we showed the computation of the prediction interval for a meta-analysis with six studies. Suppose that the meta-analysis included more studies (24, 60, or 1002) with the same pattern as in the first six. In other words, we have the same within-study error and the same pattern of dispersion but a more precise estimate of the mean effect size and of the true between-studies dispersion.

In Figure 17.4 we illustrate what the confidence interval and the prediction interval would be for these four hypothetical analyses. While the *specific* pattern shown here is unique to this analysis, the general trend will apply to any analysis.

With six studies the confidence interval (the diamond) is quite wide, but with 60 studies its width is cut by about half, and with 1002 studies its width is trivial. This follows from the formula for a confidence interval, which is

$$CI_{M^*} = M^* \pm Z\sqrt{V_{M^*}}. \tag{17.9}$$

The confidence interval reflects only error (V_{M^*}), and so we see a consistent decline in the confidence interval width as the number of studies goes from 6 to 1002. With an infinite number of studies the error would approach zero, and so the width of the confidence interval would approach zero.

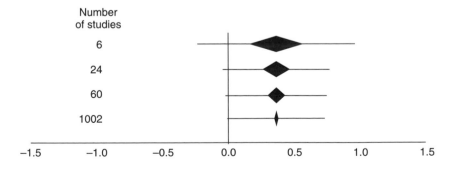

Figure 17.4 Impact of number of studies on confidence interval and prediction interval.

By contrast, the width of the prediction interval (the line) drops sharply as the number of studies goes from 6 to 24 but shows almost no change beyond that point. This follows from the formula for a prediction interval, which is

$$PI = M^* \pm t\sqrt{T^2 + V_{M^*}}. \tag{17.10}$$

The interval is based on error in estimating the mean (V_{M^*}), which is dependent on the number of studies. The interval is based also on the variance of the studies, T^2, which is not affected by the number of studies. In this example, as the number of studies increases from 6 to 24, V_{M^*} decreases and therefore the interval narrows. Beyond that point the decrease in V_{M^*} is trivial (and T^2 remains constant), so the prediction interval shows little change. With an infinite number of studies, the interval would approach μ plus/minus 1.96 τ.

SUMMARY POINTS

- For a random-effects analysis we want to know both the mean effect size and also how the true effects are distributed about the mean.
- The precision of the mean is addressed by the confidence interval. Since the confidence interval reflects only error of estimation of the mean, with an infinite number of studies its width would approach zero.
- The distribution of true effect sizes is addressed by the prediction interval. Since the prediction interval incorporates true dispersion as well as error, with an infinite number of studies it will approach the actual dispersion of true effect sizes.
- The summary effect in a forest plot has traditionally been represented by a diamond which corresponds to the confidence interval. For random-effects analyses we can modify this to display both the confidence interval and the prediction interval.

CHAPTER 18

Worked Examples (Part 2)

Introduction
Worked example for continuous data (Part 2)
Worked example for binary data (Part 2)
Worked example for correlational data (Part 2)

INTRODUCTION

In Chapter 14 we presented worked examples for computing a summary effect using continuous binary, and correlational data. Here, we continue with the same three data sets and show how to compute the measures of heterogeneity discussed in Chapters 16 and 17.

These computations are also included in Excel spreadsheets that can be downloaded from the book's web site.

WORKED EXAMPLE FOR CONTINUOUS DATA (PART 2)

On page 87 we showed how to compute the effect size and variance for each study. Here, we proceed from that point.

Using results in Table 18.1, the summary effect is given by

$$M = \frac{101.171}{244.215} = 0.4143,$$

which value is used in the column labeled *Mean* in Table 18.2.

Then, using (16.1) we sum the values in the final column of Table 18.2,

$$Q = \sum_{i=1}^{k} W_i (Y_i - M)^2 = 12.0033.$$

Introduction to Meta-Analysis   M. Borenstein, L. V. Hedges, J. P. T. Higgins, H. R. Rothstein
© 2009, John Wiley & Sons, Ltd

Table 18.1 Dataset 1 – Part D (intermediate computations).

Study	Effect	Variance	Weight	Calculated quantities			
	Y	V_Y	W	WY	WY^2	W^2	W^3
Carroll	0.095	0.033	30.352	2.869	0.271	921.21	27960.25
Grant	0.277	0.031	32.568	9.033	2.505	1060.68	34544.41
Peck	0.367	0.050	20.048	7.349	2.694	401.93	8058.00
Donat	0.664	0.011	95.111	63.190	41.983	9046.01	860371.10
Stewart	0.462	0.043	23.439	10.824	4.999	549.37	12876.47
Young	0.185	0.023	42.698	7.906	1.464	1823.12	77843.29
Sum			244.215	101.171	53.915	13802.33	1021653.52

Table 18.2 Dataset 1 – Part E (variance computations).

Study	Effect	Variance	Weight	Mean	Calculated Quantities	
	Y	V_Y	W	M	$(Y-M)^2$	$W(Y-M)^2$
Carroll	0.095	0.033	30.352	0.414	0.102	3.103
Grant	0.277	0.031	32.568	0.414	0.019	0.610
Peck	0.367	0.050	20.048	0.414	0.002	0.046
Donat	0.664	0.011	95.111	0.414	0.063	5.950
Stewart	0.462	0.043	23.439	0.414	0.002	0.053
Young	0.185	0.023	42.698	0.414	0.052	2.241
Sum						12.003

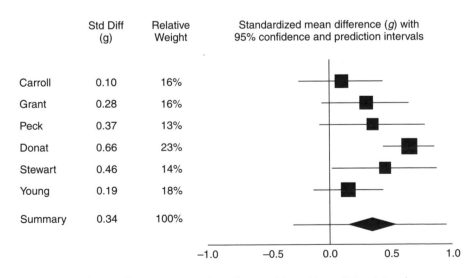

Figure 18.1 Forest plot of Dataset 1 – random-effects weights with prediction interval.

Or, using (12.3) and results in Table 18.1,

$$Q = 53.915 - \frac{(101.171)^2}{244.215} = 12.0033.$$

Under the assumption that all studies share a common effect, the expected value of Q is given by

$$df = 6 - 1 = 5$$

where k is the number of studies. The difference,

$$12.003 - 5 = 7.0033,$$

is the excess value which we attribute to differences in the true effect sizes.

The p-value for $Q = 12.003$ with $df = 5$, is 0.035. In Excel, the function =CHIDIST(12.003,5) returns 0.035. If we are using 0.10 or 0.05 as the criterion for statistical significance, we would reject the null hypothesis that all the studies share a common effect size, and accept the alternative, that the true effect is not the same in all studies.

Then, using formulas (16.6), (16.5), (16.8), and (16.9),

$$C = 244.215 - \left(\frac{13802.33}{244.215} \right) = 187.6978,$$

$$T^2 = \frac{12.003 - 5}{187.698} = 0.0373,$$

$$T = \sqrt{0.0373} = 0.1932,$$

and

$$I^2 = \left(\frac{12.003 - 5}{12.003} \right) \times 100\% = 58.34\%.$$

To compute the standard error of T^2 (from (16.11) to (16.13)), we have $sw1 = 244.215$, $sw2 = 13,802.33$, and $sw3 = 1,021,653.52$, so that

$$A = \left[df + 2 \left(244 - \frac{13802}{244} \right) 0.0373 + \left(13802 - 2 \left(\frac{1021653}{244} \right) + \frac{(13802)^2}{(244)^2} \right) 0.0373^2 \right]$$

$$= 31.0202.$$

Then, the variance of T^2 is

$$V_{T^2} = 2 \times \left(\frac{31.020}{187.698^2} \right) = 0.0018,$$

and its standard error is given by

$$SE_{T^2} = \sqrt{0.0018} = 0.0420.$$

Since $Q = 12.003 > 6 = (df + 1)$, we compute, from (16.14) to (16.19),

$$B = 0.5 \times \frac{\ln(12.0033) - \ln(5)}{\sqrt{2 \times 12.0033} - \sqrt{2 \times 5 - 1}} = 0.2305.$$

Then compute intermediate values

$$L = \text{Exp}\left(0.5 \times \ln\left(\frac{12.003}{5}\right) - 1.96 \times 0.2305\right) = 0.9862$$

and

$$U = \text{Exp}\left(0.5 \times \ln\left(\frac{12.003}{5}\right) + 1.96 \times 0.2305\right) = 2.4343.$$

Finally, the 95% confidence intervals for τ^2 may be obtained as

$$LL_{T^2} = \frac{5 \times (0.9862^2 - 1)}{187.698} = -0.0007,$$

which is set to zero, and

$$UL_{T^2} = \frac{5 \times (2.4343^2 - 1)}{187.698} = 0.1312.$$

The 95% confidence interval for τ may be obtained by taking the square roots of the confidence limits for τ^2, namely

$$LL_T = \sqrt{0.0} = 0.0,$$

and

$$UL_T = \sqrt{0.1312} = 0.3622.$$

Confidence intervals for I^2

Since $12.003 > (5 + 1)$ we compute, using formulas (16.20) through (16.25),

$$B = 0.5 \times \frac{\ln(12.003) - \ln(5)}{\sqrt{2 \times 12.003} - \sqrt{2 \times 5 - 1}} = 0.2305.$$

Compute intermediate values

$$L = \exp\left(0.5 \times \ln\left(\frac{12.003}{5}\right) - 1.96 \times 0.2305\right) = 0.9862$$

and

$$U = \exp\left(0.5 \times \ln\left(\frac{12.003}{5}\right) + 1.96 \times 0.2305\right) = 2.4343.$$

The 95% confidence intervals may then be obtained as

$$LL_{I^2} = \left(\frac{0.9862^2 - 1}{0.9862^2} \right) \times 100\% = -2.82\%,$$

which is set to zero, and

$$UL_{I^2} = \left(\frac{2.4343^2 - 1}{2.4343^2} \right) \times 100\% = 83.12.\%.$$

To obtain a 95% predictive interval for the true standardized mean difference in a future study, we use the random-effects weighted mean and its variance computed in (14.1) and (14.2), $M^* = 0.3582$ and $V_{M^*} = 0.0111$ and compute, from (17.7) and (17.8),

$$t_4^{0.05} = 2.7764,$$

$$LL_{pred} = 0.3582 - 2.7764 \times \sqrt{0.0373 + 0.0111} = -0.2525,$$

and

$$UL_{pred} = 0.3582 + 2.7764 \times \sqrt{0.0373 + 0.0111} = 0.9690.$$

This prediction interval is plotted is in Figure 18.1.

WORKED EXAMPLE FOR BINARY DATA (PART 2)

On page 92 we showed how to compute the effect size (here, the log odds ratio) and variance for each study. Here, we proceed from that point.

Using results in Table 18.3, the summary effect is given by

$$M = \frac{-30.594}{42.248} = -0.7241,$$

which value is used in the column labeled *Mean* in Table 18.4.

Then, using (16.1) we sum the values in the final column of Table 18.4,

$$Q = \sum_{i=1}^{k} W_i (Y_i - M)^2 = 10.5512.$$

Or, using (12.3) and results in Table 18.3,

$$Q = 32.705 - \frac{(-30.594)^2}{42.248} = 10.5512.$$

Table 18.3 Dataset 2 – Part D (intermediate computations).

Study	Effect	Variance	Weight	Calculated quantities			
	Y	V_Y	W	WY	WY^2	W^2	W^3
Saint	−0.366	0.185	5.402	−1.978	0.724	29.18	157.66
Kelly	−0.288	0.290	3.453	−0.993	0.286	11.92	41.18
Pilbeam	−0.384	0.156	6.427	−2.469	0.948	41.30	265.42
Lane	−1.322	0.058	17.155	−22.675	29.971	294.30	5048.71
Wright	−0.417	0.282	3.551	−1.480	0.617	12.61	44.76
Day	−0.159	0.160	6.260	−0.998	0.159	39.19	245.33
Sum			42.248	−30.594	32.705	428.50	5803.06

Table 18.4 Dataset 2 – Part E (variance computations).

Study	Effect	Variance	Weight	Mean	Calculated Quantities	
	Y	V_Y	W	M	$(Y-M)^2$	$W(Y-M)^2$
Saint	−0.366	0.185	5.402	−0.724	0.128	0.692
Kelly	−0.288	0.290	3.453	−0.724	0.191	0.658
Pilbeam	−0.384	0.156	6.427	−0.724	0.116	0.743
Lane	−1.322	0.058	17.155	−0.724	0.357	6.127
Wright	−0.417	0.282	3.551	−0.724	0.094	0.335
Day	−0.159	0.160	6.260	−0.724	0.319	1.996
Sum						10.551

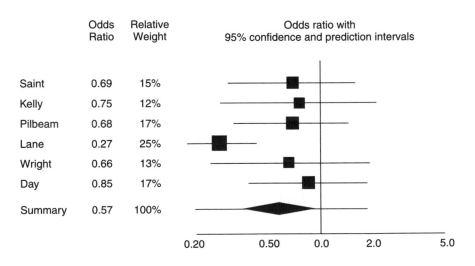

Figure 18.2 Forest plot of Dataset 2 – random-effects weights with prediction interval.

Under the assumption that all studies share a common effect, the expected value of Q is given by

$$df = 6 - 1 = 5,$$

where k is the number of studies. The difference,

$$10.5512 - 5 = 5.5512$$

is the excess value which we attribute to differences in the true effect sizes.

The p-value for $Q = 10.551$ with $df = 5$, is 0.0610. In Excel, the function $=$CHIDIST(10.551,5) returns 0.0610. If we are using 0.10 as the criterion for statistical significance, we would reject the null hypothesis that all the studies share a common effect size, and accept the alternative, that the true effect is not the same in all studies. If we are using 0.05 as the criterion, we would not have sufficient evidence to reject the null (but would not conclude that the effects are homogeneous, since the nonsignificant p-value could be due to inadequate statistical power).

Then, using formulas (16.6), (16.5), (16.8), and (16.9),

$$C = 42.248 - \left(\frac{428.50}{42.248} \right) = 32.1052,$$

$$T^2 = \frac{10.5512 - 5}{32.1052} = 0.1729,$$

$$T = \sqrt{0.1729} = 0.4158,$$

and

$$I^2 = \left(\frac{10.5512 - 5}{10.5512} \right) \times 100 = 52.61\%.$$

To compute the standard error of T^2 (from (16.11) to (16.13)), we have $sw1 = 42.25$, $sw2 = 428.5$, and $sw3 = 5,803.1$, so that

$$A = \left[df + 2\left(42.25 - \frac{428.5}{42.25} \right)0.1729 + \left(428.5 - 2\left(\frac{5803.1}{42.25} \right) + \frac{(428.5)^2}{(42.25)^2} \right)0.1729^2 \right]$$
$$= 23.7754.$$

Then, the variance of T^2 is

$$V_{T^2} = 2 \times \left(\frac{23.7754}{32.1052^2} \right) = 0.0461$$

and its standard error is given by

$$SE_{T^2} = \sqrt{0.0461} = 0.2148.$$

Since $Q = 10.5512 > 6 = (df + 1)$, we compute, from (16.14) to (16.19),

$$B = 0.5 \times \frac{\ln(10.5512) - \ln(5)}{\sqrt{2 \times 10.5512} - \sqrt{2 \times 5 - 1}} = 0.2343.$$

Then compute intermediate values

$$L = \mathrm{Exp}\left(0.5 \times \ln\left(\frac{10.5512}{5}\right) - 1.96 \times 0.2343\right) = 0.9178$$

and

$$U = \mathrm{Exp}\left(0.5 \times \ln\left(\frac{10.5512}{5}\right) + 1.96 \times 0.2343\right) = 2.2993.$$

Finally, the 95% confidence intervals for τ^2 may then be obtained as

$$LL_{T^2} = \frac{5 \times (0.9178^2 - 1)}{32.1052} = -0.0246,$$

which is set to zero, and

$$UL_{T^2} = \frac{5 \times (2.2993^2 - 1)}{32.1052} = 0.6676.$$

The 95% confidence interval for τ may be obtained by taking the square roots of the confidence limits for τ^2, namely

$$LL_T = \sqrt{0.0} = 0.0,$$

and

$$UL_T = \sqrt{0.6676} = 0.8171.$$

Confidence intervals for I^2

Since $10.5512 > (5 + 1)$ we compute, using formulas (16.20) through (16.25),

$$B = 0.5 \times \frac{\ln(10.5512) - \ln(5)}{\sqrt{2 \times 10.5512} - \sqrt{2 \times 5 - 1}} = 0.2343,$$

then compute intermediate values

$$L = \mathrm{Exp}\left(0.5 \times \ln\left(\frac{10.5512}{5}\right) - 1.96 \times 0.2343\right) = 0.9178$$

and

$$U = \mathrm{Exp}\left(0.5 \times \ln\left(\frac{10.5512}{5}\right) + 1.96 \times 0.2343\right) = 2.2993.$$

The 95% confidence intervals may then be obtained as

$$LL_{I^2} = \left(\frac{0.9178^2 - 1}{0.9178^2} \right) \times 100\% = -18.72\%,$$

which is set to zero, and

$$UL_{I^2} = \left(\frac{2.2993^2 - 1}{2.2993^2} \right) \times 100\% = 81.09\%.$$

To obtain a 95% predictive interval for the true log odds ratio in a future study, we use the random-effects weighted mean and its variance computed in (14.3) and (14.4), $M^* = -0.5663$ and $V_{M^*} = 0.0570$ and compute, from (17.7) and (17.8),

$$t_4^{0.05} = 2.7764,$$

$$LL_{pred} = -0.5663 - 2.7764 \times \sqrt{0.1729 + 0.0570} = -1.8977,$$

and

$$UL_{pred} = -0.5663 + 2.7764 \times \sqrt{0.1729 + 0.0570} = 0.7651.$$

These limits are computed on a log scale. We can convert the limits to the odds ratio scale using

$$LL_{pred} = \exp(-1.8977) = 0.1499$$

and

$$UL_{pred} = \exp(0.7651) = 2.1492.$$

This prediction interval is plotted in Figure 18.2.

WORKED EXAMPLE FOR CORRELATIONAL DATA (PART 2)

On page 97 we showed how to compute the effect size (here, the Fisher's z transformation of the correlation coefficient) and variance for each study. Here, we proceed from that point.

Using results in Table 18.5, the summary effect is given by

$$M = \frac{242.650}{647.000} = 0.3750,$$

which value is used in the column labeled *Mean* in Table 18.6.

Then, using (16.1) we sum the values in the final column of Table 18.6,

$$Q = \sum_{i=1}^{k} W_i (Y_i - M)^2 = 36.1437.$$

Or, using (12.3) and results in Table 18.5,

$$Q = 127.147 - \frac{(242.650)^2}{647.000} = 36.1437.$$

Table 18.5 Dataset 3 – Part D (intermediate computations).

Study	Effect	Variance	Weight	Calculated quantities			
	Y	V_Y	W	WY	WY^2	W^2	W^3
Fonda	0.549	0.027	37.000	20.324	11.164	1369.00	50653.00
Newman	0.693	0.011	87.000	60.304	41.799	7569.00	658503.00
Grant	0.424	0.045	22.000	9.320	3.949	484.00	10648.00
Granger	0.203	0.003	397.000	80.485	16.317	157609.00	62570773.00
Milland	0.867	0.018	57.000	49.436	42.876	3249.00	185193.00
Finch	0.485	0.021	47.000	22.781	11.042	2209.00	103823.00
Sum			647.000	242.650	127.147	172489.00	63579593.00

Table 18.6 Dataset 3 – Part E (variance computations).

Study	Effect	Variance	Weight	Mean	Calculated Quantities	
	Y	V_Y	W	M	$(Y-M)^2$	$W(Y-M)^2$
Fonda	0.549	0.027	37.000	0.375	0.030	1.124
Newman	0.693	0.011	87.000	0.375	0.101	8.804
Grant	0.424	0.045	22.000	0.375	0.002	0.052
Granger	0.203	0.003	397.000	0.375	0.030	11.787
Milland	0.867	0.018	57.000	0.375	0.242	13.812
Finch	0.485	0.021	47.000	0.375	0.012	0.565
Sum						36.144

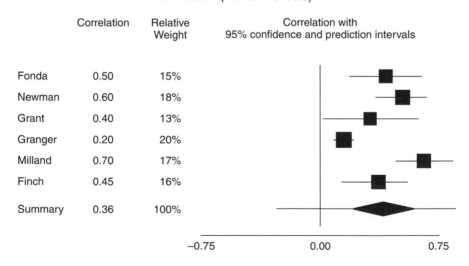

Correlation (Random effects)

	Correlation	Relative Weight	Correlation with 95% confidence and prediction intervals
Fonda	0.50	15%	
Newman	0.60	18%	
Grant	0.40	13%	
Granger	0.20	20%	
Milland	0.70	17%	
Finch	0.45	16%	
Summary	0.36	100%	

−0.75 0.00 0.75

Figure 18.3 Forest plot of Dataset 3 – random-effects weights with prediction interval.

Under the assumption that all studies share a common effect, the expected value of Q is given by

$$df = 6 - 1 = 5,$$

where k is the number of studies. The difference,

$$36.1437 - 5 = 31.1437,$$

is the excess value which we attribute to differences in the true effect sizes.

The p-value for $Q = 36.1437$ with $df = 5$, is less than 0.0001. In Excel, the function =CHIDIST(36.1437,5) returns < 0.0001. If we are using 0.10 or 0.05 as the criterion for statistical significance, we would reject the null hypothesis that all the studies share a common effect size, and accept the alternative, that the true effect is not the same in all studies.

Then, using formulas (16.6), (16.5), (16.8), and (16.9),

$$C = 647.000 - \left(\frac{172489.00}{647.000} \right) = 380.4019,$$

$$T^2 = \frac{36.1437 - 5}{380.4019} = 0.0819,$$

$$T = \sqrt{0.0819} = 0.28613,$$

and

$$I^2 = \left(\frac{36.1437 - 5}{36.1437} \right) \times 100 = 86.17\%.$$

To compute the standard error of T^2 (from (16.11) to (16.13)), we have $sw1 = 647.00$, $sw2 = 172489.00$, and $sw3 = 63,579,593.00$, so that

$$A = \left[df + 2 \left(647.00 - \frac{172489}{647.00} \right) 0.0819 \right.$$

$$\left. + \left(172489 - 2 \left(\frac{63579593}{647.00} \right) + \frac{(172489)^2}{(647.00)^2} \right) 0.0819^2 \right] = 382.4983.$$

Then, the variance of T^2 is

$$V_{T^2} = 2 \times \left(\frac{382.4983}{380.4019^2} \right) = 0.0053,$$

and its standard error is given by

$$SE_{T^2} = \sqrt{0.0053} = 0.0727.$$

Since $Q = 36.1437 > 6 = (df + 1)$, we compute, from (16.14) to (16.19),

$$B = 0.5 \times \frac{\ln(36.1437) - \ln(5)}{\sqrt{2 \times 36.1437} - \sqrt{2 \times 5 - 1}} = 0.1798.$$

Then compute intermediate values

$$L = \mathrm{Exp}\left(0.5 \times \ln\left(\frac{36.1437}{5}\right) - 1.96 \times 0.1798\right) = 1.8903$$

and

$$U = \mathrm{Exp}\left(0.5 \times \ln\left(\frac{36.1437}{5}\right) + 1.96 \times 0.1798\right) = 3.8242.$$

Finally, the 95% confidence intervals for τ^2 may then be obtained as

$$LL_{T^2} = \frac{5 \times \left(1.890^2 - 1\right)}{380.4019} = 0.0338$$

and

$$UL_{T^2} = \frac{5 \times \left(3.8242^2 - 1\right)}{380.4019} = 0.1791.$$

The 95% confidence interval for τ may be obtained by taking the square roots of the confidence limits for τ^2, namely

$$LL_T = \sqrt{0.0338} = 0.1839,$$

and

$$UL_T = \sqrt{0.1791} = 0.4232.$$

Confidence intervals for I^2

Since $Q = 36.1437 > 6 = (df + 1)$, we compute, from (16.20),

$$B = 0.5 \times \frac{\ln(36.1437) - \ln(5)}{\sqrt{2 \times 36.1437} - \sqrt{2 \times 5 - 1}} = 0.1798,$$

then compute intermediate values

$$L = \mathrm{Exp}\left(0.5 \times \ln\left(\frac{36.1437}{5}\right) - 1.96 \times 0.1798\right) = 1.8903$$

and

$$U = \text{Exp}\left(0.5 \times \ln\left(\frac{36.1437}{5}\right) + 1.96 \times 0.1798\right) = 3.8242.$$

The 95% confidence intervals may then be obtained as

$$LL_{I^2} = \left(\frac{1.8903^2 - 1}{1.8903^2}\right) \times 100\% = 72.01\%,$$

and

$$UL_{I^2} = \left(\frac{3.8241^2 - 1}{3.8241^2}\right) \times 100\% = 93.16\%.$$

To obtain a 95% predictive interval for the true Fisher's z in a future study, we use the random-effects weighted mean and its variance computed in (14.5) and (14.6), $M^* = 0.5328$ and $V_{M*} = 0.0168$ and compute, from (17.7) and (17.8),

$$t_4^{0.05} = 2.7764,$$

$$LL_{pred} = 0.5328 - 2.7764 \times \sqrt{0.0819 + 0.0168} = -0.3396,$$

and

$$UL_{pred} = 0.5328 + 2.7764 \times \sqrt{0.0819 + 0.0168} = 1.4051.$$

These limits are in the Fisher's z metric. We can convert the limits to the correlation scale using

$$LL_{pred} = \frac{e^{(2 \times -0.3396)} - 1}{e^{(2 \times -0.3396)} + 1} = -0.3271$$

and

$$UL_{pred} = \frac{e^{(2 \times 1.4051)} - 1}{e^{(2 \times 1.4051)} + 1} = 0.8865.$$

This prediction interval is plotted in Figure 18.3.

SUMMARY POINTS

- This chapter includes worked examples showing how to compute the summary effect using fixed-effect and random-effects models.
- For the standardized mean difference we work with the effect sizes directly.
- For ratios we work with the log transformed data.
- For correlations we work with the Fisher's z transformed data.
- These worked examples are available as Excel files on the book's web site.

CHAPTER 19

Subgroup Analyses

Introduction
Fixed-effect model within subgroups
Computational models
Random effects with separate estimates of τ^2
Random effects with pooled estimate of τ^2
The proportion of variance explained
Mixed-effects model
Obtaining an overall effect in the presence of subgroups

INTRODUCTION

To this point our focus has been primarily on estimating the mean effect, and in that context variation in effect sizes served primarily to qualify the mean effect. For example, we used the variation to assign weights for computing the mean effect, and to make projections about the distribution of true effect sizes about the mean effect.

Now, our focus shifts from the mean effect to the variation itself. In this chapter we show how meta-analysis can be used to compare the mean effect for different subgroups of studies (akin to analysis of variance in a primary study). In the next chapter we show how meta-analysis can be used to assess the relationship between study-level covariates and effect size (akin to multiple regression in primary studies).

Consider the following examples.

- We anticipate that a class of drugs reduces the risk of death in patients with cardiac arrhythmia, but we hypothesize that the magnitude of the effect depends on whether the condition is acute or chronic. We want to determine whether the drug is effective for each kind of patient, and also to determine whether the effect differs in the two.
- Our meta-analysis includes 10 studies that used proper randomization techniques and 10 that did not. Before computing a summary effect across all 20 studies we want to compute the effect for each group of 10, and determine if the effect size is related to the kind of randomization employed in the study.

Introduction to Meta-Analysis M. Borenstein, L. V. Hedges, J. P. T. Higgins, H. R. Rothstein
© 2009, John Wiley & Sons, Ltd

- We anticipate that forest management reduces the destruction of tree stands by insect pests, but we hypothesize that the magnitude of the effect depends on the diversity of trees in the stand. We want to determine whether forest management is effective in reducing destruction for both single species and mixed stands, and also to determine whether the effect differs in the two.
- We have data from ten studies that looked at the impact of tutoring on math scores of ninth-grade students. Five of the studies used one variant of the intervention while five used another variant. We anticipate that both variants are effective, and our primary goal in the analysis is to determine whether one is *more effective* than the other.

We shall pursue the last of these examples (the impact of tutoring on math) throughout this chapter. The effect size in this example is the standardized mean difference between groups (Hedges' g) but the same formulas would apply for any effect size index. As always, if we were working with odds ratios or risk ratios all values would be in log units, and if we were working with correlations all values would be in Fisher's z units.

Assume all the studies used the same design, with some students assigned to be tutored and others to a control condition. In some studies (here called A) students were tutored once a week while in the others (B) students were tutored twice a week. Our goal is to compare the impact of the two protocols to see if either intervention is more effective than the other.

Note. In this example we will be comparing the effect in one subgroup of studies versus the effect in a second subgroup of studies. The ideal scenario would be to have studies that directly compare the two variants of the intervention, since this would remove the potential for confounds and also reduce the error term. We assume that such studies are not available to us.

How this chapter is organized

We present three computational *models*. These are (a) fixed-effect, (b) random-effects using separate estimates of τ^2, and (c) random-effects using a pooled estimate of τ^2.

For each of the three models we present three *methods* for comparing the subgroups. These are (1) the Z-test, (2) a Q-test based on analysis of variance, and (3) a Q-test for heterogeneity.

The three statistical *models*, crossed with the three computational *methods*, yield a total of nine possible combinations. These are shown in Box 19.1, which serves as a roadmap for this chapter. Readers who want to get a sense of the issues quickly may find it easier to read the introduction and method 1 for each model, and return later to methods 2 and 3.

The dataset and all computations are available on the book's web site.

BOX 19.1   ROADMAP

	Introduction	Method 1	Method 2	Method 3
Model		Z-test	Q-test based on ANOVA	Q-test for heterogeneity
Fixed-effect	Page 151	Page 156	Page 157	Page 158
Random-effects with separate estimates of τ^2	Page 164	Page 167	Page 169	Page 170
Random-effects with pooled estimate of τ^2	Page 171	Page 176	Page 177	Page 178

FIXED-EFFECT MODEL WITHIN SUBGROUPS

A forest plot of the Tutoring studies is shown in Figure 19.1. The five A studies (at the top) have effect sizes (Hedges' g) in the approximate range of 0.10 to 0.50. The five B studies (below) have effect sizes in the approximate range of 0.45 to 0.75.

The combined effect for the A studies (represented by the first diamond) is 0.32 with a 95% confidence interval of plus/minus 0.11. The combined effect for the B studies (represented by the second diamond) is 0.61 with a 95% confidence interval of plus/minus 0.12. Our goal, then, is to compare these two effects.

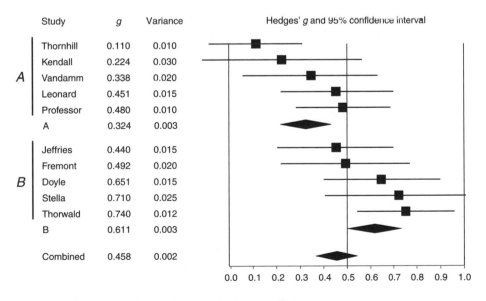

Figure 19.1 Fixed-effect model – studies and subgroup effects.

If we were working with a primary study (with Thornhill, Kendall, etc. being persons in treatment A, and Jeffries, Fremont, etc. being persons in treatment B), we would compute the mean and variance for each treatment, and our options for comparing these means would be clear. For example, we could perform a t-test to assess the difference between means relative to the standard error of the difference. Or, we could use analysis of variance to assess the variance among groups means relative to the variance within groups.

In meta-analysis we are working with subgroups of *studies* rather than groups of *subjects*, but will follow essentially the same approach, using a variant of the t-test or a variant of analysis of variance to compare the subgroup means. For this purpose we need to perform two tasks.

- Compute the mean effect and variance for each subgroup.
- Compare the mean effect across subgroups.

Computing the summary effects

In Table 19.1 the data for the A studies are displayed at the top, and data for the B studies are displayed toward the bottom.

To compute the summary effects we use the same formulas that we introduced for a single group (11.2) to (11.10). The summary effect for subgroup A is computed using values from the row marked *Sum A*. The summary effect for subgroup B is computed using values from the row marked *Sum B*. The summary effect for all studies is computed using values from the row marked *Sum*.

Table 19.1 Fixed effect model – computations.

	Study	Effect size Y	Variance Within V_Y	Variance Between T^2	Variance Total V	Weight W	Calculated quantities		
							WY	WY^2	W^2
	Thornhill	0.110	0.0100	0.0000	0.0100	100.000	11.000	1.210	10000.000
	Kendall	0.224	0.0300	0.0000	0.0300	33.333	7.467	1.673	1111.111
A	Vandamm	0.338	0.0200	0.0000	0.0200	50.000	16.900	5.712	2500.000
	Leonard	0.451	0.0150	0.0000	0.0150	66.667	30.067	13.560	4444.444
	Professor	0.480	0.0100	0.0000	0.0100	100.000	48.000	23.040	10000.000
	Sum A					350.000	113.433	45.195	28055.556
	Jefferies	0.440	0.0150	0.0000	0.0150	66.667	29.333	12.907	4444.444
	Fremont	0.492	0.0200	0.0000	0.0200	50.000	24.600	12.103	2500.000
B	Doyle	0.651	0.0150	0.0000	0.0150	66.667	43.400	28.253	4444.444
	Stella	0.710	0.0250	0.0000	0.0250	40.000	28.400	20.164	1600.000
	Thorwald	0.740	0.0120	0.0000	0.0120	83.333	61.667	45.633	6944.444
	Sum B					306.667	187.400	119.061	19933.333
	Sum					656.667	300.833	164.255	47988.889

Computations (fixed effect) for the A studies

$$M_A = \frac{113.433}{350.000} = 0.3241,$$

$$V_{M_A} = \frac{1}{350.000} = 0.0029,$$

$$SE_{M_A} = \sqrt{0.0029} = 0.0535,$$

$$LL_{M_A} = 0.3241 - 1.96 \times 0.0535 = 0.2193,$$

$$UL_{M_A} = 0.3241 + 1.96 \times 0.0535 = 0.4289,$$

$$Z_A = \frac{0.3241}{0.0535} = 6.0633,$$

$$p(Z_A) < 0.0001,$$

$$Q_A = 45.195 - \left(\frac{113.433^2}{350.000} \right) = 8.4316 \tag{19.1}$$

$$p(Q = 8.4316, \ df = 4) = 0.0770,$$

$$C_A = 350.000 - \frac{28055.556}{350.000} = 269.8413,$$

$$T_A^2 = \frac{8.4316 - 4}{269.8413} = 0.0164,$$

and

$$I_A^2 = \left(\frac{8.4316 - 4}{8.4316} \right) \times 100 = 52.5594.$$

Computations (fixed effect) for the B studies

$$M_B = \frac{187.400}{306.667} = 0.6111,$$

$$V_{M_B} = \frac{1}{306.667} = 0.0033,$$

$$SE_{M_B} = \sqrt{0.0033} = 0.0571,$$

$$LL_{M_B} = 0.6111 - 1.96 \times 0.0571 = 0.4992,$$

$$UL_{M_B} = 0.6111 + 1.96 \times 0.0571 = 0.7230,$$

$$Z_B = \frac{0.6111}{0.0571} = 10.7013,$$

$$p(Z_B) < 0.0001,$$

$$Q_B = 119.011 - \left(\frac{187.400^2}{306.667}\right) = 4.5429, \tag{19.2}$$

$$p(Q = 4.5429, df = 4) = 0.3375,$$

$$C_B = 306.667 - \frac{19933.333}{306.667} = 241.667,$$

$$T_B^2 = \frac{4.5429 - 4}{241.667} = 0.0022,$$

and

$$I_B^2 = \left(\frac{4.5429 - 4}{4.5429}\right) \times 100 = 11.9506.$$

Computations (fixed effect) for all ten studies

$$M = \frac{300.833}{656.667} = 0.4581, \tag{19.3}$$

$$V_M = \frac{1}{656.667} = 0.0015, \tag{19.4}$$

$$SE_M = \sqrt{0.0015} = 0.0390,$$

$$LL_M = 0.4581 - 1.96 \times 0.0390 = 0.3816,$$

$$UL_M = 0.4581 + 1.96 \times 0.0390 = 0.5346,$$

$$Z = \frac{0.4581}{0.0390} = 11.7396,$$

$$p(Z) < 0.0001,$$

$$Q = 164.255 - \left(\frac{300.833^2}{656.667}\right) = 26.4371, \tag{19.5}$$

$$p(Q = 26.4371, df = 9) = 0.0017,$$

$$C = 656.667 - \frac{47988.889}{656.667} = 583.5871,$$

$$T^2 = \frac{26.4371 - 9}{538.5871} = 0.0299,$$

and

$$I^2 = \left(\frac{26.4371 - 9}{26.4371} \right) \times 100 = 65.96.$$

The statistics computed above are summarized in Table 19.2.

Table 19.2 Fixed-effect model – summary statistics.

	A	B	Combined
Y	0.3241	0.6111	0.4581
V	0.0029	0.0033	0.0015
SE_Y	0.0535	0.0571	0.0390
LL_Y	0.2193	0.4992	0.3816
UL_Y	0.4289	0.7230	0.5346
Z	6.0633	10.7013	11.7396
$p2$	0.0000	0.0000	0.0000
Q	8.4316	4.5429	26.4371
df	4.0000	4.0000	9.0000
p-value	0.0770	0.3375	0.0017
Numerator	4.4316	0.5429	17.4371
C	269.8413	241.6667	583.5871
T^2	0.0164	0.0022	0.0299
I^2	52.5594	11.9506	65.9569

Comparing the effects

If we return to Figure 19.1 and excerpt the diamonds for the two subgroups we get Figure 19.2. The mean effect size for subgroups A and B are 0.324 and 0.611, with variances of 0.003 and 0.003.

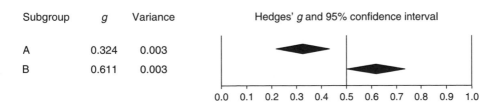

Figure 19.2 Fixed-effect – subgroup effects.

Our goal is to compare these two mean effects, and we describe three ways that we can proceed. These approaches are algebraically equivalent, and (it follows) yield the same p-value. Our goal in presenting three approaches is to provide insight into the process.

Comparing A versus B: a Z-test (Method 1)

Since there are only two subgroups here, we can work directly with the mean difference in effect sizes. In a primary study, if we wanted to compare the means in two groups we would perform a t-test. In meta-analysis the mean and variance are based on *studies* rather than *subjects* but the logic of the test is the same.

Concretely, let θ_A and θ_B be the true effects underlying groups A and B, let M_A and M_B be the estimated effects, and let V_{M_A} and V_{M_B} be their variances. If we use *Diff* to refer to the difference between the two effects, and elect to subtract the mean of A from the mean of B,

$$Diff = M_B - M_A,$$

the test statistic to compare the two effects is

$$Z_{Diff} = \frac{Diff}{SE_{Diff}}, \tag{19.6}$$

where

$$SE_{Diff} = \sqrt{V_{M_A} + V_{M_B}}. \tag{19.7}$$

Under the null hypothesis that the true effect size θ is the same for both groups,

$$H_0 : \theta_A = \theta_B, \tag{19.8}$$

Z_{Diff} would follow the normal distribution. For a two-tailed test, the p-value is given by

$$p = 2[1 - (\Phi(|Z|))], \tag{19.9}$$

where $\Phi(Z)$ is the standard normal cumulative distribution.

In the running example,

$$Diff = 0.6111 - 0.3241 = 0.2870,$$

$$SE_{Diff} = \sqrt{0.0029 + 0.0033} = 0.0782,$$

$$Z_{Diff} = \frac{0.2870}{0.0782} = 3.6691,$$

and

$$p = 2[1 - (\Phi(|3.6691|))] = 0.0002.$$

The two-tailed p-value corresponding to $Z_{Diff} = 3.6691$ is 0.0002. This tells us that the treatment effect is probably not the same for the A studies as for the B studies. In Excel, the function to compute a 2-tailed p-value for Z is $=(1-(NORMSDIST (ABS(Z))))*2$. Here, $=(1-(NORMSDIST(ABS(3.6691))))*2$ will return the value 0.0002.

Comparing A with B: a Q-test based on analysis of variance (Method 2)

In a primary study, the t-test can be used to compare the means in *two* groups, but to compare means in more than two groups we use analysis of variance. Concretely, we partition the total variance (of all subjects about the grand mean) into variance within groups (of subjects about the means of their respective groups) and variance between groups (of group means about the grand mean). We then test these various components of variance for statistical significance, with the last (variance between groups) addressing the hypothesis that effect size differs as function of group membership.

In meta-analysis the means are based on *studies* rather than *subjects* but the logic of the test is the same. Specifically, we compute the following quantities (where SS is the sum of squared deviations).

- Q_A, the weighted SS of all A studies about the mean of A.
- Q_B, the weighted SS of all B studies about the mean of B.
- Q_{within}, the sum of Q_A and Q_B.
- Q_{bet}, the weighted SS of the subgroup means about the grand mean.
- Q, the weighted SS of all effects about the grand mean.

We may write $Q_{within} = Q_A + Q_B$, to represent the sum of within-group weighted SS, or more generally, for p subgroups,

$$Q_{within} = \sum_{j=1}^{p} Q_j. \qquad (19.10)$$

In the running example

$$Q_{within} = 8.4316 + 4.5429 = 12.9745. \qquad (19.11)$$

The weighted SS are additive, such that $Q = Q_{within} + Q_{bet}$. Therefore, Q_{bet} can be computed as

$$Q_{bet} = Q - Q_{within}. \qquad (19.12)$$

Under the null hypothesis that the effect size θ is the same for all groups, 1 to p, Q_{bet} would be distributed as chi-squared with degrees of freedom equal to $p - 1$.

In the running example,

$$Q_{bet} = 26.4371 - 12.9745 = 13.4626. \qquad (19.13)$$

Table 19.3 Fixed-effect model – ANOVA table.

	Q	df	p	Formula
A	8.4316	4	0.0770	19.1
B	4.5429	4	0.3375	19.2
Within	12.9745	8	0.1127	19.11
Between	13.4626	1	0.0002	19.13
Total	26.4371	9	0.0017	19.5

Each Q statistic is evaluated with respect to the corresponding degrees of freedom. In the running example (Table 19.3),

- The 'Total' line tells us that for the full group of ten studies the variance is statistically significant ($Q = 26.4371$, $df = 9$, $p = 0.0017$).
- The 'Within' line tells us that the variance within groups (averaged across groups) is not statistically significant ($Q_{within} = 12.9745$, $df = 8$, $p = 0.1127$).
- The 'Between' line tells us that the difference between groups (the combined effect for A versus B) is statistically significant ($Q_{bet} = 13.4626$, $df = 1$, $p = 0.0002$), which means that the effect size is related to the frequency of tutoring.
- At a finer level of detail, neither the variance within subgroup A ($Q_A = 8.4316$, $df = 4$, $p = 0.0770$) nor within subgroup B ($Q_B = 4.5429$, $df = 4$, $p = 0.3375$) is statistically significant.

As always, the absence of statistical significance (here, within subgroups) means only that we cannot rule out the hypothesis that the studies share a common effect size, and it does not mean that this hypothesis has been proven.

In Excel, the function to compute a p-value for Q is =CHIDIST(Q,df). For the test of A versus B, =CHIDIST(13.4626,1) returns 0.0002.

Comparing A versus B: a Q-test for heterogeneity (Method 3)

The test we just described can be derived in a different way. We can think of the effect sizes for subgroups A and B as single studies (if we extract the two subgroup lines and the total line from Figure 19.1 and replace the diamonds with squares, to represent these as if they were studies, we get Figure 19.3). Then, we can test these 'studies' for heterogeneity, using precisely the same formulas that we introduced earlier (Chapter 16) to test the dispersion of single studies about the summary effect.

Concretely, we start with two 'studies' with effect sizes of 0.324 and 0.611, and variance of 0.003 and 0.003. Then, we apply the usual meta-analysis methods to compute Q (see Table 19.4).

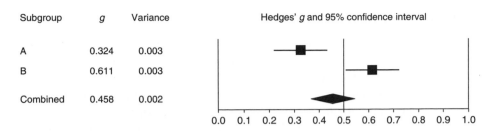

Subgroup	g	Variance	Hedges' g and 95% confidence interval
A	0.324	0.003	
B	0.611	0.003	
Combined	0.458	0.002	

Figure 19.3 Fixed-effect model – treating subgroups as studies.

Table 19.4 Fixed-effect model – subgroups as studies.

Study	Effect size Y	Variance Within V_Y	Variance Between T^2	Variance Total V	Weight W	Calculated quantities		
						WY	WY^2	W^2
A	0.3241	0.0029	0.0000	0.0029	350.000	113.433	36.763	122500.000
B	0.6111	0.0033	0.0000	0.0033	306.667	187.400	114.518	94044.444
					656.667	300.833	151.281	216544.444

In this example,

$$M = \frac{300.833}{656.667} = 0.4581, \qquad (19.14)$$

$$V_M = \frac{1}{656.667} = 0.0015, \qquad (19.15)$$

$$Q = 151.281 - \left(\frac{300.833^2}{656.667} \right) = 13.4626,$$

$$df = 2 - 1 = 1,$$

and

$$p(Q = 13.4626, df = 1) = 0.0002,$$

where Q represents the weighted sum of squares for studies A and B about the grand mean. For $Q = 13.4626$ and $df = 1$, the p-value is 0.0002.

In Excel, the function to compute a p-value for Q is =CHIDIST(Q,df), and =CHIDIST(13.4626,1) returns 0.0002.

Summary

We presented three methods for comparing the effect size across subgroups. One method was to use a Z-test to compare the two effect sizes directly. Another was to use a Q-test to partition the variance, and test the between-subgroups portion of the variance. A third was to use a Q-test to assess the dispersion of the summary effects about the combined effect. All the methods assess the difference in subgroup effects relative to the precision of the difference (or the variance across subgroups effects relative to the variance within subgroups).

As noted earlier, the methods are mathematically equivalent. The two methods that report Q, report the same value for Q (13.4626). When there is one degree of freedom (so that we can use either a Z-test or a Q-test) Z is equal to the square root of Q. In our example, the method that reports Z, reports a value of $Z = 3.6691$, which is equal to the square root of Q. All three methods yield a p-value of 0.0002.

Quantify the magnitude of the difference

The Z-test and the Q-tests address the question of *statistical*, rather than *clinical* significance. In addition to reporting the test of significance, one should generally report an estimate of the effect size, which in this context is the difference in mean effect between the two subgroups. For subgroups A and B, if we elect to subtract the mean of A from the mean of B, the difference is

$$Diff = M_B - M_A. \tag{19.16}$$

The 95% confidence interval is estimated by

$$LL_{Diff} = Diff - 1.96 \times SE_{Diff} \tag{19.17}$$

and

$$UL_{Diff} = Diff + 1.96 \times SE_{Diff}, \tag{19.18}$$

where the standard error was defined in (19.7). If we had more than two subgroups, we could repeat this procedure for all pairs of subgroups. In the running example the difference in effects (which we have defined as B minus A) and its 95% confidence interval are estimated as

$$Diff = 0.6111 - 0.3241 = 0.2870,$$

$$SE_{Diff} = \sqrt{0.0029 + 0.0033} = 0.0782,$$

$$LL_{Diff} = 0.2870 - 1.96 \times 0.0782 = 0.1337,$$

and

$$UL_{Diff} = 0.2870 + 1.96 \times 0.0782 = 0.4403.$$

In words, the true difference between the effect in the subgroup A studies, as opposed to the subgroup B studies, probably falls in the range of 0.13 to 0.44.

COMPUTATIONAL MODELS

In Part 3 of this volume we discussed the difference between a fixed-effect model and a random-effects model. Under the fixed-effect model we assume that the true effect is the same in all studies. By contrast, under the random-effects model we allow that the true effect may vary from one study to the next. This difference has implications for the way that weights are assigned to the studies, which affects both the summary effect and its standard error.

When we introduced these two models we were working with a single set of studies. Now, we are working with more than one subgroup of studies (in the running example, A and B) but the same issues apply. Under the fixed-effect model we assume that all studies in subgroup A share a common effect size and that all studies in subgroup B share a common effect size. By contrast, under the random-effects model we allow that there may be some true variation of effects within the A studies and within the B studies.

When we initially discussed the fixed-effect model we used the example of a pharmaceutical company that enrolled 1000 patients for a clinical trial and divided them among ten cohorts of 100 patients each (page 83). These ten cohorts were known to be identical in all important respects, and so it was reasonable to assume that the true effect would be the same for all ten studies. When we presented this example we noted that the conditions described (of all the studies being performed by the same researchers using the same population and methods) are rare in systematic reviews, and that in most cases the random-effects model will be more plausible than the fixed-effect.

We can expand the pharmaceutical example to apply to subgroups if we assume that five of the studies will compare *Drug A* versus placebo, and the other five will compare *Drug B* versus placebo. Within the five *Drug A* studies and within the five *Drug B* studies there should be a single true effect size, and so in this case it would be correct to use the fixed-effect model within subgroups. However, the same caveat applies here, in that this kind of systematic review, where all studies are performed by the same researchers using the same population and methods, is very rare. In the vast majority of systematic reviews these conditions will not hold, and a random-effects analysis would be a better fit for the data.

For example, in the tutoring analysis it seems plausible that the distinction between the two interventions (one hour versus two hours a week) captures some, *but not all*, of the true variation among effects. Within either subgroup of studies (A or B) there are probably differences from study to study in the motivation of the students, or the dedication of the teachers, the details of the protocol, or other factors, such that the true effect differs from study to study. If these differences do exist, and can have an impact on the effect size, then the random-effects model is a better match than the fixed-effect.

When we use the random-effects model, the impact on the summary effect within subgroups will be the same as it had been when we were working with a single population. The weights assigned to each study will be more moderate than they had been under the fixed-effect model (large studies will lose impact while small studies gain impact). And, the variance of the combined effect will increase.

T^2 should be computed within subgroups

To apply the random-effects model we need to estimate the value of τ^2, the variance of true effect sizes across studies. Since τ^2 is defined as the true variance in effect size among a set of studies, its value will differ depending on how we define the set.

If we were to define the set as all studies irrespective of which subgroup they belong to, with τ^2 based on the dispersion of all studies from the grand mean, τ^2 would tend to be relatively large. By contrast, if we define the set as all studies *within* a subgroup, with τ^2 based on the dispersion of the A studies from the mean of A and of the B studies from the mean of B, τ^2 would tend to be relatively small (especially if the A studies and the B studies do represent distinct clusters, as we have hypothesized).

Since our goal is to estimate the mean and sampling distribution of subgroup A, and to do the same for subgroup B, it is clearly the variance *within* subgroups that is relevant in the present context. Put simply, if some of the variance in effect sizes can be explained by the type of intervention, then this variance is not a factor in the sampling distribution of studies within a subgroup (where only one intervention was used). Therefore, we always estimate τ^2 within subgroups.

To pool or not to pool

When we estimate τ^2 within subgroups of studies, the estimate is likely to differ from one subgroup to the next. In the running example, the estimate of τ^2 in subgroup A was 0.016, while in subgroup B it was 0.002. We have the option to pool the within-group estimates of τ^2 and apply this common estimate to all studies. Alternatively, we can apply each subgroup's estimate of τ^2 to the studies in that subgroup.

Note. As a shorthand we refer to pooling the estimates of τ^2. In fact, though, what we actually pool are Q, df, and C, and then estimate τ^2 from these pooled values (see (19.38)).

The decision to pool (or not) depends on the following. If we assume that the true study-to-study dispersion is the same within all subgroups, then observed differences in T^2 must be due to sampling variation alone. In this case, we should pool the information to yield a common estimate, and then apply this estimate to all subgroups. This seems like a plausible expectation in the running example, where the study-to-study variation in effect size is likely to be similar for subgroups A and B.

On the other hand, if we anticipate that the true between-studies dispersion may actually differ from one subgroup to the next, then we would estimate τ^2 within subgroups and use a separate estimate of τ^2 for each subgroup. For example, suppose that we are assessing an intervention to reduce recidivism among juvenile delinquents, and comparing the effect in subgroups of studies where the delinquents did, or did not, have a history of violence. We might expect to see a wider range of effect sizes in one subgroup than the other.

There is one additional caveat to consider. If we do anticipate that τ^2 will vary from one subgroup to the next, so that the correct approach is to use separate estimates of τ^2, we still need to be sure that there are enough studies within each subgroup to yield an acceptably accurate estimate of τ^2. Generally, if there are only a few studies within subgroups (say, five or fewer), then the estimates of τ^2 within subgroups are likely to be imprecise. In this case, it makes more sense to use a pooled estimate, since the increased accuracy that we get by pooling more studies is likely to exceed any real differences between groups in the true value of τ^2.

Summary

The logic outlined above is encapsulated in the flowchart shown in Figure 19.4. If the studies within each subgroup share a common effect size, then we use the fixed-effect model to assign weights to each study (and τ^2 is zero). Otherwise, we use the random-effects model.

Under random effects we always estimate τ^2 within subgroups. If we believe that the true value of τ^2 is the same for all subgroups, then the correct procedure is to pool the estimates obtained within subgroups. If we believe that the true value of τ^2 varies from one subgroup to the next, the correct procedure is to use a separate

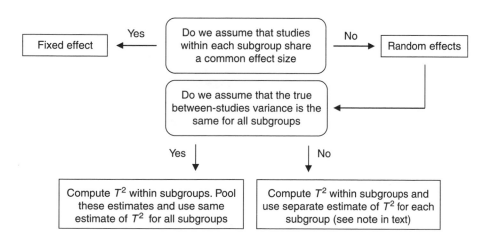

Figure 19.4 Flowchart for selecting a computational model.

estimate for each subgroup. However, if we have only a few studies within subgroups these estimates may be imprecise and therefore it may be preferable to pool the estimates.

RANDOM EFFECTS WITH SEPARATE ESTIMATES OF τ^2

Here, we proceed through the same set of computations as we did for the fixed-effect model, but this time using random-effects weights, with a separate estimate of τ^2 for each subgroup.

Computing the effects

Figure 19.5 is a forest plot of the studies in subgroups A and B. The studies are identical to those in the fixed-effect forest plot (Figure 19.2) but the summary effects, represented by the diamonds, are now based on random-effects weights. The mean effect size for subgroups A and B are 0.325 and 0.610, with variances of 0.006 and 0.004.

Computations are based on the values in Table 19.5. These values are similar to those in Table 19.1, except that the variance for each study now includes the within-study variance and the between-study variance. We did not assume a common value of τ^2 and therefore used a separate estimate of τ^2 for each subgroup. In Figure 19.5 this is indicated by the symbols at the right, where we have one value for T_A^2 and another for T_B^2. In Table 19.5, the column labeled T^2 shows 0.0164 for the A studies and 0.0022 for the B studies.

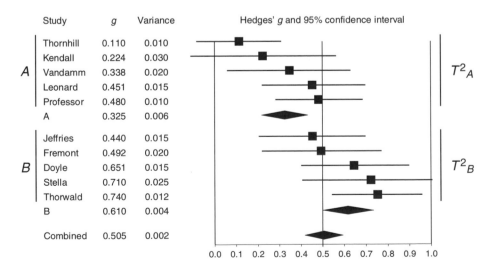

Figure 19.5 Random-effects model (separate estimates of τ^2) – studies and subgroup effects.

Table 19.5 Random-effects model (separate estimates of τ^2) – computations.

Study	Effect size Y	Variance Within V_Y	Variance Between T^2	Variance Total V	Weight W	Calculated quantities		
						WY	WY^2	W^2
Thornhill	0.110	0.0100	0.0164	0.0264	37.846	4.163	0.458	1432.308
Kendall	0.224	0.0300	0.0164	0.0464	21.541	4.825	1.081	464.017
A Vandamm	0.338	0.0200	0.0164	0.0364	27.455	9.280	3.137	753.788
Leonard	0.451	0.0150	0.0164	0.0314	31.824	14.353	6.473	1012.757
Professor	0.480	0.0100	0.0164	0.0264	37.846	18.166	8.720	1432.308
Sum A					156.512	50.787	19.868	5095.179
Jefferies	0.440	0.0150	0.0022	0.0172	57.983	25.512	11.225	3362.002
Fremont	0.492	0.0200	0.0022	0.0222	44.951	22.116	10.881	2020.582
B Doyle	0.651	0.0150	0.0022	0.0172	57.983	37.747	24.573	3362.002
Stella	0.710	0.0250	0.0022	0.0272	36.702	26.058	18.501	1347.034
Thorwald	0.740	0.0120	0.0022	0.0142	70.193	51.943	38.438	4927.012
Sum B					267.811	163.376	103.619	15018.633
Sum					424.323	214.163	123.487	20113.812

Computations (random effects, separate estimates of τ^2) for the A studies

$$M_A^* = \frac{50.787}{156.512} = 0.3245,$$

$$V_{M_A^*} = \frac{1}{156.512} = 0.0064,$$

$$SE_{M_A^*} = \sqrt{0.0064} = 0.0799,$$

$$LL_{M_A^*} = 0.3245 - 1.96 \times 0.0799 = 0.1678,$$

$$UL_{M_A^*} = 0.3245 + 1.96 \times 0.0799 = 0.4812,$$

$$Z_A^* = \frac{0.3245}{0.0799} = 4.0595,$$

$$p(Z_A^*) < 0.0001,$$

and

$$Q_A^* = 19.868 - \left(\frac{50.787^2}{156.512}\right) = 3.3882. \tag{19.19}$$

Note. The $Q*$ statistic computed here, using random-effects weights, is used *only* for the analysis of variance, to partition $Q*$ into its various components. Therefore, we do not show a *p*-value for $Q*$. Rather, the Q statistic computed using fixed-effect weights (Table 19.2) is the one that reflects the between-studies dispersion, provides a test of homogeneity for the studies within subgroup A, and is used to estimate T^2.

Computations (random effects, separate estimates of τ^2) for the B studies

$$M_B^* = \frac{163.376}{267.811} = 0.6100,$$

$$V_{M_B^*} = \frac{1}{267.811} = 0.0037,$$

$$SE_{M_B^*} = \sqrt{0.0037} = 0.0611,$$

$$LL_{M_B^*} = 0.6100 - 1.96 \times 0.0611 = 0.4903,$$

$$UL_{M_B^*} = 0.6100 + 1.96 \times 0.0611 = 0.7298,$$

$$Z_B^* = \frac{0.6100}{0.0611} = 9.9833,$$

$$p(Z_B^*) < 0.0001,$$

and

$$Q_B^* = 103.619 - \left(\frac{163.376^2}{267.811} \right) = 3.9523. \tag{19.20}$$

Computations (random effects, separate estimates of τ^2) for all ten studies
The statistics here are computed using the same value of T^2 as was used within groups (in this case, *not* pooled).

$$M^* = \frac{214.163}{424.323} = 0.5047, \tag{19.21}$$

$$V_{M^*} = \frac{1}{424.323} = 0.0024, \tag{19.22}$$

$$SE_{M^*} = \sqrt{0.0024} = 0.0485,$$

$$LL_{M^*} = 0.5047 - 1.96 \times 0.0485 = 0.4096,$$

$$UL_{M^*} = 0.5047 + 1.96 \times 0.0485 = 0.5999,$$

$$Z^* = \frac{0.5047}{0.0485} = 10.3967,$$

$$p(Z^*) < 0.0001,$$

and

$$Q^* = 123.487 - \left(\frac{214.163^2}{424.323}\right) = 15.3952. \qquad (19.23)$$

Statistics (random-effects) are summarized in Table 19.6.

Table 19.6 Random-effects model (separate estimates of τ^2) – summary statistics.

	A	B	Combined
Y	0.3245	0.6100	0.5047
V	0.0064	0.0037	0.0024
SE_Y	0.0799	0.0611	0.0485
LL_Y	0.1678	0.4903	0.4096
UL_Y	0.4812	0.7298	0.5999
Z	4.0595	9.9833	10.3967
$p2$	0.0000	0.0000	0.0000
Q	3.3882	3.9523	15.3952

Comparing the effects

If we return to Figure 19.5 and excerpt the diamonds for the two subgroups we get Figure 19.6.

The mean effect size for subgroups A and B are 0.325 and 0.610, with variances of 0.006 and 0.004.

Our goal is to compare these two mean effects, and there are several ways that we can proceed. These approaches are algebraically equivalent, and (it follows) yield the same p-value. Our goal in presenting several approaches is to provide insight into the process.

Comparing A versus B: a Z-test (Method 1)

We can use a simple Z-test to compare the mean effect for subgroups A versus B. The formulas are identical to those used earlier, but we change two symbols to

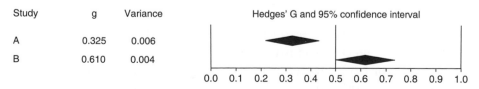

Study	g	Variance	Hedges' G and 95% confidence interval
A	0.325	0.006	
B	0.610	0.004	

Figure 19.6 Random-effects model (separate estimates of τ^2) – subgroup effects.

reflect the random-effects model. First, we use a (*) to indicate that the statistics are based on random-effects weights rather than fixed-effect weights. Second, the null hypothesis is framed as $\mu_A = \mu_B$, reflecting the fact that these are mean values, rather than $\theta_A = \theta_B$, which we used to refer to common values when we were working with the fixed-effect model.

Let μ_A and μ_B be the true mean effects underlying subgroups A and B, let M_A^* and M_B^* be the estimated effects, and let $V_{M_A^*}$ and $V_{M_B^*}$ be their variances. If we use $Diff^*$ to refer to the difference between the two effects and elect to subtract the mean of A from the mean of B,

$$Diff^* = M_B^* - M_A^*. \tag{19.24}$$

The test statistic to compare the two effects is

$$Z_{Diff}^* = \frac{Diff^*}{SE_{Diff^*}}, \tag{19.25}$$

where

$$SE_{Diff^*} = \sqrt{V_{M_A^*} + V_{M_B^*}}. \tag{19.26}$$

Under the null hypothesis that the true mean effect size μ is the same for both groups,

$$H_0^* : \mu_A^* = \mu_B^*, \tag{19.27}$$

Z_{Diff}^* would follow the normal distribution. For a two-tailed test the p-value is given by

$$p^* = 2\left[1 - \left(\Phi\left(|Z_{Diff}^*|\right)\right)\right], \tag{19.28}$$

where $\Phi(Z)$ is the standard normal cumulative distribution.

In the running example

$$Diff^* = 0.6100 - 0.3245 = 0.2856,$$

$$SE_{Diff^*} = \sqrt{0.0064 + 0.0037} = 0.1006,$$

and

$$Z_{Diff^*} = \frac{0.2856}{0.1006} = 2.8381.$$

The two-tailed p-value corresponding to $Z_{Diff}^* = 2.8381$ is 0.0045. This tells us that the mean treatment effect is probably not the same for the A studies as for the B studies. In Excel, the function to compute a 2-tailed p-value for Z is = (1-(NORMSDIST(ABS(Z))))*2. Here, =(1-(NORMSDIST(ABS(2.8381))))*2 will return the value 0.0045.

Comparing A with B: a Q-test based on analysis of variance (Method 2)

We use the same formulas as we did for method 2 under the fixed-effect model, but now apply random-effects weights. Note that this approach only works if we use the same weights to compute the overall effect as we do to compute the effects within groups. In Table 19.5, studies from subgroup A use the T^2 value of 0.0164 both for computing the subgroup mean and for computing the overall mean. Similarly, studies from subgroup B use the T^2 value of 0.0022 both for computing the subgroup mean and for computing the overall mean.

We compute the following quantities (where SS is the sum of squared deviations).

- Q_A^*, the weighted SS of all A studies about the mean of A.
- Q_B^*, the weighted SS of all B studies about the mean of B.
- Q_{within}^*, the sum of Q_A^* and Q_B^*.
- Q_{bet}^*, the weighted SS of the subgroup means about the grand mean.
- Q^*, the weighted SS of all effects about the grand mean.

We may write $Q_{within}^* = Q_A^* + Q_B^*$, to represent the sum of within-group weighted SS, or more generally, for p subgroups,

$$Q_{within}^* = \sum_{j=1}^{p} Q_j^*. \tag{19.29}$$

In the running example

$$Q_{within}^* = 3.3882 + 3.9523 = 7.3406. \tag{19.30}$$

The weighted SS are additive, such that $Q^* = Q_{within}^* + Q_{bet}^*$. Therefore, Q_{bet}^* can be computed as

$$Q_{bet}^* = Q^* - Q_{within}^*. \tag{19.31}$$

Under the null hypothesis that the effect sizes μ are the same for all groups, 1 to p, Q_{bet}^* would be distributed as chi-squared with degrees of freedom equal to $p - 1$.

In the running example

$$Q_{bet}^* = 15.3952 - 7.3406 = 8.0547. \tag{19.32}$$

Results are summarized in Table 19.7. Note that the only Q statistic that we interpret here is the one *between groups*. In the running example, the *Between* line tells us

Table 19.7 Random-effects model (separate estimates of τ^2) – ANOVA table.

	Q^*	df	p	Formula
A	3.3882			19.19
B	3.9523			19.20
Within	7.3406			19.30
Between	8.0547	1.0	0.0045	19.32
Total	15.3952			19.23

that the difference between groups (the combined effect for A versus B) is statistically significant ($Q^*_{bet} = 8.0547$, $df = 1$, $p = 0.0045$), which means that the effect size *is* related to the frequency of tutoring. In Excel, the function to compute a p-value for Q is $= CHIDIST(Q,df)$. For the test of A versus B, $=CHIDIST(8.0547,1)$ returns 0.0045.

To address the statistical significance of the total variance or the variance within groups, we use the statistics reported using the fixed-effect weights (see Table 19.3) rather than using Q^* (total), Q^*_A, Q^*_B or Q^*_{within}.

Comparing A versus B: a Q-test for heterogeneity (Method 3)

Finally, we could treat the subgroups as if they were studies and perform a test for heterogeneity across studies. If we extract the two subgroup lines and the total line from Figure 19.5 and replace the diamonds with squares we get Figure 19.7.

Concretely, we start with two *studies* with effect sizes of 0.324 and 0.610, and variances of 0.006 and 0.004. Then, we apply the usual meta-analysis methods to compute Q. Concretely, using the values in Table 19.8, and applying (11.2) and subsequent formulas, we compute

and

$$M^* = \frac{214.163}{424.323} = 0.5047, \tag{19.33}$$

$$V_M{}^* = \frac{1}{424.323} = 0.0024. \tag{19.34}$$

$$Q = 116.146 - \left(\frac{214.163^2}{424.323} \right) = 8.0547,$$

and

$$df = 2 - 1 = 1,$$

$$p(Q = 8.0547, df = 1) = 0.0045,$$

where Q represents the weighted sum of squares for Studies A and B about the grand mean. For $Q = 8.0547$ and $df = 1$, the p-value is 0.0045.

In Excel, the function to compute a p-value for Q is $=CHIDIST(Q,df)$. For the test of A versus B, $=CHIDIST(8.0547,1)$ returns 0.0045.

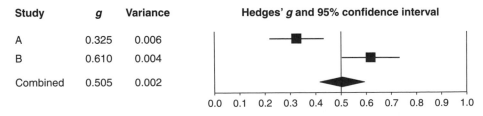

Study	g	Variance	Hedges' g and 95% confidence interval
A	0.325	0.006	
B	0.610	0.004	
Combined	0.505	0.002	

Figure 19.7 Random-effects model (separate estimates of τ^2) – treating subgroups as studies.

Table 19.8 Random-effects model (separate estimates of τ^2) – subgroups as studies.

Study	Effect size Y	Variance Within V_Y	Variance Between T^2	Variance Total V	Weight W	Calculated quantities		
						WY	WY^2	W^2
A	0.3245	0.0064	0.0000	0.0064	156.512	50.787	16.480	24495.944
B	0.6100	0.0037	0.0000	0.0037	267.811	163.376	99.666	71722.774
					424.323	214.163	116.146	96218.718

Quantify the magnitude of the difference

The difference and confidence interval are given by (19.17) and (19.18):

$$Diff^* = 0.6100 - 0.3245 = 0.2856,$$

$$SE_{Diff^*} = \sqrt{0.0064 + 0.0037} = 0.1006,$$

$$LL_{Diff^*} = 0.2856 - 1.96 \times 0.1006 = 0.0883,$$

and

$$UL_{Diff^*} = 0.2856 + 1.96 \times 0.1006 = 0.4828.$$

In words, the true difference between the effect in the A studies, as opposed to the B studies, probably falls in the range of 0.09 to 0.48.

RANDOM EFFECTS WITH POOLED ESTIMATE OF τ^2

Here, we show the computation of summary effects within subgroups, using a random-effects model with a pooled estimate of τ^2, which we refer to as τ^2_{within}. We illustrate the procedure in Figure 19.8. Note the common value of τ^2_{within} is assumed to apply to both subgroups.

Formula for estimating a pooled T^2

To estimate the pooled τ^2, proceed as follows. Recall (12.2) to (12.5) that to estimate τ^2 for a single collection of studies we use

$$T^2 = \frac{Q - df}{C}, \tag{19.35}$$

where

$$df = k - 1, \tag{19.36}$$

where k is the number of studies, and

$$C = \sum W_i - \frac{\sum W_i^2}{\sum W_i}. \tag{19.37}$$

In these equations, $Q - df$ is the excess (observed minus expected) sum of squared deviations from the weighted mean, and C is a scaling factor.

Similarly, to yield a pooled estimate of τ^2 we sum each element (Q, df, and C) across subgroups and then perform the same computation. Concretely,

$$T^2_{within} = \frac{\sum_{j=1}^{p} Q_j - \sum_{j=1}^{p} df_j}{\sum_{j=1}^{p} C_j}. \tag{19.38}$$

While the true value of τ^2_{within} cannot be less than zero (a variance cannot be negative), this method of estimating τ^2_{within} can yield a negative value due to sampling issues (when the observed dispersion is less than we would expect by chance). In this case, the estimate T^2_{within} is set to zero.

Computing the effects

Subgroup A yielded an estimate of 0.0164 while subgroup B yielded an estimate of 0.0122, represented in Figure 19.8 as T^2_A and T^2_B. We will pool these two estimates to yield a pooled value, represented as T^2_{within}, of 0.0097 (see (19.39)). This is the value used to assign weights in Table 19.10.

In the running example, the values within each group were computed earlier for A and B. Table 19.9 shows the values needed to calculate a pooled estimate T^2_{within} for the running example.

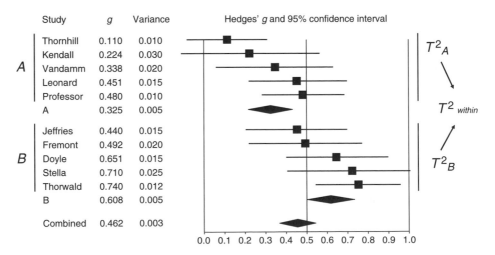

Figure 19.8 Random-effects model (pooled estimate of τ^2) – studies and subgroup effects.

Table 19.9 Statistics for computing a pooled estimate of τ^2.

Group	Q	df	C
A	8.4316	4	269.8413
B	4.5429	4	241.6667
Sum	12.9745	8	511.5079

Then,

$$T^2_{within} = \frac{12.9745 - 8}{511.508} = 0.00974. \tag{19.39}$$

Computations below are based on the values in Table 19.10. These are similar to Table 19.5, except that we now assume that all groups have the same τ^2, and use a common estimate. In Table 19.10 the same estimate of τ^2 (0.0097) is applied to all ten studies.

Table 19.10 Random-effects model (pooled estimate of τ^2) – computations.

	Study	Effect size Y	Variance Within V_Y	Variance Between T^2	Variance Total V	Weight W	Calculated quantities		
							WY	WY^2	W^2
A	Thornhill	0.110	0.0100	0.0097	0.0197	50.697	5.577	0.613	2570.150
	Kendall	0.224	0.0300	0.0097	0.0397	25.173	5.639	1.263	633.678
	Vandamm	0.338	0.0200	0.0097	0.0297	33.642	11.371	3.843	1131.752
	Leonard	0.451	0.0150	0.0097	0.0247	40.445	18.241	8.226	1635.767
	Professor	0.480	0.0100	0.0097	0.0197	50.697	24.334	11.681	2570.150
	Sum A					200.652	65.161	25.627	8541.498
B	Jefferies	0.440	0.0150	0.0097	0.0247	40.445	17.796	7.830	1635.767
	Fremont	0.492	0.0200	0.0097	0.0297	33.642	16.552	8.143	1131.752
	Doyle	0.651	0.0150	0.0097	0.0247	40.445	26.329	17.140	1635.767
	Stella	0.710	0.0250	0.0097	0.0347	28.798	20.446	14.517	829.299
	Thorwald	0.740	0.0120	0.0097	0.0217	46.030	34.062	25.206	2118.721
	Sum B					189.358	115.185	72.837	7351.306
	Sum					390.010	180.346	98.463	15892.804

Computations (random effects, pooled estimate of τ^2) for the A studies

$$M_A^* = \frac{65.161}{200.652} = 0.3247,$$

$$V_{M_A^*} = \frac{1}{200.652} = 0.0050,$$

$$SE_{M_A^*} = \sqrt{0.0050} = 0.0706,$$

$$LL_{M_A^*} = 0.3247 - 1.96 \times 0.0706 = 0.1864,$$

$$UL_{M_A^*} = 0.3247 + 1.96 \times 0.0706 = 0.4631,$$

$$Z_A^* = \frac{0.3247}{0.0706} = 4.6601,$$

$$p(Z_A^*) < 0.0001,$$

and

$$Q_A^* = 25.627 - \left(\frac{65.161^2}{200.652}\right) = 4.4660. \tag{19.40}$$

Note. The Q^* statistic computed here, using random-effects weights, is used *only* for the analysis of variance, to partition Q^* into its various components. Therefore, we do not show a p-value for Q^*. Rather, the Q statistic computed using fixed-effect weights (above) is the one that reflects the between-studies dispersion, provides a test of homogeneity for the studies within subgroup A, and is used to estimate τ_{within}^2.

Computations (random effects, pooled estimate of τ^2) for the B studies

$$M_B^* = \frac{115.185}{189.358} = 0.6083,$$

$$V_{M_B^*} = \frac{1}{189.358} = 0.0053,$$

$$SE_{M_B^*} = \sqrt{0.0053} = 0.0727,$$

$$LL_{M_B^*} = 0.6083 - 1.96 \times 0.0727 = 0.4659,$$

$$UL_{M_B^*} = 0.6083 + 1.96 \times 0.0727 = 0.7507,$$

$$Z_B^* = \frac{0.6083}{0.0727} = 8.3705,$$

$$p(Z_B^*) < 0.0001,$$

and

$$Q_B^* = 72.837 - \left(\frac{115.185^2}{189.358}\right) = 2.7706. \tag{19.41}$$

Computations (random effects, pooled estimate of τ^2) for all ten studies
The statistics here are computed using the same value of T^2 as was used within groups (in this case, the pooled estimate, T^2_{within}).

$$M^* = \frac{180.346}{390.010} = 0.4624, \tag{19.42}$$

$$V_{M^*} = \frac{1}{390.010} = 0.0026, \tag{19.43}$$

$$SE_{M^*} = \sqrt{0.0026} = 0.0506,$$

$$LL_{M^*} = 0.4624 - 1.96 \times 0.0506 = 0.3632,$$

$$UL_{M^*} = 0.4624 + 1.96 \times 0.0506 = 0.5617,$$

$$Z^* = \frac{0.4624}{0.0506} = 9.1321,$$

$$p(Z^*) < 0.0001,$$

and

$$Q^* = 98.463 - \left(\frac{180.346^2}{390.010} \right) = 15.0690. \tag{19.44}$$

The statistics computed above are summarized in Table 19.11.

Table 19.11 Random-effects model (pooled estimate of τ^2) – summary statistics.

	A	B	Combined
Y	0.3247	0.6083	0.4624
V	0.0050	0.0053	0.0026
SE_Y	0.0706	0.0727	0.0506
LL_Y	0.1864	0.4659	0.3632
UL_Y	0.4631	0.7507	0.5617
Z	4.6001	8.3705	9.1321
$p2$	0.0000	0.0000	0.0000
Q	4.4660	2.7706	15.0690

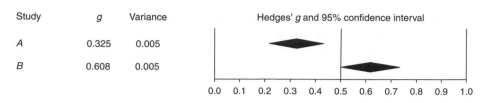

Figure 19.9 Random-effects model (pooled estimate of τ^2) – subgroup effects.

Comparing the effects

If we return to Figure 19.8 and excerpt the diamonds for the two subgroups we get Figure 19.9. The mean effect size for subgroups A and B are 0.325 and 0.608, with variances of 0.005 and 0.005.

Our goal is to compare these two mean effects, and there are several ways that we can proceed. These approaches are algebraically equivalent, and (it follows) yield the same p-value.

Comparing A versus B: a Z-test (Method 1)

We can use a Z-test to compare the mean effect for subgroups A versus B. The null hypothesis and formulas are the same as those for the prior case (where we did not assume a common value for τ^2). If we elect to subtract the mean of A from the mean of B,

$$Diff^* = M_B^* - M_A^*, \tag{19.45}$$

the test statistic to compare the two effects is

$$Z_{Diff}^* = \frac{Diff^*}{SE_{Diff^*}}, \tag{19.46}$$

where

$$SE_{Diff^*} = \sqrt{V_{M_A^*} + V_{M_B^*}}. \tag{19.47}$$

Under the null hypothesis that the true mean effect size μ_i is the same for both groups,

$$H_0 : \mu_A = \mu_B, \tag{19.48}$$

Z_{Diff}^* would follow the normal distribution. For a two-tailed test the p-value is given by

$$p^* = 2\left[1 - \left(\Phi\left(|Z_{Diff}^*|\right)\right)\right], \tag{19.49}$$

where $\Phi(Z)$ is the standard normal cumulative distribution.

In the running example

$$Diff^* = 0.6083 - 0.3247 = 0.2835,$$

$$SE_{Diff^*} = \sqrt{0.0050 + 0.0053} = 0.1013,$$

and

$$Z^*_{Diff} = \frac{0.2835}{0.1013} = 2.7986.$$

The two-tailed p-value corresponding to $Z^*_{Diff} = 2.7986$ is 0.0051. This tells us that the mean effect is probably not the same for the A studies as for the B studies. In Excel, the function to compute a 2-tailed p-value for Z is $=(1\text{-}(NORMSDIST(ABS(Z))))^*2$. Here, $=(1\text{-}(NORMSDIST(ABS(2.7986))))^*2$ will return the value 0.0045.

Comparing A with B: a Q-test based on analysis of variance (Method 2)

Again, we apply the same formulas as we did for the prior case, but this time using the random-effects weights based on a pooled estimate of τ^2. Note that this approach only works if we use the same weights to compute the overall effect as we do to compute the effects within groups. In Table 19.10 we used a T^2 value of 0.0097 for all ten studies, and this is the value used to sum *within* subgroups and also to sum *across* subgroups.

We compute the following quantities (where SS is the sum of squared deviations).

- Q^*_A, the weighted SS of all A studies about the mean of A.
- Q^*_B, the weighted SS of all B studies about the mean of B.
- Q^*_{within}, the sum of Q^*_A and Q^*_B.
- Q^*_{bet}, the weighted SS of the subgroup means about the grand mean.
- Q^* the weighted SS of all effects about the grand mean.

We may write $Q^*_{within} = Q^*_A + Q^*_B$, to represent the sum of within-group weighted SS, or more generally, for p subgroups,

$$Q^*_{within} = \sum_{j=1}^{p} Q^*_j. \tag{19.50}$$

In the running example,

$$Q^*_{within} = 4.4660 + 2.7706 = 7.2366. \tag{19.51}$$

The weighted SS are additive, such that $Q^* = Q^*_{within} + Q^*_{bet}$. Therefore, Q^*_{bet} can be computed as

$$Q^*_{bet} = Q^* - Q^*_{within}. \tag{19.52}$$

Under the null hypothesis that the true man effect size μ is the same for all groups, 1 to p, Q^*_{bet} would be distributed as chi-squared with degrees of freedom equal to $p - 1$.

In the running example

$$Q^*_{bet} = 15.0690 - 7.2366 = 7.8324. \tag{19.53}$$

Table 19.12 Random-effects model (pooled estimate of τ^2) – ANOVA table.

	Q^*	df	p	Formula
A	4.4660			19.40
B	2.7706			19.41
Within	7.2366			19.51
Between	7.8324	1	0.0051	19.53
Total	15.0690			19.44

The only Q statistic that we interpret here is the one between groups. In the running example, the *Between* line tells us that the difference between groups (the combined effect for A versus B) is statistically significant ($Q^*_{bet} = 7.8324 \, df = 1, p = 0.0051$), which means that the effect size is related to the frequency of tutoring. In Excel, the function to compute a p-value for Q is =CHIDIST(Q,df). For the test of A versus B, =CHIDIST(7.8324,1) returns 0.0051.

To address the statistical significance of the total variance or the variance within groups, we use the statistics reported using the fixed-effect weights (Table 19.3) rather than using $Q^*_{total}, Q^*_A, Q^*_B$ or Q^*_{within}.

Comparing *A* versus *B*: a *Q*-test for heterogeneity (Method 3)

Finally, we could treat the subgroups as if they were studies and perform a test for heterogeneity across studies. If we extract the two subgroup lines and the total line from Figure 19.8 and replace the diamonds with squares we obtain Figure 19.10.

Concretely, we start with two *studies* with effect sizes of 0.325 and 0.608, and variances of 0.005 and 0.005. Then, we apply the usual meta-analysis methods to compute Q. Concretely, using the values in Table 19.13, and applying (11.2) and subsequent formulas, we compute

$$M^* = \frac{180.346}{390.010} = 0.4624, \tag{19.54}$$

$$V_M{}^* = \frac{1}{390.010} = 0.0026, \tag{19.55}$$

$$Q = 91.227 - \left(\frac{180.346^2}{390.010} \right) = 7.8324,$$

$$df = 2 - 1 = 1,$$

and

$$p(Q = 7.8324, df = 1) = 0.0051.$$

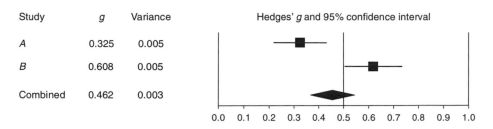

Study	g	Variance
A	0.325	0.005
B	0.608	0.005
Combined	0.462	0.003

Figure 19.10 Random-effects model (pooled estimate of τ^2) – treating subgroups as studies.

Table 19.13 Random-effects model (pooled estimate of τ^2) – subgroups as studies.

Study	Effect size Y	Variance Within V_Y	Variance Between T^2	Variance Total V	Weight W	Calculated quantities		
						WY	WY^2	W^2
A	0.3247	0.0050	0.0000	0.0050	200.652	65.161	21.161	40261.386
B	0.6083	0.0053	0.0000	0.0053	189.358	115.185	70.066	35856.405
					390.010	180.346	91.227	76117.791

where Q represents the weighted sum of squares for Studies A and B about the grand mean. For $Q = 7.8324$ and $df = 1$, the p-value is 0.0051.

In Excel, the function to compute a p-value for Q is =CHIDIST(Q,df). For example, =CHIDIST(7.8324,1) returns 0.0051.

Quantify the magnitude of the difference

The difference and confidence interval are given by (19.17) and (19.18):

$$Diff^* = 0.6083 - 0.3247 = 0.2835,$$

$$SE_{Diff^*} = \sqrt{0.0050 + 0.0053} = 0.1013,$$

$$LL_{Diff^*} = 0.2835 - 1.96 \times 0.1013 = 0.0850,$$

and

$$UL_{Diff^*} = 0.2835 + 1.96 \times 0.1013 = 0.4821.$$

In words, the true difference between the effect in the A studies, as opposed to the B studies, probably falls in the range of 0.09 to 0.48.

THE PROPORTION OF VARIANCE EXPLAINED

In primary studies, a common approach to describing the impact of a covariate is to report the proportion of variance explained by that covariate. That index, R^2, is defined as the ratio of explained variance to total variance,

$$R^2 = \frac{\sigma^2_{explained}}{\sigma^2_{total}} \tag{19.56}$$

or, equivalently,

$$R^2 = 1 - \left(\frac{\sigma^2_{unexplained}}{\sigma^2_{total}} \right). \tag{19.57}$$

This index is intuitive because it can be interpreted as a ratio, with a range of 0 to 1 (or expressed as a percentage in the range of 0% to 100%). Many researchers are familiar with this index, and have a sense of what proportion of variance is likely to be explained by different kinds of covariates or interventions.

This index cannot be applied directly to meta-analysis for the following reason. In a primary study, a covariate that explains all of the variation in the dependent variable will reduce the error to zero (and R^2, the proportion of variance explained, would reach 100%).

For example, Figure 19.11 depicts a primary study with 10 participants. All those in group A have the same score (0.3) and all those in group B have the same score (0.7). Since the variance *within* each subgroup is 0.0, group membership explains 100% of the original variance, and R^2 is 100%. In a real study, of course, there would be some variance within groups and R^2 would be less than 100%, but the fact that R^2 can potentially reach 100% is part of what makes this index intuitive.

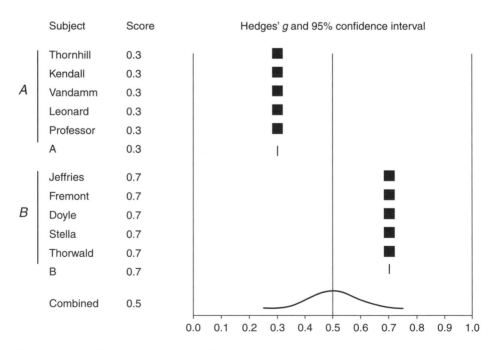

Figure 19.11 A primary study showing subjects within groups.

By contrast, consider what happens in a meta-analysis if we have two subgroups of studies. We assume that there are five studies in each subgroup, with a *true* summary effect (say, a standardized mean difference) of 0.30 for each study in subgroup A and of 0.70 for each study in subgroup B. However, while the true effect is identical for each study within its subgroup, the observed effects will differ from each other because of random error.

Thus, the variance within groups, while smaller than the variance between groups, can never approach zero. If the within-study error is a substantial portion of the total variance observed (say, 75%), then the upper limit of R^2 would be only 25%. As such, two important qualities of the index (the fact that it has a natural scale of 0% to 100% and the fact that it has the same range across studies) would no longer apply.

Since the problem with using R^2 is the fact that study-level covariates in a meta-analysis can address only the true variance τ^2 (and not the within-study variance v), the logical solution is to redefine R^2 (or to define a new index) that is based solely on the true variance. Rather than defining R^2 as the proportion of *total* variance explained by the covariates, we will define it as the proportion of *true* variance explained by the covariates. Since the true variance is estimated as T^2, this gives us

$$R^2 = \frac{T^2_{explained}}{T^2_{total}},\qquad(19.58)$$

or

$$R^2 = 1 - \left(\frac{T^2_{unexplained}}{T^2_{total}}\right).\qquad(19.59)$$

In the context of subgroups, the numerator in (19.59) is the between-studies variance within subgroups, and the denominator is the total between-studies variance (within-subgroups plus between-subgroups). Therefore, the equation can be written

$$R^2 = 1 - \left(\frac{T^2_{within}}{T^2_{total}}\right).\qquad(19.60)$$

In the running example, T^2 for the full set of studies was 0.0299 (see page 155), and T^2 computed by working within subgroups and then pooling across subgroups was 0.0097 (see page 173). This gives us

$$R^2 = 1 - \left(\frac{0.0097}{0.0299}\right) = 0.6745.\qquad(19.61)$$

In Figure 19.12 we have superimposed a normal curve for the distribution of true effects within each subgroup of studies, and also across all ten studies. The relatively narrow dispersion within groups is based on the T^2 of 0.0097, while the relatively wide dispersion across groups is based on the T^2 of 0.0299, and R^2 captures this change.

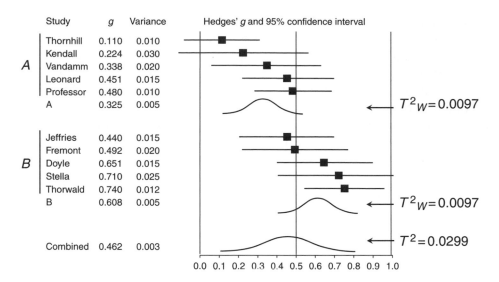

Figure 19.12 Random-effects model – variance within and between subgroups.

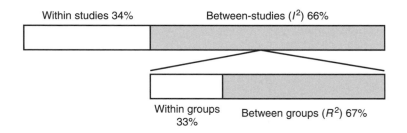

Figure 19.13 Proportion of variance explained by subgroup membership.

The same idea is shown from another perspective in Figure 19.13. On the top line, 34% of the total variance was within studies and 66% was between studies (which is also the definition of I^2). The within-studies variance cannot be explained by study-level covariates, and so is removed from the equation and we focus on the shaded part. On the bottom line, the type of intervention is able to explain 67% of the *relevant* variance, leaving 33% unexplained. Critically, the 67% and 33% sum to 100%, since we are concerned only with the variance between studies.

Note 1. While the R^2 index has a range of 0 to 1 (0% to 100%) in the population, it is possible for sampling error to yield an observed value of R^2 that falls outside of this range. In that case, the value is set to either 0 (0%) or 1 (100%).

Note 2. The R^2 index only makes sense if we are using a random-effects model, which allows us to think about explaining some of the between-studies variance. Under the fixed-effect model the between-studies variance is set at zero and cannot be changed. Also, the computational model proposed here for estimating R^2 only works for the case where we assume that τ^2 is the same for all subgroups.

MIXED-EFFECTS MODEL

In this volume we have been using the term fixed effect to mean that the effect is identical (*fixed*) across all relevant studies (within the full population, or within a subgroup).

In fact the use of the term *fixed effect* in connection with meta-analysis is at odds with the usual meaning of *fixed effects* in statistics. A more suitable term for the fixed-effect meta-analysis might be a *common-effect* meta-analysis. The term *fixed effects* is traditionally used in another context with a different meaning. Concretely, we can talk about the subgroups as being *fixed* in the sense of fixed rather than random. For example, if we want to compare the treatment effect for a subgroup of studies that enrolled only males versus a subgroup of studies that enrolled only females, then we would assume that the subgroups are *fixed* in the sense that anyone who wanted to perform this analysis would need to use these same two subgroups (male and female). By contrast, if we have subgrouping of studies by country, then we might prefer to treat the subgroups as random. A random-effects assumption across subgroups of studies in the US, UK, Japan, Australia and Sweden would allow us to infer what the effect might be in a study in Israel, by assuming it comes from the same random-effects distribution. In this chapter we assume that when we are interested in comparing subgroups we make an assumption of the first type, which means that anyone who performs this comparison must use the same set of subgroups.

We mention this here for two reasons. One is to alert the reader that in the event that the subgroups have been sampled at random from a larger pool (as in the example of countries), then we are able to take this additional source of variability into account. The mechanism for doing so is beyond the scope of an introductory book.

The other reason is to explain the meaning of the term *mixed model*, which is sometimes used to describe subgroup analyses. As explained in this chapter the summary effect *within subgroups* can be computed using either a fixed-effect model or a random-effects model. As outlined immediately above, the difference *across subgroups* can be assessed using either a fixed-effects model or a random-effects model (although the meaning of *fixed* is different here). This leads to the following nomenclature.

If we use a fixed-effect model within subgroups and also across subgroups, the analysis is called a fixed-effects analysis. If we use a random-effects model within subgroups and a fixed-effect model across subgroups (the approach that we generally advocate), the model is called a mixed-effects model. We have the further possibility of assuming random effects both within and across subgroups; such a model is called a random-effects (or fully random-effects) model.

OBTAINING AN OVERALL EFFECT IN THE PRESENCE OF SUBGROUPS

In the tables and forest plots presented in this chapter we presented a summary effect for each subgroup and also for the total population. Since our primary concern has been with looking at difference between subgroups we paid little attention to the value for the total population. Here, we consider if that value should be reported at all, and if so, how it should be computed.

Should we report a summary effect across all subgroups?

The question of whether or not we should report a summary effect across all subgroups depends on our goals and also on the nature of the data.

Suppose the primary goal of the analysis is to see if a treatment is more effective among acute patients than among chronic patients, and it emerges that the treatment is very effective in one group but harmful in the other. In this case, the take-home message should be that we need to look at each group separately. To report that the treatment is moderately effective (on average) would be a bad idea since this is true for neither group and misrepresents the core finding. In this case, it would be better to report the effect for the separate subgroups only.

By contrast, if it turns out that the treatment is equally effective (or nearly so) in both subgroups, then it might be helpful to report a combined effect to serve as a summary. This would probably be the case also if there are minor differences among groups, but the substantive implication of the treatment (or the relationship) is the same for all groups. This is especially true if there are many subgroups, and the reader will be looking for a single number that is easy to recall.

If we do decide to report a combined effect across subgroups, we need to be clear about what this value represents, since this determines how it will be computed. The basic options are explained below.

Option 1. Combine subgroup means and ignore between-subgroup variance

One option is to compute the weighted mean of the subgroup means. In other words, we treat each subgroup as a study and perform a fixed-effect analysis using the mean effect and variance for each subgroup. In this chapter, we showed three versions of this approach.

These computations were shown for the fixed-effect model in (19.14) and (19.15) and where we computed the weighted mean of the two subgroups. Note that we would get the identical values if we worked with the original ten studies and weighted each by its fixed-effect weight (see (19.3) and (19.4)).

These computations were shown for the random-effects model with separate estimates of τ^2 in (19.33) and (19.34), where we computed the weighted mean of the two subgroups. Note that we would get the identical values if we worked with the original ten studies and weighted each by its random-effects weight, with a separate estimate of τ^2 for each subgroup (see (19.21) and (19.22)).

These computations were shown for the random-effects model with a pooled estimate of τ^2 in (19.54) and (19.55), where we computed the weighted mean of the two subgroups. Note that we would get the identical values if we worked with the original ten studies and weighted each by its random-effects weight, with a pooled estimate of τ^2 (see (19.42) and (19.43)).

In all three cases, the combined effect refers to no actual population but is rather the average of two different populations. If the subgroups were male and female then the combined effect is the expected effect in a population that included both males and females (in the same proportions as in the subgroups). As always, the standard error of the mean speaks to the precision of the mean, and not to the dispersion of effects across subgroups (which is treated as zero).

Option 2. Combine subgroup means, and model the between-subgroup variance

A second option is to assume a random-effects model across subgroups. In other words, all the formulas and concepts discussed in Chapter 12 are applied here, except that the unit of analysis is the subgroup rather than the study. This would make sense if the subgroups have been sampled at random from a larger group of relevant subgroups. For example, we have the mean effect of a treatment in the US and in Australia, but we want to estimate what the mean effect of that treatment would be across all relevant countries.

In this case we need to address precisely the same kinds of issues we addressed when discussing heterogeneity in Chapter 12. First, we compute a measure of between-subgroups dispersion, T^2_{bet}. Then, we compute a weighted mean of the subgroups, where the weights are based on the within-subgroup error and the between-subgroups variance. To the extent that the subgroup means differ from each other, the standard error of the combined effect will be increased (but this additional error will be diminished as additional subgroups are added).

We can also focus on the dispersion itself (as in Chapters 16 and 17). For example, we can use the estimate of τ^2_{bet} to build a prediction interval that gives us the expected range of effect sizes for the next country (in our example) selected at random.

Option 3. Perform a separate random-effects analysis on the full set of studies.

If we want to report a combined effect across subgroups, then a third option is simply to perform a separate random-effects meta-analysis including all of the studies, and ignoring subgroup membership. Rather than estimate τ^2 within subgroups (as we did before) we estimate it across all studies, and so it will tend to be larger.

Comparing the options

When our primary goal is to assess differences among subgroups, and use an analysis of variance table as part of the process, the combined effects across subgroups are computed using option 1. This yields a set of internally consistent data.

If we really care about the combined effect across subgroups then options 2 and 3 are the more logical choices. If the subgroups really have been selected at random from a larger set, then option 2 allows us to model the different sources of error separately and obtain a better estimate of the true confidence interval for the combined effect (as well as discuss prediction intervals for a future subgroup), and is probably the better choice. This assumes, of course, that we have sufficient information to obtain a reasonably precise estimate of the variance among subgroups. By contrast, if the subgrouping is not of major importance, or if multiple different subgroupings of the studies are being considered, then option 3 is the more logical choice.

SUMMARY POINTS

- Just as we can use t-tests or analysis of variance in primary studies to assess the relationship between group membership and outcome, we can use analogs of these procedures in meta-analysis to assess the relationship between subgroup membership and effect size.
- We presented three methods that can be used to compare the mean effect across subgroups. To compare the mean effect in two groups we can use a Z-test. To compare the mean effect in two or more groups we can use analysis of variance (modified for use with subgroups) or the Q-test of homogeneity. All three procedures are mathematically equivalent.
- These analyses may be performed using either the fixed-effect or the random-effects model within groups, but in most cases the latter is appropriate.
- In primary studies we use R^2 to reflect the proportion of variance explained by group membership. An analogous index, which reflects the proportion of true variance explained by subgroup membership, can be used for meta-analysis.

CHAPTER 20

Meta-Regression

Introduction
Fixed-effect model
Fixed or random effects for unexplained heterogeneity
Random-effects model

INTRODUCTION

In primary studies we use regression, or multiple regression, to assess the relation-ship between one or more covariates (moderators) and a dependent variable. Essentially the same approach can be used with meta-analysis, except that the covariates are at the level of the study rather than the level of the subject, and the dependent variable is the effect size in the studies rather than subject scores. We use the term *meta-regression* to refer to these procedures when they are used in a meta-analysis.

The differences that we need to address as we move from primary studies to meta-analysis for regression are similar to those we needed to address as we moved from primary studies to meta-analysis for subgroup analyses. These include the need to assign a weight to each study and the need to select the appropriate model (fixed versus random effects). Also, as was true for subgroup analyses, the R^2 index, which is used to quantify the proportion of variance explained by the covariates, must be modified for use in meta-analysis.

With these modifications, however, the full arsenal of procedures that fall under the heading of multiple regression becomes available to the meta-analyst. We can work with sets of covariates, such as three variables that together define a treatment, or that allow for a nonlinear relationship between covariates and the effect size. We can enter covariates into the analysis using a pre-defined sequence and assess the impact of any set, over and above the impact of prior sets, to control for confounding variables. We can incorporate both categorical (for example, dummy-coded) and continuous variables as covariates. We can use these procedures both to assess the

Introduction to Meta-Analysis   M. Borenstein, L. V. Hedges, J. P. T. Higgins, H. R. Rothstein
© 2009, John Wiley & Sons, Ltd

impact of covariates and also to predict the effect size in studies with specific characteristics.

Multiple regression incorporates a wide array of procedures, and we cannot cover these fully in this volume. Rather, we assume that the reader is familiar with multiple regression in primary studies, and our goal here is to show how the same techniques used in primary studies can be applied to meta-regression.

As is true in primary studies, where we need an appropriately large ratio of *subjects* to covariates in order for the analysis be to meaningful, in meta-analysis we need an appropriately large ratio of *studies* to covariates. Therefore, the use of meta-regression, especially with multiple covariates, is not a recommended option when the number of studies is small. In primary studies some have recommended a ratio of at least ten subjects for each covariate, which would correspond to ten studies for each covariate in meta-regression. In fact, though, there are no hard and fast rules in either case.

FIXED-EFFECT MODEL

As we did when discussing subgroup analysis, we start with the fixed-effect model, which is simpler, and then move on to the random-effects model, which is generally more appropriate.

The BCG data set

Various researchers have published studies that assessed the impact of a vaccine, known as BCG, to prevent the development of tuberculosis (TB). With the re-emergence of TB in the United States in recent years (including many drug-resistant cases), researchers needed to determine whether or not the BCG vaccine should be recommended. For that reason, Colditz *et al.* (1994) reported a meta-analysis of these studies, and Berkey *et al.* (1995) showed how meta-regression could be used in an attempt to explain some of the variance in treatment effects.

The forest plot is shown in Figure 20.1. The effect size is the risk ratio, with a risk ratio of 0.10 indicating that the vaccine reduced the risk of TB by 90%, a risk ratio of 1.0 indicating no effect, and risk ratios higher than 1.0 indicating that the vaccine increased the risk of TB. Studies are sorted from most effective to least effective. As always for an analysis of risk ratios, the analysis was performed using log transformed values and then converted back to risk ratios for presentation.

Using a fixed-effect analysis the risk ratio for the 13 studies is 0.650 with a confidence interval of 0.601 to 0.704, which says that the vaccine decreased the risk of TB by at least 30% and possibly by as much as 40%. In log units the risk ratio is -0.430 with a standard error of 0.040. The Z-value is -10.625 ($p < 0.0001$), which allows us to reject the null hypothesis of no effect.

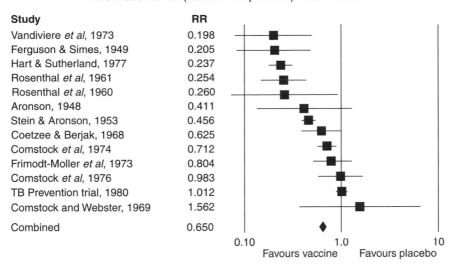

Figure 20.1 Fixed-effect model – forest plot for the BCG data.

At least as interesting, however, is the substantial variation in the treatment effects, which ranged from a risk ratio of 0.20 (an 80% reduction in risk) to 1.56 (a 56% *increase* in risk). While some of this variation is due to within-study error, some of it reflects variation in the true effects. The Q-statistic is 152.233 with $df = 12$ and $p < 0.0001$. T^2 is 0.309, which yields a prediction interval of approximately 0.14 to 1.77, meaning that the true effect (risk ratio) in the next study could fall anywhere in the range of 0.14 to 1.77. The value of I^2 is 92.12, which means that 92% of the observed variance comes from real differences between studies and, as such, can potentially be explained by study-level covariates.

The next issue for the authors was to try and explain some of this variation. There was reason to believe that the drug was more effective in colder climates. This hypothesis was based on the theory that persons in colder climates were less likely to have a natural immunity to TB. It was also based on the expectation that the drug would be more potent in the colder climates (in warmer climates the heat would cause the drug to lose potency, and direct exposure to sunlight could kill some of the bacteria that were required for the vaccine to work properly).

In the absence of better predictor variables (such as the actual storage conditions used for the vaccine) Berkey *et al.* (1995) used absolute distance from the equator as a surrogate for climate (i.e. geographical regions in the Northern US would be colder than those in the tropics), and used regression to look for a relationship between *Distance* and treatment effect. Given the *post hoc* nature of this analysis, a positive finding would probably not be definitive, but would suggest a direction for additional research. (See also Sutton *et al.*, 2000; Egger *et al.*, 2001.)

Assessing the impact of the slope

Table 20.1 shows the data for each study (events and sample size, effect size and latitude). Table 20.2 shows the results for a meta-regression using absolute latitude to predict the log risk ratio.

The regression coefficient for latitude is -0.0292, which means that every one degree of latitude corresponds to a decrease of 0.0292 units in effect size. In this case, the effect size is the log risk ratio, and (given the specifics of this example) this corresponds to a more effective vaccination.

If we were working with a primary study and wanted to test the coefficient for significance we might use a t-test of the form

$$t = \frac{B}{SE_B},\qquad(20.1)$$

In meta-analysis the coefficient for any covariate (B) and its standard error are based on groups of *studies* rather than groups of *subjects* but the same logic applies. Historically, in meta-regression the test is based on the Z-distribution, and that is the

Table 20.1 The BCG dataset.

	Vaccinated		Control					
	TB	Total	TB	Total	RR	ln RR	V_{lnRR}	Latitude
Vandiviere et al, 1973	8	2545	10	629	0.198	−1.621	0.223	19
Ferguson & Simes, 1949	6	306	29	303	0.205	−1.585	0.195	55
Hart & Sutherland, 1977	62	13598	248	12867	0.237	−1.442	0.020	52
Rosenthal *et al*, 1961	17	1716	65	1665	0.254	−1.371	0.073	42
Rosenthal *et al*, 1960	3	231	11	220	0.260	−1.348	0.415	42
Aronson, 1948	4	123	11	139	0.411	−0.889	0.326	44
Stein & Aaronson, 1953	180	1541	372	1451	0.456	−0.786	0.007	44
Coetzee & Berjak, 1968	29	7499	45	7277	0.625	−0.469	0.056	27
Comstock *et al*, 1974	186	50634	141	27338	0.712	−0.339	0.012	18
Frimodt-Moller *et al*, 1973.	33	5069	47	5808	0.804	−0.218	0.051	13
Comstock *et al*, 1976	27	16913	29	17854	0.983	−0.017	0.071	33
TB Prevention Trial, 1980	505	88391	499	88391	1.012	0.012	0.004	13
Comstock & Webster, 1969	5	2498	3	2341	1.562	0.446	0.533	33

Table 20.2 Fixed-effect model – Regression results for BCG.

	Fixed effect, Z-Distribution					
	Point estimate	Standard error	95% Lower	95% Upper	Z-value	p-Value
Intercept	0.34356	0.08105	0.18471	0.50242	4.23899	0.00002
Latitude	−0.02924	0.00265	−0.03444	−0.02404	−11.02270	0.00000

Table 20.3 Fixed-effect model – ANOVA table for BCG regression.

	Analysis of variance		
	Q	df	p-Value
Model (Q_{model})	121.49992	1	0.00000
Residual (Q_{resid})	30.73309	11	0.00121
Total (Q)	152.23301	12	0.00000

approach presented here (however, see notes at the end of this chapter about other approaches). The statistic to test the significance of the slope is

$$Z = \frac{B}{SE_B} . \qquad (20.2)$$

Under the null hypothesis that the coefficient is zero, Z would follow the normal distribution.

In the running example the coefficient for latitude is -0.02924 with standard error 0.00265, so

$$Z = \frac{-0.02924}{0.00265} = -11.0227.$$

The two-tailed p-value corresponding to $Z = -11.0227$ is < 0.00001. This tells us that the slope is probably not zero, and the vaccination is more effective when the study is conducted at a greater distance from the equator.

The Z-test can be used to test the statistical significance of any single coefficient but when we want to assess the impact of several covariates simultaneously we need to use the Q-test. (This is analogous to the situation in primary studies where we use a t-test to assess the impact of one coefficient but an F-test to assess the impact of two or more.)

As we did when working with analysis of variance we can divide the sum of squares into its component parts, and create an analysis of variance table as follows.

As before, Q is defined as a weighted sum of squares, which we can partition into its component parts. Q reflects the total dispersion of studies about the grand mean. Q_{resid} reflects the distance of studies from the regression line. Q_{model} is the dispersion explained by the covariates.

Each Q statistic is evaluated with respect to its degrees of freedom, as follows.

- Q is 152.2330, with 12 degrees of freedom and $p < 0.00001$ (this is the same value presented for the initial meta-analysis with no covariates). This means that the amount of total variance is more than we would expect based on within-study error.
- Q_{model} is 121.4999 with 1 degree of freedom and $p < 0.00001$. This means that the relationship between latitude and treatment effect is stronger than we would expect by chance.

- Q_{resid} is 30.7331 with 11 degrees of freedom and $p < 0.0001$. This means that even with latitude in the model, some of the between-studies variance (reflected by the distance between the regression line and the studies) remains unexplained.

Q_{model} here is analogous to Q_{bet} for subgroup analysis, and Q_{resid} is analogous to Q_{within} for subgroup analysis. If the covariates are coded to represent subgroups, then Q_{model} will be identical to Q_{bet}, and Q_{resid} will be identical to Q_{within}.

The Z-test and the Q-test

In this example there is only one covariate and so we have the option of using either the Z-test or the Q-test to test its relationship with effect size. It follows that the two tests should yield the same results, and they do. The Z-value is -11.0227, with a corresponding p-value of <0.0001. The Q-value is 121.4999 with a corresponding p-value of <0.0001 (with 1 df). Finally, Q should be equal to Z^2 (since Q squares each difference while Z does not) and in fact -11.0227^2 is equal to 121.4999.

When we have more than one covariate the Q statistic serves as an omnibus test of the hypothesis that all the B's are zero. The Z-test can be used to test any coefficient, with the others held constant.

Quantify the magnitude of the relationship

The Z-test, like all tests of significance, speaks to the question of statistical, rather than substantive, significance. Therefore, in addition to reporting the test of significance, one should always report the magnitude of the relationship. Here, the relationship of latitude to effect (expressed as a log risk ratio) is

$$\ln(RR) = 0.3435 - 0.0292(X)$$

where X is the absolute latitude. Figure 20.2 shows the plot of log risk ratio on latitude.

In the graph, each study is represented by a circle that shows the actual coordinates (observed effect size by latitude) for that study. The size (specifically, the area) of each circle is proportional to that study's weight in the analysis. Since this analysis is based on the fixed-effect model, the weight is simply the inverse of the within-study variance for each study.

The center line shows the predicted values. A study performed relatively close to the equator (such as the study performed in Madras, India, latitude 13) would have an expected effect near zero (corresponding to a risk ratio of 1.0, which means that the vaccination has no impact on TB). By contrast, a study at latitude 55 (Saskatchewan) would have an expected effect near -1.20 (corresponding to a risk ratio near 0.30, which means that the vaccination is expected to decrease the risk of TB by about 70%).

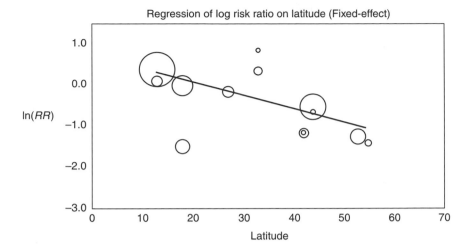

Figure 20.2 Fixed-effect model – regression of log risk ratio on latitude.

The 95% confidence interval for B is given by

$$LL_B = B - 1.96 \times SE_B \tag{20.3}$$

and

$$UL_B = B + 1.96 \times SE_B. \tag{20.4}$$

In the BCG example

$$LL_B = (-0.0292) - 1.96 \times 0.0027 = -0.0344$$

and

$$UL_B = (-0.0292) + 1.96 \times 0.0027 = -0.0240.$$

In words, the true coefficient could be as low as -0.0344 and as high as -0.0240. These limits can be used to generate confidence intervals on the plot.

FIXED OR RANDOM EFFECTS FOR UNEXPLAINED HETEROGENEITY

In Part 3 we discussed the difference between a fixed-effect model and a random-effects model. Under the fixed-effect model we assume that the true effect is the same in all studies. By contrast, under the random-effects model we allow that the true effect may vary from one study to the next.

When we were working with a single population the difference in models translated into one true effect versus a distribution of true effects for all studies. When we were working with subgroups (analysis of variance) it translated into one true effect versus a distribution of effects for all studies within a subgroup (for example, studies that used Intervention *A* or studies that used Intervention *B*).

For meta-regression it translates into one true effect versus a distribution of effects for studies with the same predicted value (for example, two studies that share the same value on all covariates). This is shown schematically in Figure 20.3 and Figure 20.4.

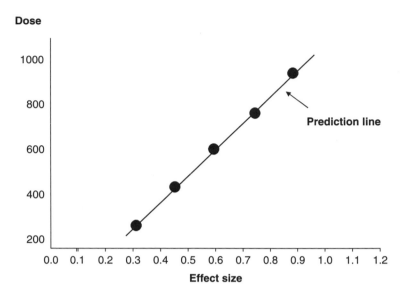

Figure 20.3 Fixed-effect model – population effects as function of covariate.

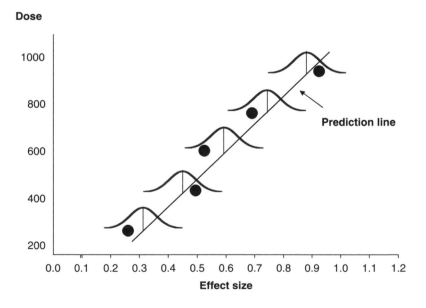

Figure 20.4 Random-effects model – population effects as a function of covariate.

Under the fixed-effect model, for any set of covariate values (that is, for any predicted value) there is one population effect size (represented by a circle in Figure 20.3). Under the random-effects model, for any predicted value there is a distribution of effect sizes (in Figure 20.4 the distribution is centered over the predicted value but the population effect size can fall to the left or right of center). (In both figures we assume that the prediction is perfect, so that the true effect (or mean effect) falls directly on the prediction line.)

As always, the selection of a method should follow the logic of how the studies were selected. When we introduced the idea of fixed versus random effects for a single population, the example we used for the fixed-effect model was a pharmaceutical company that planned a series of ten trials that were identical for all intents and purposes (page 83). When we moved on to analysis of variance we extended the same example, and assumed that five cohorts would be used to test placebo versus *Drug A*, while five would be used to test placebo versus *Drug B* (page 161). We can extend this example, and use it to create an example where a fixed-effect analysis would be appropriate for meta-regression. As before, we'll assume a total of 10 studies, five for placebo versus *Drug A* and five for placebo versus *Drug B*. This time we'll assume that each study used either 10, 20, 40, 80, or 160 mg. of the drug and we will use regression to assess the impact of Drug and Dose. The fixed-effect model makes sense here because the studies are known to be identical on all other factors.

As before, we note that this example is not representative of most systematic reviews. In the vast majority of cases, especially when the studies are performed by different researchers and then culled from the literature, it is more plausible that the impact of the covariates captures some, *but not all*, of the true variation among effects. In this case, it is the random-effects model that reflects the nature of the distribution of true effects, and should therefore be used in the analyses. Also as before, if the study design suggests that the random-effects model is appropriate, then this model should be selected *a priori*. It is a mistake to start with the fixed-effect model and move on to random effects only if the test for heterogeneity is statistically significant.

Since the meaning of a summary effect size is different for fixed versus random effects, the null hypothesis being tested also differs. Both test a null hypothesis of no linear relationship between the covariates and the effect size. The difference is that under the fixed-effect model that effect size is the common effect size for all studies with a given value of the covariates. Under the random-effects model that effect size is the mean of the true effect sizes for all studies with a given value of the covariates. This is important, because the different null hypotheses reflect different assumptions about the sources of error. This means that different error terms are used to compute tests of significance and confidence intervals under the two models.

Computationally, the difference between fixed effect and random effects is in the definition of the variance. Under the fixed-effect model the variance is the variance within studies, while under the random-effects model it is the variance within studies plus the variance between studies (τ^2). This holds true for one population, for multiple subgroups, and for regression, but the mechanism used to estimate τ^2 depends on the context. When we are working with a single population, τ^2 reflects the dispersion of true effects across all studies, and is therefore computed for the full set of studies. When we are working with subgroups, τ^2 reflects the dispersion of true effects within a subgroup, and is therefore computed within subgroups. When we are working with regression, τ^2 reflects the dispersion of true effects for studies with the same predicted value (that is, the same value on the covariates) and is therefore computed for each point on the prediction slope. As a practical matter, of course, most points on the slope have only a single study, and so this computation is less transparent than that for the single population (or subgroups) but the concept is the same. The computational details are handled by software and will not be addressed here.

The practical implications of using a random-effects model rather than a fixed-effect model for regression are similar to those that applied to a single population and to subgroups. First, the random-effects model will lead to more moderate weights being assigned to each study. As compared with a fixed-effect model, the random-effects model will assign more weight to small studies and less weight to large studies. Second, the confidence interval about each coefficient (and slope) will be wider than it would be under the fixed-effect model. Third, the *p*-values corresponding to each coefficient and to the model as a whole are less likely to meet the criterion for statistical significance.

As always, the selection of a model must be based on the context and characteristics of the studies. In particular, if there is heterogeneity in true effects that is not explained by the covariates, then the random-effects model is likely to be more appropriate.

RANDOM-EFFECTS MODEL

We return now to the BCG example and apply the random-effects model (Figure 20.5).

Using a random effects analysis the risk ratio for the 13 studies is 0.490 with a confidence interval of 0.345 to 0.695, which says that the *mean effect* of the vaccine was to decrease the risk of TB by at least 30% and possibly by as much as 65% (see Figure 20.5). In log units the risk ratio is -0.714 with a standard error of 0.179, which yields a Z-value of -3.995 ($p < 0.001$) which allows us to reject the null hypothesis of no effect.

At least as interesting, however, is the substantial variation in the treatment effects, which ranged from a risk ratio of 0.20 (vaccine *reduces* the risk by 80%) to 1.56 (vaccine *increases* the risk by 56%). The relevant statistics were presented when we discussed the fixed-effect model.

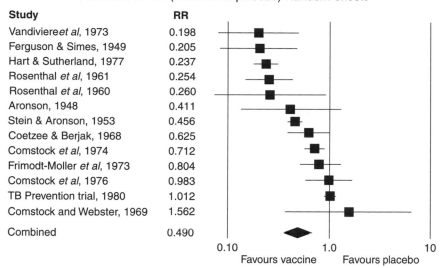

Figure 20.5 Random-effects model – forest plot for the BCG data.

Assessing the impact of the slope

A meta-regression using the random-effect model (method of moments) yields the results shown in Table 20.4.

This has the same format as Table 20.2, showing the coefficients for predicting the log risk ratio from latitude and related statistics. We use an asterisk (*) to indicate that these statistics are based on the random-effects model. With that distinction, the interpretation of the slope(s) is the same as that for the fixed-effect model. Concretely,

$$Z^* = \frac{B^*}{SE_{B^*}}. \tag{20.5}$$

Under the null hypothesis that the coefficient is zero, Z^* would follow the normal distribution.

In the running example the coefficient for latitude is -0.0923 with standard error 0.00673, so

$$Z = \frac{-0.02923}{0.00673} = -4.3411.$$

Table 20.4 Random-effects model – regression results for BCG.

			Random effects, Z-Distribution			
	Point estimate	Standard error	95% Lower	95% Upper	Z-value	p-Value
Intercept	0.25954	0.23231	−0.19577	0.71486	1.11724	0.26389
Latitude	−0.02923	0.00673	−0.04243	−0.01603	−4.34111	0.00001

Table 20.5 Random-effects model – test of the model.

Test of the model:
Simultaneous test that all coefficients (excluding intercept) are zero
$Q^*_{model} = 18.8452$, $df = 1$, $p = 0.00001$
Goodness of fit: Test that unexplained variance is zero
$T^2 = 0.063$, $SE = 0.055$, $Q_{resid} = 30.733$, $df = 11$, $p = 0.00121$

(In this example the slope happens to be almost identical under the fixed-effect and random-effects models, but this is not usually the case.) The two-tailed p-value corresponding to $Z^* = -4.3411$ is 0.00001. This tells us that the slope is probably not zero, and the vaccination is more effective when the study is conducted at a greater distance from the equator.

Under the null hypothesis that none of the covariates 1 to p is related to effect size, Q^*_{model} would be distributed as chi-squared with degrees of freedom equal to p. In the running example, $Q^*_{model} = 18.8452$, $df = 1$, and $p = 0.00001$ (see Table 20.5).

In this example there is only one covariate (latitude) and so we have the option of using either the Z-test or the Q-test to assess the impact of this covariate. It follows that the two tests should yield the same results, and they do. The Z-value is -4.3411, with a corresponding p-value of 0.00001. The Q-value is 18.8452 with a corresponding p-value of 0.00001. Finally, Q^*_{model} should be equal to Z^{*2} and in fact 18.8452 equals -4.3411^2.

The goodness of fit test addresses the question of whether there is heterogeneity that is not explained by the covariates. Q_{resid} can also be used to estimate (and test) the variance, τ^2, of this unexplained heterogeneity. This Q_{resid} is the weighted residual SS from the regression using fixed-effect weights (see Table 20.3)

Q^*_{model} here is analogous to Q^*_{bet} for subgroup analysis, and Q_{resid} is analogous to Q_{within} for subgroup analysis. If the covariates represent subgroups, then Q^*_{model} is identical to Q^*_{bet} and Q_{resid} is identical to Q_{within}. If there are no predictors then Q_{resid} here is the same as Q for the original meta-analysis.

When working with meta-regression with the fixed-effect model we were able to partition the total variance into a series of components, with Q_{model} plus Q_{resid} summing to Q. This was possible with the fixed-effect model because the weight assigned to each study was determined solely by the within-study error, and was therefore the same for all three sets of calculations. By contrast, under the random-effects model the weight assigned to each study incorporates between-studies variance also, and this varies from one set of calculations to the next. Therefore, the variance components are not additive. For that reason, we display an analysis of variance table for the fixed-effect analysis, but not for the random-effects analysis.

Quantify the magnitude of the relationship

The relationship of latitude to effect (expressed as a log risk ratio) is

$$\ln (RR) = 0.2595 - 0.0292(X)$$

where X is the absolute latitude. We can plot this in Figure 20.6.

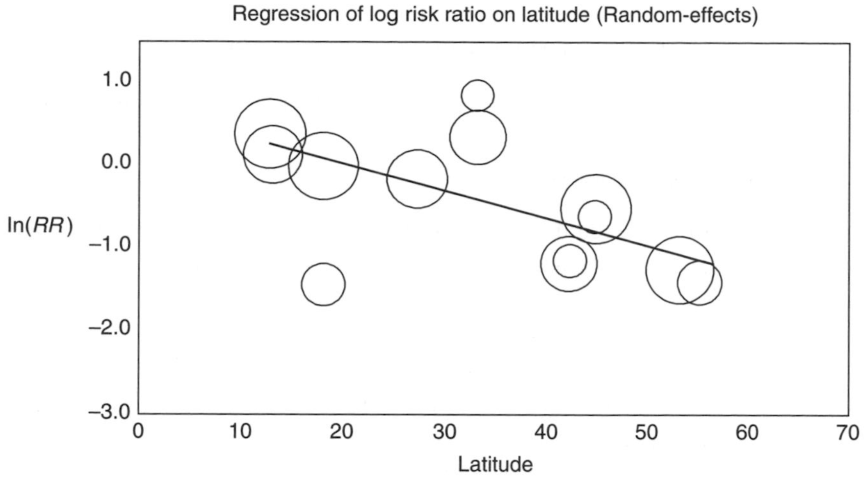

Figure 20.6 Random-effects model – regression of log risk ratio on latitude.

In this Figure, each study is represented by a circle that shows the actual coordinates (observed effect size by latitude) for that study. The size (specifically, the area) of each circle is proportional to that study's weight in the analysis. Since this analysis is based on the random-effects model, the weight is the total variance (within-study plus T^2) for each study.

Note the difference from the fixed-effect graph (Figure 20.2). When using random effects, the weights assigned to each study are more similar to one another. For example, the TB prevention trial (1980) study dominated the graph under the fixed-effect model (and exerted substantial influence on the slope) while Comstock and Webster (1969) had only a trivial impact (the relative weights for the two studies are 41% and 0.3% respectively). Under random effects the two are more similar (14% and 1.6% respectively).

The center line shows the predicted values. A study performed relatively close to the equator (latitude of 10) would have an expected effect near zero (corresponding to a risk ratio of 1.0, which means that the vaccination has no impact on TB). By contrast, a study at latitude 55 (Saskatchewan) would have an expected effect near -1.50 (corresponding to a risk ratio near 0.20, which means that the vaccination decreased the risk of TB by about 80%).

The 95% confidence interval for B is given by

$$LL_{B^*} = B^* - 1.96 \times SE_{B^*} \qquad (20.6)$$

and

$$UL_{B^*} = B^* + 1.96 \times SE_{B^*}. \qquad (20.7)$$

In the running example

$$LL_{B^*} = (-0.0292) - 1.96 \times 0.0067 = -0.0424$$

and

$$UL_{B^*} = (-0.0292) + 1.96 \times 0.0067 = -0.0160.$$

In words, the true coefficient could be as low as -0.0424 and as high as -0.0160.

The proportion of variance explained

In Chapter 19 we introduced the notion of the proportion of variance explained by subgroup membership in a random-effects analysis. The same approach can be applied to meta-regression.

Consider Figure 20.7, which shows a set of six studies with no covariate. Since there is no covariate the prediction slope is simply the mean (the intercept, if we were to compute a regression), depicted by a vertical line. The normal distribution at the bottom of the figure reflects T^2, and is needed to explain why the dispersion *from the prediction line* (the mean) exceeds the within-study error.

Now, consider Figure 20.8, which shows the same size studies with a covariate X, and the prediction slope depicted by a line that reflects the prediction equation. The normal distribution at each point on the prediction line reflects the value of T^2, and is needed to explain why the dispersion *from the prediction line* (this time, the slope) exceeds the within study error. Because the covariate explains some of the between-studies variance, the T^2 in Figure 20.8 is smaller than the one in Figure 20.8., and the ratio of the two can be used to quantify the proportion of variance explained.

Note 1. Normally, we would plot the effect size on the Y axis and the covariate on the X axis (see, for example, Figure 20.6). Here, we have transposed the axes to maintain the parallel with the forest plot.

Note 2. For clarity, we plotted the true effects for each figure. In practice, of course, we observe estimates of the true effects, remove the portion of variance attributed to within-study error, and impute the amount of variance remaining.

In primary studies, a common approach to describing the impact of a covariate is to report the proportion of variance explained by that covariate. That index, R^2, is defined as the ratio of explained variance to total variance,

$$R^2 = \frac{\sigma^2_{explained}}{\sigma^2_{total}} \tag{20.8}$$

or, equivalently,

$$R^2 = 1 - \left(\frac{\sigma^2_{unexplained}}{\sigma^2_{total}} \right). \tag{20.9}$$

This index is intuitive as it can be interpreted as a ratio, with a range of 0 to 1, or of 0% to 100%. Many researchers are familiar with this index, and have a sense of what proportion of variance is likely to be explained by different kinds of covariates or interventions.

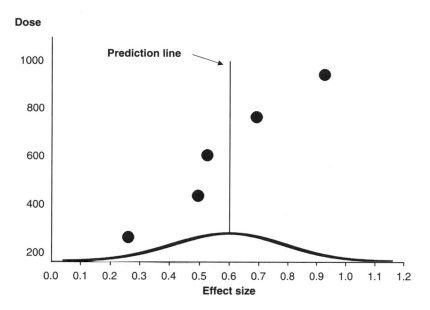

Figure 20.7 Between-studies variance (T^2) with no covariate.

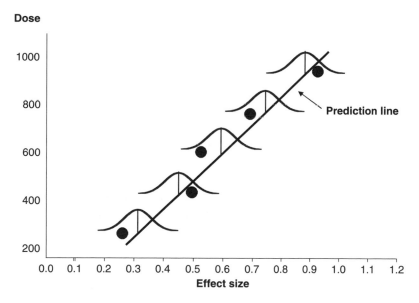

Figure 20.8 Between-studies variance (T^2) with covariate.

This index cannot be applied directly to meta-analysis. The reason is that in meta-analysis the total variance includes both variance within studies and between studies. The covariates are study-level covariates, and as such they can potentially explain only the between-studies portion of the variance. In the running illustration, even if

Table 20.6 Random-effects model – comparison of model (latitude) versus the null model.

Comparison of model with latitude versus the null model

Total between-study variance (intercept only)
T^2_{total} = 0.309, SE = 0.230, Q_{resid} = 152.233, df = 12, p = 0.00000

Unexplained between-study variance (with latitude in model)
$T^2_{unexplained}$ = 0.063, SE = 0.055, Q_{resid} = 30.733, df = 11, p = 0.0012

Proportion of total between-study variance explained by the model
R^2 analog = 1−(0.063/0.309) 79.50%

the *true* effect for each study fell directly on the prediction line the proportion of variance explained would not approach 1.0 because the *observed* effects would fall at some distance from the prediction line.

Therefore, rather than working with this same index we use an analogous index, defined as the *true* variance explained, as a proportion of the total *true* variance. Since the true variance is the between-studies variance, τ^2, we compute

$$R^2 = \frac{T^2_{explained}}{T^2_{total}} \tag{20.10}$$

or

$$R^2 = 1 - \left(\frac{T^2_{unexplained}}{T^2_{total}} \right). \tag{20.11}$$

In the running example T^2_{total} for the full set of studies was 0.309, and $T^2_{unexplained}$ for the equation with latitude is 0.063. This gives us

$$R^2 = 1 - \left(\frac{0.063}{0.309} \right) = 0.7950. \tag{20.12}$$

This is shown schematically for the running example (see Figure 20.9). In Figure 20.9, the top line shows that 8% of the total variance was within studies and 92%

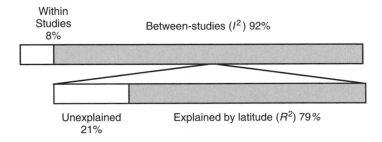

Figure 20.9 Proportion of variance explained by latitude.

was between studies (which is also the definition of I^2). The within-studies variance cannot be explained by a study-level moderator, and so is removed from the equation and we focus on the shaded part.

On the bottom line, the type of intervention is able to explain 79% of the relevant variance, leaving 21% unexplained. Critically, the 79% and 21% sum to 100%, since we are concerned only with the variance between-studies.

While the R^2 index has a range of 0 to 1 in the population, it is possible for sampling error to yield a value of R^2 that falls outside of this range. In that case, the value is set to either 0 (if the estimate falls below 0) or to 1 (if it falls above 1).

SUMMARY POINTS

- Just as we can use multiple regression in primary studies to assess the relationship between subject-level covariates and an outcome, we can use meta-regression in meta-analysis to assess the relationship between study-level covariates and effect size.
- Meta-regression may be performed under the fixed-effect or the random-effects model, but in most cases the latter is appropriate.
- In addition to testing the impact of covariates for statistical significance, it is important to quantify the magnitude of their relationship with effect size. For this purpose we can use an index based on the percent reduction in true variance, analogous to the R^2 index used with primary studies.

CHAPTER 21

Notes on Subgroup Analyses and Meta-Regression

Introduction
Computational model
Multiple comparisons
Software
Analyses of subgroups and regression analyses are observational
Statistical power for subgroup analyses and meta-regression

INTRODUCTION

In this chapter we address a number of issues that are relevant to both subgroup analyses (analysis of variance) and to meta-regression.

COMPUTATIONAL MODEL

The researcher must always choose between a fixed-effect model and a random-effects model. When we are working with a single set of studies the fixed-effect analysis assumes that all studies share a common effect size. When we are working with subgroups, it assumes that all studies within a subgroup share a common effect size. When we are working with meta-regression, it assumes that all studies which have the same values on the covariates share a common effect size.

These kinds of assumption can sometimes be justified, as in the pharmaceutical example that we used on pages 83, 161 and 195. In most cases, however, especially when the studies for the review have been culled from the literature, it is more plausible to assume that the subgroup membership or the covariates explain *some*, but *not all*, of the dispersion in effect sizes. Therefore, the random-effects model is more likely to fit the data, and is the model that should be selected.

Introduction to Meta-Analysis   M. Borenstein, L. V. Hedges, J. P. T. Higgins, H. R. Rothstein
© 2009, John Wiley & Sons, Ltd

Mistakes to avoid in selecting a model

When we introduced the idea of a random-effects model in Chapter 12 we noted that researchers sometimes start with a fixed-effect model and then move to a random-effects model if there is empirical evidence of heterogeneity (a statistically significant p-value). In the case of subgroup analysis this approach would suggest that we start by using the fixed-effect model within groups, and then move to the random-effects model only if Q within groups was statistically significant. In the case of meta-regression it would suggest that we start by using the fixed-effect model, and then move to the random-effects model only if the Q for the residual error was statistically significant.

We explained that this approach was problematic when working with a single set of studies, and it continues to be a bad idea here, for the same reasons. If substantive considerations suggest that the effect size is likely to vary (within the full set of studies, within subgroups, or for studies with a common set of covariate values) then we should be using the corresponding model even if the test for heterogeneity fails to yield a significant p-value. This lack of significance means only that we have failed to meet a certain threshold of proof (possibly because of low statistical power) and does not prove that the studies share a common effect size.

Practical differences related to the model

Researchers often ask about the practical implications of using a random-effects model rather than a fixed-effect model. The random-effects model will apportion the study weights more evenly, so that a large study has less impact on the summary effect (or regression line) than it would have under the fixed-effect model, and a small study has more impact that it would have under the fixed-effect model. Also, confidence intervals will tend to be wider under the random-effects model than under the fixed-effect model. While this tells us what the impact will be of using the fixed-effect or random-effects model, it says nothing about which model we should use. The only issue relevant to that decision is the question of which model fits the data.

The null hypothesis under the different models

Since the meaning of a summary effect size is different for fixed versus random effects, the null hypothesis being tested also differs under the two models.

Recall that when we are working with a single group, under the fixed-effect model the summary effect size represents the common effect size for all the studies. The null hypothesis is that the common effect size is equal to a nil value (0.00 for a difference, or 1.00 for a ratio). By contrast, under the random-effects model the summary effect size represents the mean of the distribution of effect sizes. The null hypothesis is that the mean of all possible studies is equal to the nil value.

In subgroup analyses, under the fixed-effect model the summary effect size for subgroups A and B each represents the common effect size for a group of studies. The null hypothesis is that the common effect for the A studies is the same as the common effect for the B studies. By contrast, under the random-effects model the effect size for subgroups A and B each represents the mean of a distribution of effect sizes. The null hypothesis is that the mean of all possible A studies is identical to the mean of all possible B studies.

In regression, under the fixed-effect model we assume that there is one true effect size for any given value of the covariate(s). The null hypothesis is that this effect size is the same for all values of the covariate(s). By contrast, under the random-effects model we assume that there is a distribution of effect sizes for any given value of the covariate(s). The null hypothesis is that this mean is the same for all values of the covariate(s).

While the distinction between a *common* effect size and a *mean* effect size might sound like a semantic nuance, it actually reflects an important distinction between the models. In the case of the fixed-effect model, because we assume that we are dealing with a common effect size, we apply an error model which assumes that the between-studies variance is zero. In the case of the random-effects model, because we allow that the effect sizes may vary, we apply an error model which makes allowance for this additional source of uncertainty. This difference has an impact on the mean (the summary effect for a single group, the summary effect within subgroups, and the slope in a meta-regression). It also has an impact on the standard error, tests of significance and confidence intervals.

Some technical considerations in random-effects meta-regression

As is the case for a standard random-effects meta-analysis in the absence of covariates, several methods are available for estimating τ^2 in meta-regression, including a moment method and maximum likelihood method. In practice, any differences among methods will usually be small.

The results we presented in this chapter used a moment estimate, which is the same as the method we used in Chapter 16 to estimate τ^2 for a single group. If we were to perform a meta-regression with no covariates, our estimate of τ^2 would be the same as the estimate we would obtain using the formulas in that chapter.

Whichever method is used to estimate τ^2, the use of a Z-test to assess the statistical significance of a covariate (or the difference between two subgroups), while common, is not strictly appropriate. When dealing with simple numerical data, to compute a confidence interval or to test the significance of a difference (or variance) we use Z if the sampling distribution is *known*. By contrast, we use t if the sampling distribution is being *estimated* from the dispersion observed in the sample (as it is, for example, when we compare means using a t-test).

Similarly, in meta-analysis, the Z-distribution is appropriate only for the fixed-effect model, where the only source of error is within studies. By contrast, when we use a random-effects model, we are estimating the dispersion across studies, and should account for this by using a t-distribution. Several methods have been proposed to address this issue, including one by Knapp and Hartung (2003) which is outlined below. While these can be applied to any use of the random-effects model (for a single group of studies, for a subgroup analysis, and for meta-regression), they have to date only been implemented in software for meta-regression.

The Knapp-Hartung method involves two modifications to the standard error for the random-effects model. First, the between-studies component of the variance is multiplied by a factor that makes it correspond to the t-distribution rather than the Z-distribution. Second, the test statistic is compared against the t-distribution rather than the Z-distribution. This has the effect of expanding the width of the confidence intervals and of moving the p-value away from zero.

Higgins and Thompson (2004) proposed an approach that bypasses the sampling distributions and instead employs a permutation test to yield a p-value. Using this approach we compute the Z-score corresponding to the observed covariate. Then, we randomly redistribute the covariates among studies and see what proportion of these yield a Z-score exceeding the one that we had obtained. This proportion may be viewed as an exact p-value.

MULTIPLE COMPARISONS

In primary studies researchers often need to address the issue of multiple comparisons. The basic problem is that if we conduct a series of analyses with alpha set at 0.05 for each, then the overall likelihood of a type I error (assuming that the null is actually true) will exceed 5%. This problem crops up when a study includes more than two groups and we compare more than one pair of means. It also arises when we perform an analysis on more than one outcome.

While there is consensus that conducting many comparisons can pose a problem, there is no consensus about how this problem should be handled. Some suggest conducting an omnibus test that asks if there are any nonzero effects, and then proceeding to look at pair-wise comparisons only if the initial test meets the criterion for significance. Others suggest going straight to the pair-wise tests but using a stricter criterion for significance (say 0.01 rather than 0.05 for five tests). Hedges and Olkin (1985) discuss this and other methods to control the error rate when using multiple tests. Some suggest that the researcher not make any formal adjustment, but evaluate the data in context. For example, one significant p-value in forty tests would not be seen as grounds for rejection of the null hypothesis.

Essentially the same issue exists in meta-analysis. In the case of subgroup analyses, if a meta-analysis includes a number of subgroups, the issue of multiple comparisons arises when we start to compare several pairs of subgroup means. In the case of meta-regression this issue arises when we include a number of covariates and want to test each one for significance. As with primary studies, while there is consensus that conducting many comparisons can pose a problem, there is no consensus about how this problem should be handled. The approaches generally used for primary studies can be applied to meta-analysis as well.

SOFTWARE

Some of the programs developed for meta-analysis are able to perform subgroup analysis as well as meta-regression (see Chapter 44). Note that programs intended for statistical analysis of primary studies should not be used to perform these procedures in meta-analysis, for two reasons. First, routines for analysis of variance or multiple regression intended for primary studies do not weight the studies, as is needed for meta-analysis. While most programs do allow the user to assign weights, this becomes a difficult procedure when we move to random-effects weights (which are usually the ones we want to use). Second, the rules for assigning degrees of freedom in the analysis of variance and meta-regression are different for meta-analysis than for primary studies, and so using the primary-study routines for a meta-analysis will yield incorrect standard errors and p-values.

ANALYSES OF SUBGROUPS AND REGRESSION ANALYSES ARE OBSERVATIONAL

In a randomized trial, participants are assigned at random to a condition (such as treatment versus placebo). Because the participants are assumed to be similar in all respects except for the treatment condition, differences that do emerge between conditions can be attributed to the treatment. By contrast, in an observational study we compare pre-existing groups, such as workers with a college education versus those who did not attend college. While we can report on differences in wages of the two groups we cannot attribute this outcome to the amount of schooling because the groups differ in various ways. For example, we are likely to find that those with a college education are paid more, but we cannot attribute this to their schooling since it could be due (at least in part) to other factors associated with higher socio-economic status.

The issue of randomized versus observational studies as it relates to meta-analysis is discussed in Chapter 40. There, we discuss the fact that randomized studies and observational studies address different questions, and for this reason it generally makes sense to include only one or the other in a given meta-analysis.

However, there is one issue that is directly relevant to the present discussion, as follows. Assume we start with a set of randomized experiments that assess the impact of an intervention. The effect in any single experiment could serve to establish causality and the summary effect can also serve to establish causality. This is because the relationship between treatment and outcome is protected by the randomization process (it *must be* due to treatment) in each study, and this protection carries over to the summary effect.

However, *even if the individual studies are randomized trials*, once we move beyond the goal of reporting a summary effect and proceed to perform a subgroup analyses or meta-regression, *we have moved out of the domain of randomized experiments, and into the domain of observational studies*. For example, suppose that half the studies used a low dose of aspirin while half used a high dose, and that the impact of the treatment was significantly stronger in the high-dose studies. It is *possible* that the difference is due to the dose, but it is also possible that the studies that used a higher dose differed in some systematic way from the other studies. Perhaps these studies used patients who were in poor health, or older, and therefore more likely to benefit from the treatment. Therefore, the difference between subgroups, or the relationship between a covariate and effect size, is *observational*. The same caveats that apply to any observational studies, in particular the fact that relationship does not imply causality, apply here too.

That said, in primary observational studies, researchers sometimes use regression analysis to try and remove the impact of potential confounders. In the aspirin example they might enter covariates in the sequence of health, age, and dose, to assess the impact of dose with health and age held constant. This is not a perfect solution since there may be other confounders of which we are not aware, but this approach can help to isolate the impact of specific factors and generate hypotheses to be tested in randomized trials. The same holds true for meta-regression. Of course, since covariate values are assigned at the study level, meta-regression can be used to adjust for potential confounders only for comparisons across studies, and not for potential confounders *within* studies.

There is one exception to the rule that subgroup analysis and regression cannot prove causality. This exception is the case where we know that the studies are identical in all respects except for the one captured by subgroup membership or by the covariate. The pharmaceutical example is a case in point. Here, we enrolled 1000 patients and assigned some to studies that would test a low dose of the drug vs. placebo, and others to studies that would test a high dose of the drug vs. placebo. Here, the assignment to subgroups *is* random. The same would apply if the patients were assigned to ten studies where the dose of drug was varied on a continuous scale, and we used meta-regression to test the relationship between dose and effect size. This set of circumstances is rarely (if ever) found in practice.

STATISTICAL POWER FOR SUBGROUP ANALYSES AND META-REGRESSION

Statistical power is the likelihood that a test of significance will reject the null hypothesis. In the case of subgroup analyses it is the likelihood that the Z-test to compare the effect in two groups, or the Q-test to compare the effects across a series of groups, will yield a statistically significant p-value. In the case of meta-regression it is the likelihood that the Z-test of a single covariate or the Q-test of a set of covariates will yield a statistically significant p-value.

Power depends on the size of the effect and the precision with which we measure the effect. For subgroup analysis this means that power will increase as the difference between (or among) subgroup means increases, and/or the standard error within subgroups decreases. For meta-regression this means that power will increase as the magnitude of the relationship between the covariate and effect size increases, and/or the precision of the estimate increases. In both cases, a key factor driving the precision of the estimate will be the total number of individual subjects across all studies and (for random effects) the total number of studies.

While there is a general perception that power for testing the main effect is consistently high in meta-analysis, this perception is not correct (see Chapter 29) and certainly does not extend to tests of subgroup differences or to meta-regression. The failure to find a statistically significant p-value when comparing subgroups or in meta-regression could mean that the effect (if any) is quite small, but could also mean that the analysis had poor power to detect even a large effect. One should never use a nonsignificant finding to conclude that the true means in subgroups are the same, or that a covariate is not related to effect size.

SUMMARY POINTS

- The selection of a computational model (fixed-effect or random-effects) should be based on our understanding of the underlying distribution. In most cases, especially when the studies have been gathered from the published literature, the random-effects model (within-subgroups) is more plausible than the fixed-effect model.
- The strategy of starting with the fixed-effect model and then moving to the random-effects (or mixed-effect) model if the test for heterogeneity is significant, is a mistake, and should be strongly discouraged.
- The problem of performing multiple tests (the fear that the actual alpha may exceed the nominal alpha) is similar in meta-analysis to the same problem in primary studies, and similar strategies are suggested for dealing with this problem.
- The relationship between effect size and subgroup membership, or between effect size and covariates, is observational, and cannot be used to prove causality. This holds true even if all studies in the analysis are randomized trials. The protection afforded by the study design carries over to the summary effect across all studies, but not to other analyses.
- Statistical power for detecting a difference among subgroups, or for detecting the relationship between a covariate and effect size, is often low, and the usual caveats apply. To wit, failure to obtain a statistically significant difference among subgroups should never be interpreted as evidence that the effect is the same across subgroups. Similarly, failure to obtain a statistically significant effect for a covariate should never be interpreted as evidence that there is no relationship between the covariate and the effect size.

Further Reading

Cohen, J., West, S.G., Cohen, P., & Aiken, L. (2002). *Applied Multiple Regression/Correlation Analysis for the Behavioral Sciences* (3rd ed). Mahwah, NJ, Lawrence Erlbaum Assoc.

Higgins, J.P.T., & Thompson, S.G (2004). Controlling the risk of spurious findings from meta-regression. *Statistics in Medicine* 23,1663–1682.

Knapp, G. & Hartung, J. (2003). Improved tests for a random effects meta-regression with a single covariate. *Statistics in Medicine* 22, 2693–2710.

Complex Data Structures

CHAPTER 22

Overview

Thus far we have assumed that each study contributes one (and only one) effect size to a meta-analysis. In this section we consider cases where studies contribute more than one effect size to the meta-analysis. These usually fall into one of the following types.

Multiple independent subgroups within a study

Sometimes a single study will report data for several cohorts of participants. For example, if researchers anticipate that the treatment effect (e.g., drug versus placebo) could vary by age, they might report the treatment effect separately for children and for adults. Similarly, if researchers anticipate that the treatment effect could vary by disease stage they might report the effect separately for patients enrolled with early-stage disease and for those enrolled with late-stage disease.

The defining feature here is that the subgroups are independent of each other, so that each provides unique information. For this reason, we can treat each subgroup as though it were a separate study, which is sometimes the preferred method. However, there are sometimes other options to consider, and we will be discussing these as well.

Multiple outcomes or time-points within a study

In some cases researchers will report data on several related, but distinct outcomes. A study that looked at the impact of tutoring might report data on math scores and also on reading scores. A study that looked at the association between diet and cardiovascular disease might report data on stroke and also on myocardial infarction. Similarly, a study that followed subjects over a period of time may report data using the same scale but at a series of distinct time-points. For example, studies that looked at the impact of an intervention to address a phobia might collect data at one month, six months, and twelve months.

The defining feature here is that *the same* participants provide data for the different outcomes (or time-points). We cannot treat the different outcomes as though they were independent as this would lead to incorrect estimates of the variance for the summary effect. We will show how to correct the variance to take account of the relationship among the outcomes.

Introduction to Meta-Analysis   M. Borenstein, L. V. Hedges, J. P. T. Higgins, H. R. Rothstein
© 2009, John Wiley & Sons, Ltd

More than one comparison group within a study

Sometimes, a study will include several treatment groups and a single control group. For example, one effect size may be defined as the difference between the placebo group and drug *A*, while another is defined as the difference between the same placebo group and drug *B*.

The defining feature here is similar to multiple outcomes, in that some participants (those in the control group) contribute information to more than one effect size. The methods proposed for dealing with this problem are similar to those proposed for multiple outcomes. They also include some options that are unique to the case of multiple comparisons.

How this Part is organized

The next three chapters address each of these cases in sequence. Within each chapter we first show how to combine data to yield a *summary* effect, and then show how to look at *differences* in effects.

The worked examples in these chapters use the fixed-effect model. We adopt this approach because it involves fewer steps and thus allows us to focus on the issue at hand, which is how to compute an effect size and variance. Once we have these effect sizes we can use them for a fixed-effect or a random-effects analysis, and the latter is generally more appropriate.

In the worked examples we deliberately use a generic effect size rather than specifying a particular effect size such as a standardized mean difference or a log odds ratio. The methods discussed here can be applied to any effect size, including those based on continuous, binary, correlational, or other kinds of data. As always, computations for risk ratios or odds ratios would be performed using log values, and computations for correlations would be performed using the Fisher's *z* transformed values.

CHAPTER 23

Independent Subgroups within a Study

Introduction
Combining across subgroups
Comparing subgroups

INTRODUCTION

The first case of a complex data structure is the case where studies report data from two or more independent subgroups.

Suppose we have five studies that assessed the impact of a treatment on a specific type of cancer. All studies followed the same design, with patients randomly assigned to either standard or aggressive treatment for two months. In each study, the results were reported separately for patients enrolled with stage-1 cancer and for those enrolled with stage-2 cancer. The stage-1 and stage-2 patients represent two independent subgroups since each patient is included in one group or the other, but not both.

If our goal was to compute the summary treatment effect for all stage-1 patients and, separately, for all stage-2 patients, then we would perform two separate analyses. In this case we would treat each subgroup as a separate study, and include the stage-1 studies in one analysis and the stage-2 studies in the other.

This chapter addresses the case where we want to use data from two or more subgroups in the *same* analysis. Specifically,

- We want to compute a summary effect for the impact of the intervention for stage-1 and stage-2 patients combined.
- Or, we want to compare the effect size for stage-1 patients versus stage-2 patients.

Introduction to Meta-Analysis   M. Borenstein, L. V. Hedges, J. P. T. Higgins, H. R. Rothstein
© 2009, John Wiley & Sons, Ltd

Table 23.1 Independent subgroups – five fictional studies.

Study	Subgroup	ES	Variance
Study 1	Stage 1	0.300	0.050
	Stage 2	0.100	0.050
Study 2	Stage 1	0.200	0.020
	Stage 2	0.100	0.020
Study 3	Stage 1	0.400	0.050
	Stage 2	0.200	0.050
Study 4	Stage 1	0.200	0.010
	Stage 2	0.100	0.010
Study 5	Stage 1	0.400	0.060
	Stage 2	0.300	0.060

COMBINING ACROSS SUBGROUPS

The defining feature of independent subgroups is that each subgroup contributes independent information to the analysis. If the sample size within each subgroup is 100, then the effective sample size across two subgroups is 200, and this will be reflected in the precision of the summary effect. However, within this framework we have several options for computing the summary effect.

We shall pursue the example of five studies that report data separately for patients enrolled with stage-1 or stage-2 cancer. The effect size and variance for each subgroup are shown in Table 23.1 and are labeled simply *ES* and *Variance* to emphasize the point that these procedures can be used with any effect size. If the outcome was continuous (means and standard deviations), the effect size might be a standardized mean difference. If the outcome was binary (for example, whether or not the cancer had metastasized), the effect size might be the log risk ratio.

Using subgroup as unit of analysis (option 1a)

One option is simply to treat each subgroup as a separate study. This is shown in Table 23.2, where each subgroup appears on its own row and values are summed across the ten rows.

Then, using formulas (11.3) to (11.5),

$$M = \frac{76.666}{413.333} = 0.1855,$$

with variance

$$V_M = \frac{1}{413.333} = 0.0024$$

Table 23.2 Independent subgroups – summary effect.

Study	Subgroup	ES	Variance	WT	ES*WT
Study 1	Stage 1	0.30	0.05	20.000	6.000
	Stage 2	0.10	0.05	20.000	2.000
Study 2	Stage 1	0.20	0.02	50.000	10.000
	Stage 2	0.10	0.02	50.000	5.000
Study 3	Stage 1	0.40	0.05	20.000	8.000
	Stage 2	0.20	0.05	20.000	4.000
Study 4	Stage 1	0.20	0.01	100.000	20.000
	Stage 2	0.10	0.01	100.000	10.000
Study 5	Stage 1	0.40	0.06	16.667	6.667
	Stage 2	0.30	0.06	16.667	5.000
Sum				413.333	76.667

and standard error

$$SE_M = \sqrt{0.0024} = 0.0492.$$

Using study as unit of analysis (option 1b)

A second option is to compute a composite score for each study and use this in the analysis, as in Figure 23.1. The unit of analysis is then the study rather than the subgroup.

Computing a combined effect across subgroups within a study

The mean and variance of the composite within a study are computed by performing a fixed-effect meta-analysis on the subgroups for that study. For study 1, this is shown in Figure 23.1 and in Table 23.3.

We apply formulas (11.3) and (11.4) to yield a mean effect

$$M = \frac{8.0000}{40.0000} = 0.2000$$

Study	Subgroup	Effect size	Variance	Mean	Variance
Study 1	Stage-1	0.30	0.05	0.200	0.025
	Stage-2	0.10	0.05		

Figure 23.1 Creating a synthetic variable from independent subgroups.

Table 23.3 Independent subgroups – synthetic effect for study 1.

Subgroup	Effect Y	Variance V_Y	Weight W	Computed WY
Stage 1	0.30	0.05	20.000	6.000
Stage 2	0.10	0.05	20.000	2.000
Sum			40.000	8.000

with variance

$$V_M = \frac{1}{40.0000} = 0.0250.$$

Note that the variance for the study (0.025) is one-half as large as the variance for either subgroup (0.050) since it is based on twice as much information.

This procedure is used to form a composite effect size and variance for each study, as shown in Table 23.4. Then, we perform a meta-analysis working solely with these study-level effect sizes and variances.

At this point we can proceed to the meta-analysis using these five (synthetic) scores. To compute a summary effect and other statistics using the fixed-effect model, we apply the formulas starting with (11.3). Using values from the line labeled *Sum* in Table 23.4,

$$M = \frac{76.667}{413.333} = 0.1855$$

with variance

$$V_M = \frac{1}{413.333} = 0.0024$$

Table 23.4 Independent subgroups – summary effect across studies.

Study	Subgroup	ES	Variance	ES	Variance	WT	ES*WT
Study 1	Stage 1	0.300	0.050	0.200	0.025	40.000	8.000
	Stage 2	0.100	0.050				
Study 2	Stage 1	0.200	0.020	0.150	0.010	100.000	15.000
	Stage 2	0.100	0.020				
Study 3	Stage 1	0.400	0.050	0.300	0.025	40.000	12.000
	Stage 2	0.200	0.050				
Study 4	Stage 1	0.200	0.010	0.150	0.005	200.000	30.000
	Stage 2	0.100	0.010				
Study 5	Stage 1	0.400	0.060	0.350	0.030	33.333	11.667
	Stage 2	0.300	0.060				
Sum						413.333	76.667

and standard error

$$SE_M = \sqrt{0.0024} = 0.0492.$$

Note that the summary effect and variance computed using study as the unit of analysis are identical to those computed using subgroup as the unit of analysis. This will always be the case when we use a fixed effect analysis to combine effects at both steps in the analysis (within studies and across studies).

However, the two methods will yield different results if we use a random effects analysis to combine effects across studies. This follows from the fact that T^2 (which is used to compute weights) may be different if based on variation in effects from study to study than if based on variation in effects from subgroup to subgroup. Therefore, the decision to use subgroup or study as the unit of analysis should be based on the context for computing T^2. Consider the following two cases.

- Case 1: Five researchers studied the impact of an intervention. Each researcher selected five schools at random, and each school is reported as an independent subgroup within the study. In this situation, between-school variation applies just as much within studies as across studies. We would therefore use subgroup as the unit of analysis (option 1a).
- Case 2: Five researchers have published papers on the impact of an intervention. Each researcher worked in a single school, and the subgroups are grade 1, grade 2, and so on. We expect the effects to be relatively consistent within a school, but to vary substantially from one school to the next. To allow for this between-school variation we should use a random-effects model only *across studies*. To properly estimate this component of uncertainty we would use study as the unit of analysis (option 1b).

Recreating the summary data for the full study (option 2)

Options 1a and 1b differ in the unit of analysis, but they have in common that the effect size is computed *within* subgroups. Another option (option 2) is to use the summary data from the subgroups to recreate the data for the study as a whole, and then use this summary data to compute the effect size and variance.

When the subgroup data are reported as 2×2 tables we can simply collapse cells to recreate the data for the full sample. That is, we sum cell A over all subgroups to yield an overall cell A, and repeat the process for cells B, C, and D.

When the subgroup data are reported as means, standard deviations, and sample size for each treatment group the combined sample size is summed across subgroup. For example, for treatment group 1,

$$n_1 = n_{11} + n_{12}, \tag{23.1}$$

the combined mean is computed as the weighted mean (by sample size) across groups,

$$\overline{X}_1 = \frac{n_{11}\,\overline{X}_{11} + n_{12}\,\overline{X}_{12}}{n_{11} + n_{12}}, \tag{23.2}$$

and the combined standard deviation is computed as

$$S_1 = \sqrt{\frac{(n_{11} - 1)\,S_{11}^2 + (n_{12} - 1)\,S_{12}^2 + \dfrac{n_{11}n_{12}}{n_{11} + n_{12}}(\overline{X}_{11} - \overline{X}_{12})^2}{n_{11} + n_{12} - 1}}, \tag{23.3}$$

where $\overline{X}_{11}$, $\overline{X}_{12}$ are the means in subgroups 1 and 2 of treatment group 1; S_{11}, S_{12} the standard deviations, and n_{11}, n_{12} the sample sizes; of subgroups 1 and 2.

When the subgroup data are reported as correlations, analogous formulas exist to recreate the correlation for the full study, but these are beyond the scope of this book.

Option 2 is sometimes used when some studies report summary data for all subjects combined, while others break down the data by subgroups. If the researcher believes that the subgroup classifications are unimportant, and wants to have a uniform approach for all studies (to compute an effect size from a single set of summary data) then this option will prove useful.

However, it is important to understand that this is a fundamentally different approach than other options. To return to the example introduced at the start of this chapter, under options 1a and 1b the effect size was computed *within* subgroups, which means that the effect size is *the impact of intervention controlling for cancer stage* (even if we then merge the effect sizes to yield an overall effect). By contrast, under option 2 we merge the summary data and *then* compute an effect size. Therefore the effect is 'the impact of intervention *ignoring* cancer stage'.

When the studies are randomized trials, the proportion of participants assigned to each treatment is typically constant from one subgroup to the next. In this case there is not likely to be a confounder between treatment and subgroup, and so either approach would be valid. By contrast, in observational studies the proportion of exposed subjects may vary from one subgroup to the next, which would yield confounding between exposure and subgroup. In this case option 2 should *not* be used. (This is the same issue discussed in Chapter 33, under the heading of Simpson's paradox.)

COMPARING SUBGROUPS

When our goal is to *compare* the effect size in different subgroups (rather than *combine* them) we have two options, as follows.

Using subgroup as unit of analysis

One option is simply to treat each subgroup as a separate study, where each study is classified (in this example) as stage 1 or stage 2. We then compute a summary effect for all the stage 1 effects, another for all the stage 2 effects, and then compare the two using a Z-test or analysis of variance as discussed in Chapter 19.

A second option is to compute the effect size within subgroups for each study, and then to compute the difference in effects within each study. In this case each study will contribute one effect to the analysis, where the effect is the difference between subgroups.

The first option is a more general approach. It allows us to work with studies that report data for any subgroup or combination of subgroups (one study has subgroups *A* and *B*, another *B* and *C*, and so on), and then to use all relevant subgroups to compute the summary effect.

The second option can only be used if all studies report data on the same two subgroups, which is relatively rare. When this option *can* be used, however, it will usually yield a more precise estimate of the difference in effects in random effects analyses, and is also desirable because differences in effects are not confounded by possible differences between studies.

SUMMARY POINTS

- When we have independent subgroups within a study, each subgroup contributes independent information. Therefore, if the sample size within each subgroup is 100, then the effective sample size across five subgroups is 500. In this sense, independent subgroups are no different than independent studies.

- To compute a summary effect we typically compute the effect within subgroups and then either use these effects as the unit of analysis, or merge effects within each study and use study as the unit of analysis. A second option is to combine the summary data from all subgroups to recreate the original study-level data, and then compute an effect size from this data. The second approach should be used only in limited circumstances.

- To compare effects across subgroups we typically use subgroup as the unit of analysis. In some cases we may also be able to compute the difference between subgroups in each study, and use study as the unit of analysis.

CHAPTER 24

Multiple Outcomes or Time-Points within a Study

Introduction
Combining across outcomes or time-points
Comparing outcomes or time-points within a study

INTRODUCTION

The second case of a complex data structure is the case where a study reports data on more than one outcome, or more than one time-point, where the different outcomes (or time-points) are based on the same participants.

For example, suppose that five studies assessed the impact of tutoring on student performance. All studies followed the same design, with students randomly assigned to either of two groups (tutoring or control) for a semester, after which they were tested for proficiency in reading and math. The effect was reported separately for the reading and the math scores, but within each study *both outcomes were based on the same students*.

Or, consider the same situation with the following difference. This time, assume that each study tests only for reading but does so at two time-points (immediately after the intervention and again six months later). The effect was reported separately for each time-point but *both measures were based on the same students*.

For our purposes the two situations (multiple outcomes for the same subjects or multiple time-points for the same subjects) are identical, and we shall treat them as such in this discussion. We shall use the term *outcomes* throughout this chapter, but the reader can substitute *time-points* in every instance.

If our goal was to compute a summary effect for the impact of the intervention on reading, and *separately* for the impact of the intervention on math scores, we would simply perform two separate meta-analyses, one using the data for reading and the other using the data for math. The issues we address in this chapter are how to

Introduction to Meta-Analysis   M. Borenstein, L. V. Hedges, J. P. T. Higgins, H. R. Rothstein
© 2009, John Wiley & Sons, Ltd

proceed when we want to incorporate both outcomes in the same analysis. Specifically,

- We want to compute a summary effect for the intervention on *Basic skills*, which combines the data from reading and math.
- Or, we want to investigate the *difference* in effect size for reading versus math.

In either case, the issue we need to address is that the data for reading and math are not independent of each other and therefore the errors are correlated.

COMBINING ACROSS OUTCOMES OR TIME-POINTS

The data for the five fictional studies are shown in Table 24.1. In study 1, for example, the effect size for reading was 0.30 with a variance of 0.05, and the effect size for math was 0.10 with a variance of 0.05.

While it might seem that we could treat each line of data as a separate study and perform a meta-analysis with ten *studies*, this is problematic for two reasons. One problem is that in computing the summary effect across studies this approach will assign more weight to studies with two outcomes than to studies with one outcome. (While this problem does not exist in our set of studies, it would be a problem if the number of outcomes varied from study to study.)

The second, and more fundamental problem, is that this approach leads to an improper estimate of the precision of the summary effect. This is because it treats the separate outcomes as providing independent information, when in fact the math and reading scores come from the same set of students and therefore are not independent of each other. If the outcomes are positively correlated (which is almost always the case with effects that we would want to combine), this approach underestimates the error (and overestimates the precision) of the summary effect.

Table 24.1 Multiple outcomes – five fictional studies.

Study	Outcome	ES	Variance
Study 1	Reading	0.300	0.050
	Math	0.100	0.050
Study 2	Reading	0.200	0.020
	Math	0.100	0.020
Study 3	Reading	0.400	0.050
	Math	0.200	0.050
Study 4	Reading	0.200	0.010
	Math	0.100	0.010
Study 5	Reading	0.400	0.060
	Math	0.300	0.060

Table 24.2 Creating a synthetic variable as the mean of two outcomes.

Study	Outcome	Effect size	Variance	Mean	Variance
Study 1	Math	0.30	0.05	0.20	?
	Reading	0.10	0.05		

Note. If the correlation between outcomes is negative, this approach will over-estimate the error (and underestimate the precision) of the summary effect. The solutions presented below will work for this case as well, but in the discussion we assume that we are dealing with a positive correlation.

To address these problems, rather than treating each outcome as a separate unit in the analysis, we'll compute the mean of the outcomes for each study, and use this synthetic score as the unit of analysis. In Table 24.2 we show this schematically for study 1.

We start with summary data for two outcomes (math and reading), and compute an effect size and variance for each. If the data are continuous (means and standard deviations on the exam) the effect size might be Hedges' g. If the data are binary (number of students passing the course) the effect size might be a log risk ratio. And so on. Then, we compute a synthetic effect size for *Basic skills* which incorporates both the math and reading effects. The method used to compute this effect size and its variance is explained below.

Since every study will be represented by one score in the meta-analysis regardless of the number of outcomes included in the mean, this approach solves the problem of more weight being assigned to studies with more outcomes. This approach also allows us to address the problem of non-independent information, since the formula for the variance of the synthetic variable will take into account the correlation among the outcomes.

Computing a combined effect across outcomes

Our notation will be to use Y_1, Y_2 etc. for effect sizes from different outcomes or time points within a study, and Y_j to refer to the jth of these. Strictly, we should use Y_{ij}, for the jth outcome (or time-point) in the ith study. However, we drop the i subscript for convenience. The effect size for *Basic skills* is computed as the mean of the reading and math scores,

$$\overline{Y} = \frac{1}{2}\,(Y_1 + Y_2). \tag{24.1}$$

This is what we would use as the effect estimate from this study in a meta-analysis. Using formulas described in Box 24.1, the variance of this mean is

$$V_{\overline{Y}} = \frac{1}{4}\,(V_{Y_1} + V_{Y_2} + 2r\sqrt{V_{Y_1}}\sqrt{V_{Y_2}}) \tag{24.2}$$

BOX 24.1 COMPUTING THE VARIANCE OF A COMPOSITE OR A DIFFERENCE

1. The variance of the sum of two correlated variables

If we know that the variance of Y_1 is V_1 and the variance of Y_2 is V_2, then

$$\text{var}(Y_1 + Y_2) = V_1 + V_2 + 2r\sqrt{V_1}\sqrt{V_2},$$

where r is the correlation coefficient that describes the extent to which Y_1 and Y_2 co-vary. If Y_1 and Y_2 are inextricably linked (so that a change in one determines completely the change in the other), then $r = 1$, and the variance of the sum is roughly twice the sum of the variances. At the other extreme, if Y_1 and Y_2 are unrelated, then $r = 0$ and the variance is just the sum of the individual variances. This is because when the variables are unrelated, knowing both gives us twice as much information, and so the variance is halved compared with the earlier case.

2. The impact of a scaling factor on the variance

If we know the variance of X, then the variance of a scalar (say c) multiplied by X is given by

$$\text{var}(cX) = c^2 \times \text{var}(X).$$

3. The variance of the mean of two correlated variables

Combining 1 with 2, we can see that the variance of the mean of Y_1 and Y_2 is

$$\text{var}\left(\frac{1}{2}(Y_1 + Y_2)\right) = \left(\frac{1}{2}\right)^2 \text{var}(Y_1 + Y_2) = \frac{1}{4}(V_1 + V_2 + 2r\sqrt{V_1}\sqrt{V_2}).$$

4. The variance of the sum of several correlated variables

If we know Y_i has variance V_i for several variables $i = 1, \ldots, m$, then the formula in 1 extends as follows:

$$\text{var}\left(\sum_{i=1}^{m} Y_i\right) = \sum_{i=1}^{m} V_i + \sum_{i \neq j}(r_{ij}\sqrt{V_i}\sqrt{V_j})$$

where r_{ij} is the correlation between Y_i and Y_j.

5. The variance of the mean of several correlated variables

Combining 4 with 2, we can see that the variance of the mean of several variables is

$$\text{var}\left(\frac{1}{m}\sum_{i=1}^{m} Y_i\right) = \left(\frac{1}{m}\right)^2 \text{var}\left(\sum_{i=1}^{m} Y_i\right) = \left(\frac{1}{m}\right)^2 \left(\sum_{i=1}^{m} V_i + \sum_{i \neq j}(r_{ij}\sqrt{V_i}\sqrt{V_j})\right).$$

6. The variance of the difference between two correlated variables

If we know that the variance of Y_1 is V_1 and the variance of Y_2 is V_2, then

$$\text{var}(Y_1 - Y_2) = V_1 + V_2 - 2r\sqrt{V_1}\sqrt{V_2},$$

BOX 24.1 CONTINUED

where r is the correlation coefficient that describes the extent to which Y_1 and Y_2 co-vary. If Y_1 and Y_2 are inextricably linked (so that a change in one determines completely the change in the other), then $r = 1$, and the variance of the difference is close to zero. At the other extreme, if Y_1 and Y_2 are unrelated, then $r = 0$ and the variance is the sum of the individual variances. If the correlation is $r = 0.5$ then the variance is approximately the average of the two variances.

---

where r is the correlation between the two outcomes. If both variances V_{Y_1} and V_{Y_2} are equal (say to V), then (24.2) simplifies to

$$V_{\bar{Y}} - \frac{1}{2}V(1 + r). \qquad (24.3)$$

In the running example, in study 1 the effect sizes for math and reading are 0.30 and 0.10, the variance for each is 0.02. Suppose we know that the correlation between them is 0.50. The composite score for *Basic skills* ($\bar{Y}$) is computed as

$$\bar{Y} = \frac{1}{2}(0.30 + 0.10) = 0.2000,$$

with variance (based on (24.2))

$$V_{\bar{Y}} = \frac{1}{4}(0.05 + 0.05 + 2 \times 0.50 \times \sqrt{0.05} \times \sqrt{0.05}) = 0.0375,$$

or, equivalently (using (24.3)),

$$V_{\bar{Y}} = \frac{1}{2} \times 0.05 \times (1 + 0.50) = 0.0375.$$

Using this formula we can see that if the correlation between outcomes was zero, the variance of the composite would be 0.025 (which is half as large as either outcome alone) because the second outcome provides entirely independent information. If the correlation was 1.0 the variance of the composite would be 0.050 (the same as either outcome alone) because all information provided by the second outcome is redundant. In our example, where the correlation is 0.50 (*some* of the information is redundant) the variance of the composite falls between these extremes. When we were working with independent subgroups (earlier in this chapter) the correlation was zero, and therefore the variance of the composite was 0.025.

These formulas are used to create Table 24.2, where the variance for each composite is based on formula (24.2) and the weight is simply the reciprocal of the variance.

At this point we can proceed to the meta-analysis using these five (synthetic) scores. To compute a summary effect and other statistics using the fixed-effect model, we apply the formulas starting with (11.3). Using values from the line labeled *Sum* in Table 24.3,

Table 24.3 Multiple outcomes – summary effect.

Study	Outcome	ES	Variance	ES	Correlation	Variance	Weight	ES*WT
Study 1	Reading	0.300	0.050	0.200	0.500	0.038	26.667	5.333
	Math	0.100	0.050					
Study 2	Reading	0.200	0.020	0.150	0.600	0.016	62.500	9.375
	Math	0.100	0.020					
Study 3	Reading	0.400	0.050	0.300	0.600	0.040	25.000	7.500
	Math	0.200	0.050					
Study 4	Reading	0.200	0.010	0.150	0.400	0.007	142.857	21.429
	Math	0.100	0.010					
Study 5	Reading	0.400	0.060	0.350	0.800	0.054	18.519	6.481
	Math	0.300	0.060					
Sum							275.542	50.118

$$M = \frac{50.118}{275.542} = 0.1819,$$

with variance

$$V_M = \frac{1}{275.542} = 0.0036.$$

The average difference between the tutored and control groups on *Basic skills* is 0.1819 with variance 0.0036 and standard error 0.060. The 95% confidence interval for the average effect is 0.064 to 0.300. The Z-value for a test of the null is 3.019 with a two-sided *p*-value of 0.003.

Working with more than two outcomes per study

These formulas can be extended to accommodate any number of outcomes. If *m* represents the number of outcomes within a study, then the composite effect size for that study would be computed as

$$\overline{Y} = \frac{1}{m}\left(\sum_{j}^{m} Y_j\right),\tag{24.4}$$

and the variance of the composite is given by

$$V_{\overline{Y}} = \left(\frac{1}{m}\right)^2 \text{var}\left(\sum_{j=1}^{m} Y_i\right) = \left(\frac{1}{m}\right)^2\left(\sum_{j=1}^{m} V_i + \sum_{j\neq k}\left(r_{jk}\sqrt{V_j}\sqrt{V_k}\right)\right)\tag{24.5}$$

as derived in Box 24.1. If the variances are all equal to *V* and the correlations are all equal to *r*, then (24.5) simplifies to

$$V_{\overline{Y}} = \frac{1}{m}V(1 + (m-1)r).\tag{24.6}$$

Impact of the correlations on the combined effect

One issue to consider is what happens as the correlation moves toward 1.0. Continuing with the simplified situation where all observations within a study have the same variance (V) and all pairs of observations within the study have the same correlation (r), if the m observations are independent of each other $(r = 0)$, the variance of the composite is V/m. If the m observations are not independent of each other, then the variance of the composite is V/m times a correction factor. We will refer to this correction factor as the *variance inflation factor (VIF)*, which is

$$VIF = 1 + (m - 1)r, \qquad (24.7)$$

where m is the number of observations and r is the correlation between each pair. An increase in either m or r (or both) will result in a higher inflation of the variance compared with treating the different outcomes as independent of each other.

In Table 24.4 we explore how the variance inflation factor depends on the value of r, the correlation coefficient. For the purposes of this illustration we assume the simplistic situation of a study having just two outcomes $(m = 2)$ with the same variance $(V = 0.2)$ for each outcome. Each column in the table (A-E) corresponds to a different correlation coefficient between these outcomes.

The variance of the composite for the study is

$$V_{\bar{Y}} = \frac{1}{m}V \times VIF. \qquad (24.8)$$

Taking as an example column C, the correlation is $r = 0.50$, and the variance inflation factor is

$$VIF = 1 + (2 - 1) \times 0.50 = 1.5000.$$

Table 24.4 Multiple outcomes – Impact of correlation on variance of summary effect.

	A	B	C	D	E
Effect size (here assumed identical for all outcomes)	0.4	0.4	0.4	0.4	0.4
Number of outcomes (m)	2	2	2	2	2
Variance of each outcome (V)	0.2	0.2	0.2	0.2	0.2
Correlation among outcomes (r)	0.000	0.250	0.500	0.750	1.000
Variance inflation factor (VIF)	1.000	1.250	1.500	1.750	2.000
Variance of composite	0.100	0.125	0.150	0.175	0.200
Standard error of composite	0.316	0.354	0.387	0.418	0.447
Standard error inflation factor	1.000	1.118	1.225	1.323	1.414
Lower limit	−0.220	−0.293	−0.359	−0.420	−0.477
Upper limit	1.020	1.093	1.159	1.220	1.277
p-value (2-tailed)	0.206	0.258	0.302	0.339	0.371

Thus, the variance of the composite score for the study is

$$V_{\bar{Y}} = \frac{1}{2} \times 0.2 \times 1.5000 = 0.150.$$

As we move from left to right in the table (from a correlation of 0.00 to 1.00) the variance inflation factor (*VIF*) and (by definition) the variance double. If the inflation factor for the variance moves from 1.00 to 2.00, it follows that the inflation factor for the standard error (which is the square root of the variance) will move from 1.00 to 1.44. Therefore, the width of the confidence interval will increase by a factor of 1.44 (and, correspondingly, the Z-value for the test of the null hypothesis for this study would decrease by a factor of 1.44).

When the correlation is unknown

This table also provides a mechanism for working with synthetic variables when we don't know the correlation among outcomes. Earlier, we assumed that the correlation between math and reading was known to be 0.50, and used that value to compute the standard error of the combined effect and the related statistics. In those cases where we don't know the correlation for the study in question, we should still be able to use other studies in the same field to identify a plausible range for the correlation. We could then perform a sensitivity analysis and might assume, for example, that if the correlation falls in the range of 0.50 to 0.75 then the standard error probably falls in the range of 0.39 to 0.42 (columns C to D in the table).

Researchers who do not know the correlation between outcomes sometimes fall back on either of two 'default' positions. Some will include both math and verbal scores in the analysis and treat them as independent. Others would use the average of the reading variance and the math variance. It is instructive, therefore, to consider the practical impact of these choices.

Treating the two outcomes as independent of each other yields the same precision as setting the correlation at 0.00 (column A). By contrast, using the average of the two variances yields the same precision as setting the correlation at 1.00 (column E). In effect, then, researchers who adopt either of these positions as a way of bypassing the need to specify a correlation, are actually adopting a correlation, albeit implicitly. And, the correlation that they adopt falls at either extreme of the possible range (either zero or 1.0). The first approach is almost certain to underestimate the variance and overestimate the precision. The second approach is almost certain to overestimate the variance and underestimate the precision. In this context, the idea of working with a *plausible* range of correlations rather than the *possible* range offers some clear advantages.

As we noted at the outset, exactly the same approach applies to studies with multiple outcomes and to studies with multiple time-points. However, there could be a distinction between the two when it comes to deciding what is a plausible range of correlations. When we are working with different outcomes at a single point in time, the plausible range of correlations will depend on the similarity of the outcomes. When we are working with the same outcome at multiple time-points, the plausible range of correlations will depend on such factors as the time elapsed between assessments and the stability of the relative scores over this time period.

One issue to consider is what happens if the correlations between multiple outcomes are higher in some studies than in others. This variation will affect the *relative weights* assigned to different studies, with *more weight* going to the study with a *lower correlation*. In the running example the variances for reading and math were the same in studies 1 and 3, but the correlation between reading and math was higher in study 3. Therefore, study 3 had a higher variance and was assigned less weight in the meta-analysis.

COMPARING OUTCOMES OR TIME-POINTS WITHIN A STUDY

We now turn to the problem of investigating *differences* between outcomes or between time-points. To extend the current example, suppose that each study reports the impact of the intervention for math and for reading and we want to know if the impact is stronger for one of these outcomes than for the other. Or, each study reports the effect at 6 months and 12 months, and we want to know if the effect changes over time.

When our goal was to compute a combined effect based on both outcomes our approach was to create a synthetic variable for each study (defined as the mean of the effect sizes) and to use this as the effect size in the analysis. We will follow the same approach here, except that the synthetic variable will be defined as the difference in effect sizes rather than their mean.

The approach is shown in Table 24.5. As before, we start with summary data for two outcomes (math and reading), and compute an effect size and variance for each. Then, we compute a synthetic effect size, which is now the *difference* between the two effects and its variance, as explained below.

This approach allows us to address the problem of correlated error, since the formula for the variance of the synthetic variable will take into account the correlation between the outcomes.

Computing a variance for correlated outcomes

Whenever we use sample data to estimate a difference, the variance reflects the error of our estimate. If we compute the difference of two *unrelated* outcomes, each with

Table 24.5 Creating a synthetic variable as the difference between two outcomes.

Study	Outcome	Effect size	Variance	Difference	Variance
Study 1	Math	0.30	0.05	0.20	?
	Reading	0.10	0.05		

variance V, then the variance of the difference is $2V$, which incorporates the two sources of error. By contrast, if we compute the difference of two (positively) related outcomes, then some of the error is redundant, and so the total error is less than $2V$. If the correlation between outcomes is 0.50, the variance of the difference would be equal to V, and as the correlation approaches 1.00, the variance of the difference would approach zero. The operating principle is that the higher the correlation between the outcomes, the lower the variance (the higher the precision) of the difference. The formula for the variance of a difference from correlated outcomes (see Box 24.1) is

$$V_{Y_{diff}} = V_{Y_1} + V_{Y_2} - 2r\sqrt{V_{Y_1}}\sqrt{V_{Y_2}}. \qquad (24.9)$$

In words, we sum the two variances and then *subtract* a value that reflects the correlated error.

Note the difference from the formula for variance of a mean, where we *added* the correlated error and included a scaling factor. When we *combine* positively correlated outcomes, a higher correlation between outcomes results in *a higher variance*. By contrast, when we compute the *difference* between positively correlated outcomes, a higher correlation between outcomes results in *a lower variance*.

To understand why, suppose that we assess patients using two different measures of depression. If a patient is having a particularly good day when the measures are taken, both scores will tend to be higher than the patient's average. If the patient is having a bad day, both will tend to be lower than the patient's average. If we compute a *combined* effect, the error will *build* as we increase the number of outcomes. If this is a *good* day, both measures will over-estimate the patient's level of functioning. By contrast, if we compute a *difference*, we *subtract* one effect from the other, and the day-to-day variation is removed.

Computing a difference between outcomes

With this as background, we can return to the running example, and discuss the computation of the synthetic effect size and its variance.

The difference between reading and math is computed as

$$Y_{diff} = Y_1 - Y_2, \qquad (24.10)$$

with variance

$$V_{Y_{diff}} = V_{Y_1} + V_{Y_2} - 2r\sqrt{V_{Y_1}}\sqrt{V_{Y_2}}. \qquad (24.11)$$

If both variances are equal to the same variance, V, then (24.11) simplifies to

$$V = 2V(1 - r). \qquad (24.12)$$

In the running example, the difference between reading and math in study 1 is computed as

$$V_{diff} = 0.30 - 0.10 = 0.2000,$$

with variance

$$V_{Y_{diff}} = 0.05 + 0.05 - 2 \times 0.50 \times \sqrt{0.05}\sqrt{0.05} = 0.05,$$

or equivalently,

$$V_{Y_{diff}} = 2(0.05)(1 - 0.50) = 0.05.$$

These formulas are used to create Table 24.6, where the variance for each composite is based on formula (24.11) and the weight is simply the reciprocal of the variance.

At this point we can proceed to the meta-analysis using these five (synthetic) scores. The scores happen to represent difference scores, but the same formulas apply. Under the fixed-effect model the formulas starting with (11.3) yield a summary effect

$$M = \frac{27.750}{232.500} = 0.1194,$$

with variance

$$V_M = \frac{1}{232.500} = 0.0043.$$

The average difference between the effect size for reading and the effect size for math is 0.1194 with variance 0.0043 and standard error 0.066. The 95% confidence interval for the average difference is -0.009 to 0.248. The Z-value for a test of the null is 1.820 with a two-sided p-value of 0.069.

Working with more than two outcomes per study

The formulas presented for a difference based on two outcomes can be extended to accommodate any number of outcomes using contrasts. For example, we could look

Table 24.6 Multiple outcomes – difference between outcomes.

		ES	Variance	ES	Correlation	Variance	Weight	ES*WT
Study 1	Reading	0.300	0.050	0.200	0.500	0.050	20.000	4.000
	Math	0.100	0.050					
Study 2	Reading	0.200	0.020	0.100	0.600	0.016	62.500	6.250
	Math	0.100	0.020					
Study 3	Reading	0.400	0.050	0.200	0.600	0.040	25.000	5.000
	Math	0.200	0.050					
Study 4	Reading	0.200	0.010	0.100	0.400	0.012	83.333	8.333
	Math	0.100	0.010					
Study 5	Reading	0.400	0.060	0.100	0.800	0.024	41.667	4.167
	Math	0.300	0.060					
Sum							232.500	27.750

at the difference between (a) math scores and (b) the mean of reading and verbal scores. However, this is beyond the scope of this volume.

Impact of the correlations on the combined effect

One issue to consider is what happens if the correlation between two outcomes is higher in some studies than in others. This variation will affect the *relative weights* assigned to different studies, with more weight going to the study with a higher correlation. In the running example the variances for reading and math were the same in studies 1 and 3, but the correlation between reading and math was higher in study 3. Therefore, study 3 had a lower variance and was assigned *more* weight in the meta-analysis. This is the opposite of what happens for a composite.

A second issue to consider is what happens as the set of correlations as a whole moves toward 1.0. Continuing with the simplified situation where both observations within a study have the same variance (V), if the two observations are independent of each other, the variance of the composite is $2V$. If the observations are not independent of each other, then the variance of the composite is $2V$ times a correction factor. We will refer to this correction factor as the *variance inflation factor* (*VIF*),

$$VIF = 1 - r, \tag{24.13}$$

where r is the correlation between the two components. An increase in r will result in a deflation of the variance compared with treating the different outcomes as independent of each other.

In Table 24.7 we explore how the variance inflation factor depends on the value of r, the correlation coefficient. For the purposes of this illustration we assume the simplistic situation of a study having the same variance ($V_Y = 0.2$) for each outcome. Each column in the table (A-E) corresponds to a different correlation coefficient between these outcomes.

The variance of the difference between the outcomes is

$$V_{Y_{diff}} = 2 \times V_Y \times VIF. \tag{24.14}$$

Taking as an example column C, the correlation is $r = 0.50$ and the variance inflation factor is

$$VIF = 1 - 0.50 = 0.5000.$$

Thus the variance of the composite score for one study is

$$V_{Y_{diff}} = 2 \times 0.20 \times 0.50 = 0.20.$$

As we move from left to right in the table (from a correlation of 0.00 to 0.75) the variance inflation factor (*VIF*) moves from 1.00 to 0.25. If the inflation factor for the variance moves from 1.00 to 0.25, it follows that the inflation factor for the standard error (which is the square root of the variance) will move from 1.00 to 0.50.

Table 24.7 Multiple outcomes – Impact of correlation on the variance of difference.

	A	B	C	D	E
Difference (Y)	0.4	0.4	0.4	0.4	0.4
Variance of each outcome (V)	0.2	0.2	0.2	0.2	0.2
Correlation between outcomes	0.000	0.250	0.500	0.750	1.000
Variance inflation factor	1.000	0.750	0.500	0.250	0.000
Variance of difference ($V_{Y_{diff}}$)	0.400	0.300	0.200	0.100	0.000
Standard error of difference	0.283	0.245	0.200	0.141	0.003
Standard error inflation factor	1.000	0.866	0.707	0.500	0.010
Lower limit	−0.155	−0.0802	0.008	0.124	0.394
Upper limit	0.955	0.8802	0.792	0.676	0.406
p-value (2-tailed)	0.158	0.103	0.046	0.005	0.000

Therefore, the confidence interval will narrow by 50 %, and the Z-value for the test of the null will double.

Note. In this example we focused on correlations in the range of 0.0 to 0.75, columns A-D in the table. As the correlation approaches 1.0 (column E) the variance will approach zero. This means that the width of the confidence interval will approach zero, the Z-value will approach infinity, and the p-value will approach zero. These apparent anomalies reflect what would happen if all error were removed from the equation. In Table 24.7, the correlation displayed as 1.000 is actually entered as 0.9999.

When the correlation is unknown

Table 24.7 also provides a mechanism for working with synthetic variables when we don't know the correlation among outcomes. Earlier, we assumed that the correlation between math and reading was known to be 0.50, and used that value to compute the standard error of the difference and related statistics. In those cases where we don't know the correlation for the study in question, we should still be able to use other studies in the same field to identify a plausible range for the correlation. We could then perform a sensitivity analysis and say, for example, that if the correlation falls in the range of 0.50 to 0.75 then the two-tailed p-value probably falls in the range of 0.046 to 0.005 (columns C to D in the table).

Researchers who do not know the correlation between outcomes sometimes treat the outcomes as coming from independent subgroups. It is instructive, therefore, to consider the practical impact of this choice. Treating the two outcomes as independent of each other yields the same precision as setting the correlation at 0.00 (column A). In effect, then, researchers who take this approach as a way of bypassing the need to specify a correlation, are actually adopting a correlation, albeit implicitly. And, the correlation that they adopt is zero. As such, it is almost certain to overestimate the variance and underestimate the precision of the difference. In this context, (as in the case of a combined effect) the idea of working with a *plausible range of correlations* offers some clear advantages.

SUMMARY POINTS

- When we have effect sizes for more than one outcome (or time-point) within a study, based on the same participants, the information for the different effects is not independent and we need to take account of this in the analysis.
- To compute a summary effect using multiple outcomes we create a synthetic effect size for each study, defined as the mean effect size in that study, with a variance that takes account of the correlation among the different outcomes. We then use this effect size and variance to compute a summary effect across studies. Higher correlations yield *less* precise estimates of the summary effect.
- To compute the difference in effects we create a synthetic effect size for each study, defined as the *difference* between effect sizes in that study, with a variance that takes account of the correlation among the different outcomes. We then use this effect size and variance to assess the difference in effect sizes. Higher correlations yield *more* precise estimates of the difference in effects.

Further Reading

Cooper, H. (1982) Scientific Guidelines for conducting integrative research reviews. *Review of Educational Research*, 52(2), 291–302.

Glaser, L. & Olkin, I. (1994) Stochastically dependent effect sizes. In Cooper, H. & Hedges, L. V., *The Handbook of Research Synthesis*. New York: Russell Sage Foundation.

CHAPTER 25

Multiple Comparisons within a Study

Introduction
Combining across multiple comparisons within a study
Differences between treatments

INTRODUCTION

The final case of a complex data structure is the case where studies use a single control group and several treatment groups. For example, suppose we are working with five studies that assessed the impact of tutoring on student performance. Each study included three groups – a control group (a free study period), intervention *A* (tutoring focused on that day's school lesson) and intervention *B* (tutoring based on a separate agenda).

If our goal was to compute a summary effect for *A* versus control and separately for *B* versus control, we would simply perform two separate meta-analyses, one using the *A* versus control comparison from each study, and one using the *B* versus control comparison from each study.

The issues we address in this chapter are how to proceed when we want to incorporate both treatment groups in the same analysis. Specifically,

- We want to compute a summary effect for the active intervention (combining *A* and *B*) versus control
- Or, we want to investigate the difference in effect size for intervention *A* versus intervention *B*

COMBINING ACROSS MULTIPLE COMPARISONS WITHIN A STUDY

The issue we need to address is that the effect for *A* versus control and the effect for *B* versus control are not independent of each other. If each group (*A*, *B* and control) has 200 participants and we treated the two effects as independent, our effective sample size would appear to be 800 (since we count the control group twice) when in fact the true sample size is 600.

Introduction to Meta-Analysis   M. Borenstein, L. V. Hedges, J. P. T. Higgins, H. R. Rothstein
© 2009, John Wiley & Sons, Ltd

The problem, and the solution, are very similar to the ones we discussed for multiple outcomes (or time-points) within a study. If our goal is to compare *any treatment* versus control, we can create a composite variable which is simply the mean of *A* versus control and *B* versus control. The variance of this composite would be computed based on the variance of each effect size as well as the correlation between the two effects. At that point, all the formulas for combining data from multiple outcomes would apply here as well.

The difference between multiple outcomes and multiple comparison groups is the following. In the case of multiple outcomes, the correlation between outcomes could fall anywhere in the range of zero (or even a negative correlation) to 1.0. We suggested that the researcher work with a range of plausible correlations, but even this approach would typically yield a nontrivial range of possible correlations (say, 0.25 to 0.75) and variances. By contrast, in the case of multiple comparison groups, the correlation can be estimated accurately based on the number of cases in each group. For example, if group *A*, group *B* and the control group each have 200 participants, the correlation between *A* versus control and *B* versus control is 0.50. (This follows from the fact that the correlation between group *A* and group *B* is 0, while the correlation between control and control is 1, yielding a combined correlation midway between the two, or 0.50.) Therefore, we can work with a correlation of 0.50 without the need to conduct a sensitivity analysis based on a range of possible correlations.

This approach can be extended for the case where the sample size differs from one group to the next. For example, we can use a weighted mean of the effects rather than a simple mean, to give more weight to the treatments with more subjects. In this case, we would also need to adjust the variance to take account of the weighting. If the sample size differs from group to group the correlation will no longer be 0.50, but can be estimated precisely based on the data, without the need to resort to external correlations.

An alternate approach for working with multiple comparison groups is to collapse data from the treatment groups and use this data to compute an effect size and variance. If we are working with binary data from one control group and two treatment groups in a 2×3 table we would collapse the two treatment groups to create a 2×2 table, and then compute the effect size from that. Or, if we are working with means and standard deviations for three groups (*A*, *B* and control) we would collapse the data from *A* and *B* to yield a combined mean and standard deviation, and then compute the effect size for the control group versus this merged group (see option 2 for independent subgroups, (23.1), (23.2), and (23.3)). This approach will yield essentially the same results as the method proposed above.

DIFFERENCES BETWEEN TREATMENTS

We now turn to the problem of investigating *differences* between treatments when the different treatments use the same comparison group. To extend the current example, suppose that we have two treatment groups (*A* and *B*) and a control group. We want to know if one of the treatments is superior to the other.

While the approach used for computing a *combined* effect with multiple comparisons was similar to that for multiple outcomes, this is not the case when we turn to *differences* among the treatments. In the case of multiple outcomes, we had an effect size for reading (defined as the difference between treated and control) and an effect size for math (the difference between treated and control). Our approach was to work with the difference between the two effect sizes. In the case of multiple comparisons the analogous approach would be to compute the effect size for *A* versus control, and the effect size for *B* versus control, and then work with the difference between the two effect sizes.

While this approach would work, a better (potentially more powerful) approach is to ignore the control group entirely, and simply define the effect size as the difference between *A* and *B*. If we are working with binary data we would create a 2 x 2 table for *A* versus *B* and use this to compute an effect size. If we are working with means and standard deviations we would compute an effect size from the summary data in these two groups, ignoring the control group entirely.

This approach will only work if all studies have the same groups (here, *A* and *B*), which allows us to create the same effect size (*A* versus *B*) for each study. In practice, we are likely to encounter problems since some studies might compare *A* versus *B*, while others compare *A* versus control and still others compare *B* versus control. Or, some studies might include more than two comparison groups. Methods developed to address these kinds of issues are beyond the scope of this book, but are covered in the further readings.

SUMMARY POINTS

- When a study uses one control group and more than one treatment group, the data from the control group is used to compute more than one effect size. Therefore, the information for these effect sizes is not independent and we need to take this into account when computing the variance.
- To compute a combined effect, ignoring differences among the treatments, we can create a synthetic effect size for each study, defined as the mean effect size in that study (say, the mean of treatment *A* versus control and of treatment *B* versus control), with a variance that takes account of the correlation among the different treatments. We can then use this synthetic effect size and variance to compute a summary effect across studies. This is the same approach used with multiple outcomes.
- To look at differences among treatments the preferred option is to perform a direct comparison of treatment *A* versus treatment *B*, removing the control group from the analysis entirely. In some cases this will not be possible for practical reasons. In this case we can revert to the synthetic effect size, or can apply advanced methods.

Further Reading

Caldwell, D.M., Ades A.E. & Higgins, J.P.T. (2005). Simultaneous comparison of multiple treatments: combining direct and indirect evidence. *BMJ* 331: 897–900.

Glass, G.V, McGaw, B., & Smith, M.L., (1981). *Meta-analysis in Social Research*. Beverly Hills: Sage Publications.

Higgins J.P.T. & Green, S. (eds) (2008). *Cochrane Handbook for Systematic Reviews of Interventions*. Chichester, UK: John Wiley & Sons, Ltd.

Salanti G, Higgins J, Ades A.E. Ioannidis J.P.A. (2008). Evaluation of networks of randomized trials. *Statistical Methods in Medical Research* 17: 279–301.

CHAPTER 26

Notes on Complex Data Structures

Introduction
Summary effect
Differences in effect

INTRODUCTION

In this Part we discussed three cases where studies provide more than one unit of data for the analysis. These are the case of multiple independent subgroups within a study, multiple outcomes or time-points based on the same subjects, and two or more treatment groups that use the same comparison group.

SUMMARY EFFECT

One issue we addressed was how to compute a summary effect using all of the data. For independent subgroups this meant looking at the impact of treatment versus no treatment, and ignoring any differences between stage-1 patients and stage-2 patients. For multiple outcomes this meant looking at the impact of the intervention on basic skills, and ignoring any differences between the impact on math versus reading. For multiple treatment groups it meant looking at the impact of treatment and control, and ignoring any differences among variants of the treatment.

In all cases, the key issue was the need to address any possible redundancy of information, since the precision of the combined effect is strongly dependent on the amount of information. To highlight the difference among the three cases, we used the same numbers in the worked examples as we moved from one chapter to the next. For example, for study 1, we assumed a variance of 0.05 between the two units of information, whether for two independent groups or for two outcomes.

Introduction to Meta-Analysis   M. Borenstein, L. V. Hedges, J. P. T. Higgins, H. R. Rothstein
© 2009, John Wiley & Sons, Ltd

The formula for the variance of a composite is the same in all cases, namely (in its simple form)

$$V_{\bar{Y}} = \frac{1}{2} V_Y(1 + r).$$ (26.1)

Consider, then, how this formula plays out for independent subgroups, for multiple outcomes, and for multiple comparisons.

- For multiple independent subgroups r is always zero, and so the variance of the composite is 0.025.
- For multiple outcomes r can take on any value. We assume that it falls somewhere in the range of 0.00 to 1.00, and assume further that the researcher can provide a range of plausible values for r. For example, we might have evidence that r is probably close to 0.50, with a plausible range of 0.25 to 0.75. In that case the variance would probably be close to 0.038, with a plausible range of 0.031 to 0.044.
- For multiple comparisons r can be determined based on the number of treatment groups and the number of subjects in each groups. If there is one control group and two treatment groups, and the subjects are divided evenly across groups, then r would be 0.50 and the variance would be 0.038. In other cases r could move either up or down, but can always be computed, and therefore we don't need to work with a range of values.

DIFFERENCES IN EFFECT

The second issue we addressed was how to look at the difference between effects.

For independent subgroups this meant looking at whether the treatment was more effective for one of the subgroups (stage-1 or stage-2 patients) than the other. For multiple outcomes this meant looking at whether the intervention had more of an impact on one outcome (reading or m ath) than the other. For multiple treatment groups it meant looking at whether one of the treatments was more effective than the other.

Again, the key issue was the need to address any possible redundancy of information, since the precision of the difference is strongly dependent on the amount of information. To highlight the difference among the three cases we used the same numbers in the worked examples as we moved from one chapter to the next. For example, we assumed a variance of 0.05 for each subgroup, or for each outcome, or for each comparison.

The formula for the variance of a difference is the same in all cases, namely (in its simple form)

$$V_{Y_{diff}} = 2V_Y(1 - r).$$ (26.2)

This formula incorporates the term $(1-r)$, which means that a higher correlation will yield a more precise estimate of the difference. This is the reverse of the case for a composite effect, where the formula incorporates the term $(1 + r)$, and a higher correlation will yield a less precise estimate.

- For multiple independent subgroups r is always zero, and so the variance of the difference is 0.100.
- For multiple outcomes r can take on any value. We assume that it falls somewhere in the range of 0.00 to 1.00, and assume further that the researcher can provide a range of plausible values for r. For example, we might have evidence that r is probably close to 0.50, with a plausible range of 0.25 to 0.75. In that case the variance would probably be close to 0.050, with a plausible range of 0.075 to 0.025.
- For multiple comparisons we have essentially the same situation as for multiple outcomes, except that we can actually compute the correlation needed for the formula. However, there are other approaches available that allow for head-to-head comparisons of the treatment groups.

PART 6

Other Issues

CHAPTER 27

Overview

The first chapter in this Part addresses the issue of vote counting. Vote counting is the name used to describe the idea of seeing how many studies yielded a significant result, and how many did not. We explain why this approach is always a bad idea. In fact, if the techniques used in meta-analysis are extensions of procedures in primary studies, then vote counting for multiple studies is an extension of a mistake that is ubiquitous in primary studies.

In the next chapter we address the issue of statistical power in meta-analysis. A meta-analysis often yields a more powerful test of the null hypothesis than any of the separate studies. Here, we explain why this is true, and offer some examples to show how important this can be. At the same time, we caution that this is not always the case. While there is a general perception that all meta-analyses have high power to yield a statistically significant effect, this is not always the case for the main effect, and is rarely the case for other tests (such as tests for heterogeneity). We discuss the factors that drive power in a meta-analysis, and compare these with the factors that drive power in a primary study.

Another chapter outlines the issue of publication bias. Several lines of evidence demonstrate that studies that yield larger effect sizes are more likely to be published, and incorporated in a meta-analysis, than similar studies that yield smaller effect sizes. We discuss the evidence for this phenomenon, and methods to assess its likely impact on any given meta-analysis.

Introduction to Meta-Analysis   M. Borenstein, L. V. Hedges, J. P. T. Higgins, H. R. Rothstein
© 2009 John Wiley & Sons, Ltd

CHAPTER 28

Vote Counting – A New Name for an Old Problem

Introduction
Why vote counting is wrong
Vote counting is a pervasive problem

INTRODUCTION

One question we often ask of the data is whether or not it allows us to reject the null hypothesis of no effect. Researchers who address this question using a narrative review need to synthesize the p-values reported by the separate studies. Since these are discrete pieces of information and the narrative review provides no statistical mechanism for synthesizing these values, narrative reviewers often resort to a process called vote counting. Under this process the reviewer counts the number of statistically significant studies and compares this with the number of statistically nonsignificant studies.

In some cases this process has been formalized, such that one actually counts the number of significant and nonsignificant p-values and picks the winner. In some variants, the reviewer would look for a clear majority rather than a simple majority. Or, the reviewer might not work directly with the p-values, but with the discussion section of the papers which are based on the p-values.

One might think that summarizing p-values through a vote-counting procedure would yield more accurate decision than any one of the single significance tests being summarized. This is not generally the case, however. In fact, Hedges and Olkin (1980) showed that the power of vote-counting considered as a statistical decision procedure can not only be lower than that of the studies on which it is based, the power of vote counting can tend toward zero as the number of studies increases. In other words, vote counting is not only misleading, it tends to be *more* misleading as the amount of evidence (the number of studies) increases!

Introduction to Meta-Analysis   M. Borenstein, L. V. Hedges, J. P. T. Higgins, H. R. Rothstein
© 2009, John Wiley & Sons, Ltd

In any event, the idea of vote counting is fundamentally flawed and the variants on this process are equally flawed (and perhaps even more dangerous, since the basic flaw is less obvious when hidden behind a more complicated algorithm or is one step removed from the p-value). Our goal in this chapter is to explain why this is so, and to provide a few examples.

WHY VOTE COUNTING IS WRONG

The logic of vote counting says that a significant finding is evidence that an effect exists, while a nonsignificant finding is evidence that an effect is absent. While the first statement is true, the second is not. While a nonsignificant finding *could* be due to the fact that the true effect is nil, it can also be due simply to low statistical power.

Put simply, the p-value reported for any study is a function of the observed effect size and the sample size. Even if the observed effect is substantial, the p-value will not be significant unless the sample size is adequate. In other words, as most of us learned in our first statistics course, *the absence of a statistically significant effect is not evidence that an effect is absent*.

For example, suppose five randomized controlled trials (RCTs) had been performed to test the impact of an intervention, and that none were statistically significant (the p-value in each case is 0.265) as illustrated in Figure 28.1. The vote count is 5 to 0 against an effect, and one might assume that the intervention has no effect.

By contrast, the meta-analysis (Figure 28.1), by combining the information into a single analysis, allows us to perform a proper test of the null. Not only is this approach valid, but the test of the summary effect is often much more powerful than tests performed on any of the separate studies. When we merge the data, the effect size stays the same, but the confidence interval narrows and no longer includes the null. The p-value for each study alone is 0.265, but the p-value for the summary effect is

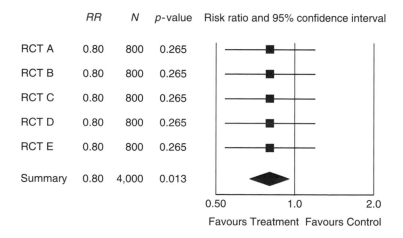

Figure 28.1 The p-value for each study is > 0.20 but the p-value for the summary effect is < 0.02.

0.013. Clearly, the absence of significance in each study is due to a lack of precision rather than a small effect.

For purposes of explaining why vote counting is a bad idea, we could end the chapter here. However, because vote counting in its various forms is so pervasive, we will expand on this idea to show how the basic mistake that underlies vote counting affects much of the literature, and how meta-analysis can help address this problem.

VOTE COUNTING IS A PERVASIVE PROBLEM

While the term vote counting is associated with narrative reviews it can also be applied to the single study, where a significant *p*-value is taken as evidence that an effect exists, and a nonsignificant *p*-value is taken as evidence that an effect does not exist. Numerous surveys in a wide variety of substantive fields have repeatedly documented the ubiquitous nature of this mistake.

In medicine, for example, Freiman, Chalmers, Smith and Kuebler (1978) surveyed reports of controlled clinical trials that had been published in a number of medical journals (primarily *The Lancet*, the *New England Journal of Medicine*, and the *Journal of the American Medical Association* during the period 1960–1977), and selected 71 that had reported negative results. The authors found that if the true drug effect had been in the region of 50% (e.g. a mortality rate of 30% for placebo vs. 15% for drug), median power would have been 60%. In other words, even if the drug cut the mortality rate in half there was still a 40% probability that the study would have failed to obtain a statistically significant result.

The authors went on to make the following point: Despite the fact that power was terribly low, in most cases the absence of statistical significance was interpreted as meaning that the drug *was not effective*. They wrote: 'The conclusion is inescapable that many of the therapies discarded as ineffective after inconclusive "negative" trials may still have a clinically meaningful effect' (p. 694). In fact, it is possible (or likely) that some of the therapies discarded on this basis might well have had very substantial therapeutic effects.

In the social sciences Cohen (1962) surveyed papers published in the *Journal of Abnormal and Social Psychology* in 1960. Mean power to detect a small, medium, or large effect, respectively, was 0.18, 0.48, and 0.83. Cohen noted that despite the low power, when the studies with *negative* results are published, readers tend to interpret the absence of statistical significance as evidence that the treatment has been proven ineffective.

In the years that followed a kind of cottage industry developed of publishing papers that documented the fact of low power in any number of journals in the area of behavioral research. Many of these are cited in Sedlmeier and Gigerenzer (1989) and Rossi (1990). Similar papers were published to document the same problem in the field of medicine (Borenstein, 1994; Hartung, Cottrell & Giffen, 1983; Phillips,

Scott, & Blasczcynski, 1983; Reed & Slaichert, 1981; Reynolds, 1980) and psychiatry (Kane & Borenstein, 1985).

Sedlmeier and Gigerenzer (1989) published a paper entitled *Do studies of statistical power have an effect on the power of statistical studies?* They found that in the 25 years since Cohen's initial survey power had not changed in any substantive way. Similarly, Rossi (1990) reviewed papers published in 1982 in the *Journals of Abnormal Psychology*, *Consulting and Clinical Psychology*, and *Personality and Social Psychology*. Mean power to detect small, medium, and large effects, respectively, was 0.17, 0.57, and 0.83.

This led one of the current authors (Borenstein, 2000) to propose four theorems, as follows.

1. Power in many fields of research is abysmally low.
2. Rule (1) appears to be impervious to change.
3. The absence of significance should be interpreted as *more information is required* but is interpreted in error as meaning *no effect exists.*
4. Rule (3) appears to be impervious to change.

In a sense, then, vote counting did not originate with the narrative review. Rather, the basic mistake has existed for decades, where it found a home in primary research. When the field moved on to narrative reviews, this basic mistake was named and codified but remained basically unchanged.

There is, however, one important difference. When we are working with a single study and we have a nonsignificant result we don't have any way of knowing whether or not the effect is real. The nonsignificant *p*-value could reflect either the fact that the true effect is nil *or* the fact that our study had low power. While we caution against accepting the former (that the true effect is nil) we cannot rule it out.

By contrast, when we use meta-analysis to synthesize the data from a series of studies we can often identify the true effect. And in many cases (for example if the true effect is substantial and is consistent across studies) we can assert that the nonsignificant *p*-value in the separate studies was due to low power rather than the absence of an effect.

In the streptokinase meta-analysis on page 10, for example, it is clear that the treatment does reduce the risk of death. It is fair to say that the reason that 27 studies had nonsignificant *p*-values was *not* because the treatment had no effect, but rather was because of low statistical power. (In the next chapter we actually compute the power for the streptokinase studies.)

Moving beyond the null

In this chapter we have shown that *if our goal* is to test the null hypothesis, then meta-analysis (unlike the narrative review) provides a statistically sound mechanism for this purpose. However, we want to emphasize that meta-analysis allows us *to move beyond a test of the null.* It allows us to assess the magnitude of the effect (which is often a more relevant question) and to determine whether or not the effect size is consistent across studies.

SUMMARY POINTS

- Vote counting is the process of counting the number of studies that are statistically significant and comparing this with the number that are not statistically significant.
- Vote counting treats a nonsignificant p-value as evidence that an effect is absent. In fact, though, small, moderate, and even large effect sizes may yield a nonsignificant p-value due to inadequate statistical power. Therefore, vote counting is never a valid approach.

CHAPTER 29

Power Analysis for Meta-Analysis

INTRODUCTION

A common goal in research (both in primary studies and in meta-analysis) is to test the null hypothesis of no effect. If that is our goal, then it is important to ensure that the study has good statistical power (a sufficiently high likelihood of yielding a statistically significant result). In this chapter we pursue two themes related to statistical power.

The first theme is conceptual. We discuss the factors that determine power and explore how the value of these factors may change as we move from a primary study to a meta-analysis. On this basis we can see why power for a meta-analyses is sometimes (but not always) higher than power in any of the included studies. Here, we address only power for a test of the main effect.

The second theme is practical. We briefly review the process of power analysis for primary studies, and then show how the same process can be extended for meta-analysis. Here, we focus primarily on power for a test of the main effect, but also include material on tests of heterogeneity.

A CONCEPTUAL APPROACH

Background

The significance test (performed *after* the study is completed) takes the form

Introduction to Meta-Analysis   M. Borenstein, L. V. Hedges, J. P. T. Higgins, H. R. Rothstein
© 2009, John Wiley & Sons, Ltd

$$Z = \frac{M}{SE_M} \qquad (29.1)$$

where Z is the test statistic, M is the effect size, and SE_M is the standard error of the effect size. The observed value of Z is then compared with the criterion alpha (α). If alpha has been set at 0.05, then a p-value lower than 0.05 (a Z-value beyond ± 1.96) will be statistically significant.

Therefore, the likelihood that the results will be statistically significant depends on the following.

- The effect size. As M increases, Z increases, and the likelihood of statistical significance increases.
- The precision of the estimate. As the precision increases (as SE_M *decreases*), Z increases, and the likelihood of statistical significance increases.
- The criterion for significance (α). As α moves away from zero, the likelihood that p will be less than α increases, and the likelihood of statistical significance increases.

The difference between the significance test and a power analysis is that we perform the significance test *after* the data have been collected, at which point M, SE_M, and α are known. By contrast, when we compute power (usually, *before* the study has been performed) we need to make an assumption about M, an educated guess about SE_M, and select a value for α. As such, we are working with projected values rather than observed values. Still, the factors that control power are the same as those that control the significance test. To wit, as the expected effect size increases, as the precision of the estimate increases, and/or as α is moved away from zero, the higher the power.

Power for meta-analyses as compared with primary studies

With this as background we can anticipate how power considerations differ between primary studies and meta-analysis. Typically, the expected effect size and the criterion for significance (α) will be the same for the primary study and for the meta-analysis. However, the precision will differ (sometimes substantially) as we move from primary studies to a meta-analysis.

To get a sense of how the precision changes as we move from the individual studies to the summary effect we can work with the confidence intervals on the forest plot. Concretely, the width of each confidence interval (the distance from the lower limit to the upper limit) is proportional to the standard error (the denominator in (29.1)).

For example, consider the Cannon *et al.* meta-analysis that we discussed in Chapter 1. The width of the confidence interval is substantially narrower for the summary effect than for any of the included studies. Therefore, power to test the summary effect in the meta-analysis is substantially higher than power to test the effect in any of the primary studies. Assuming a risk ratio of 85% and a baseline risk of 9.4%

(the mean values actually observed in these studies), power for the four studies (Prove-it, A to Z, TNT, Ideal) was 36%, 39%, 70%, and 65%, respectively. Therefore, it is not surprising that three of the studies failed to meet the criterion for significance, with only one (TNT) yielding a p-value under 0.05. By contrast, if we synthesize the effects in a meta-analysis, the combined sample size is 13,774, the statistical power is 83%, and the observed p-value is < 0.0001.

Similarly, in Chapter 2 we discussed a meta-analysis of 33 trials that tested the impact of streptokinase (versus placebo) to prevent death following a heart attack. Again, the confidence interval is narrower for the summary effect than for any of the included studies, and (except for the largest primary studies) the difference is substantial. Assuming that streptokinase actually reduces the risk of death by some 20% (which is the summary risk ratio for this data), then based on the sample size and event rates in the studies we can determine that only three had power exceeding 80%. Of the remaining 30 studies, none had power in the range of 60% to 80%, 3 had power in the range of 40% to 60%, 6 had power in the range of 20% to 40%, and 21 had power of less than 20%. Therefore, it is not surprising that only six of the 33 studies were statistically significant. By contrast, when we combine the effects from these studies in a meta-analysis the power for the summary effect exceeds 99.9% and the p-value for the summary effect is 0.0000008.

The fact that a meta-analysis will often have high power is important because (as in these examples) primary studies often suffer from low power. While researchers are encouraged to design studies with power of at least 80%, this goal is often elusive. Many studies in medicine, psychology, education and an array of other fields have power substantially lower than 80% to detect large effects, and substantially lower than 50% to detect smaller effects that are still important enough to be of theoretical or practical importance. By contrast, a meta-analysis based on multiple studies will have a higher total sample size than any of the separate studies and the increase in power can be substantial.

The problem of low power in the primary studies is especially acute when looking for adverse events. The problem here is that studies to test new drugs are *powered* to find a treatment effect for the drug, and do not have adequate power to detect side effects (which have a much lower event rate, and therefore lower power). For example, a recent meta-analysis synthesized data from 44 studies and suggested that *Avandia* may increase the risk of death or myocardial infarction (MI). Because the risk of death or MI is very low, power in the individual studies was quite low. Two of the studies had power of 15% and 18%. The other 42 studies had power of less than 8%. (These computations are based on the event rates and effect sizes combined across the 44 studies.) By contrast, the meta-analysis had power of 66% and a p-value that either met or approached the 0.05 criterion (this depends on the method used in the analysis).

While the examples such as the streptokinase analysis and the statins analysis, where the meta-analysis had high power, are representative of *many* meta-analyses, they are not representative of *all* meta-analyses. Assuming a nontrivial effect size, power is primarily a function of the precision, and so to understand why some meta-analyses will have high power while others (with a similar effect size) will not, we need to consider the factors that control precision, as follows.

Power under the fixed-effect model

When we are working with a fixed-effect analysis, precision for the summary effect is always higher than it is for any of the included studies. Under the fixed-effect analysis precision is largely determined by the total sample size (accumulated over all studies in the analysis), and it follows the total sample size will be higher across studies than within studies. If the analysis includes a large number of small studies, the difference in power can be substantial.

Consider a meta-analysis of k studies with the simplest design, such that each study comprises a single sample of n observations with standard deviation σ. When the effect size *is consistent* across studies we saw in Chapter 13 that the standard error of the mean, SE_M, is given by (Box 13.1)

$$SE_M = \sqrt{\frac{\sigma^2}{k \times n}}\,. \tag{29.2}$$

Because k (the number of studies) and n (the sample size in each study) appear together, SE_M (and therefore the power) of a fixed-effect meta-analysis will depend only on the total sample size $k \times n$. The power will be the same for a meta-analysis with 10 studies of 100 persons each, as it would be for one primary study with 1000 persons.

As the term $k \times n$ approaches infinity the standard error will approach zero and (provided that the effect size is nonzero) power will approach 100%.

Power under the random-effects model

By contrast, when we move to a random-effects analysis we need to deal with two sources of error. One is the error within studies, and the other is the variance between studies. (The latter is *real* variance, but we refer to it here as error in the sense that it leads to uncertainty in the value of the mean effect.) Now, we can no longer use sample size as a surrogate for precision. Rather, we need to compute the precision based on both components.

Under the random-effects model we saw in Chapter 13 that the standard error of the summary effect is given by

$$SE_{M^*} = \sqrt{\frac{\sigma^2}{k \times n} + \frac{\tau^2}{k}}\,. \tag{29.3}$$

The first term is identical to that for the fixed-effect model and, again, with a large enough sample size (either enough studies or a large enough sample within studies), this term will approach zero. By contrast, the second term (which reflects the between-studies variance) will only approach zero if the estimated value of τ^2 is zero, or as the number of *studies* approaches infinity.

These formulas do not apply exactly in practice, but the conceptual point does. Concretely, in a random-effects meta-analysis, power depends on within-study error and between-studies variation. If the effect sizes are reasonably consistent from study to study, and/or if the analysis includes a substantial number of studies, then the second of these will tend to be small, and power will be driven by the cumulative sample size. In this case the meta-analysis will tend to have higher power than any of the included studies. This was the case for the statins analysis and for the streptokinase analysis. However, if the effect size varies substantially from study to study, and the analysis includes only a few studies, then this second aspect will limit the potential power of the meta-analysis. In this case, power could be limited to some low value even if the analysis includes tens of thousands of persons.

Above, we suggested that one can get a sense for the power of the summary effect (as compared with power for the included studies) by comparing the confidence interval width in the two. The same logic extends to the difference in power between fixed-effect and random-effects analyses. If the width of the confidence interval is roughly the same in the two, then power will be roughly the same. By contrast, if the random-effects interval is substantially wider then power will be lower and, depending on the effect size, may not approach acceptable levels.

IN CONTEXT

Power to test main effects

There is a general perception that meta-analyses have high power to detect main effects, probably stemming from some well known meta-analyses that did include large numbers of studies and therefore had high power. The Cannon *et al.* and the streptokinase studies are two examples. A number of recent reviews in the social sciences (e.g. Wilson *et al.*, 2003a, 2003b) have included more than 200 studies each.

However, most meta-analyses have far fewer studies than this. The Cochrane Database of Systematic Reviews is a database of systematic reviews, primarily of randomized trials, for medical interventions in all areas of healthcare, and currently includes over 3000 reviews. In this database, the median number of trials included in a review is six. When a review includes only six studies, power to detect even a moderately large effect, let alone a small one, can be well under 80%. While the median number of studies in a review differs by the field of research, in almost any field we do find some reviews based on a small number of studies, and so we cannot simply assume that power is high.

Power for tests comparing subgroups, and for meta-regression

Even when power to test the main effect is high, many meta-analyses are not concerned with the main effect at all, but are performed solely to assess the impact of covariates (or moderator variables). For example, we might know that an intervention increases the survival time for patients with a specific form of cancer. The question to be addressed is not whether the treatment works, but whether one variant of the treatment is more effective than another variant.

The test of a moderator variable in a meta-analysis is akin to the test of an interaction in a primary study, and both suffer from the same factors that tend to decrease power. First, the *effect size* is actually the difference between the two effect sizes and so is almost invariably smaller than the main effect size. Second, the sample size within groups is (by definition) smaller than the total sample size. Therefore, power for testing the moderator will often be very low (Hedges and Pigott, 2004). The fact of low power for tests of the effects of covariates is especially important because these kinds of analyses are often carried out in order to demonstrate that the moderator variables don't have an effect – i.e. to *accept* the null hypothesis. The logic of accepting the null is based on the assumption of high power, and that assumption is rarely tested.

Power for tests of homogeneity, or goodness of fit

Typically, an analysis that looks at the main effect is accompanied by a test of homogeneity. Here, a nonsignificant *p*-value might be taken to mean that the treatment effect is consistent across studies. Similarly, an analysis that looks at covariates (by comparing subgroups or using meta-regression) is often followed by a test for goodness of fit, and a nonsignificant *p*-value is taken to mean that the covariates explain all the variance. In fact, though, these kinds of analyses routinely suffer from low power. Power analysis could help researchers to recognize this fact, and refrain from drawing (possibly incorrect) conclusions based on the fact that the results are not statistically significant.

WHEN TO USE POWER ANALYSIS

In primary studies, power analysis is used primarily to determine an appropriate sample size, since this is largely under the control of the investigators. For example, researchers might modify the sample size by changing the planned enrollment period, or the number of sites, or by changing the inclusion criteria for the study. In meta-analysis the issues are rather different because the studies already exist, but there are some parallels. We have some control over the number of studies, since the inclusion criteria could be modified to include more or fewer studies. For example, if it looks as if we will not be able to obtain enough studies to yield adequate power we might consider widening the inclusion criteria, to include studies with a wider range of types of participants. Conversely, if there appears to be an abundance of studies we may elect to narrow the inclusion criteria. Altering the inclusion criteria changes the question being addressed by the review, however, and in most situations it is more appropriate to answer the original question than to adjust it because of power considerations.

While most meta-analyses are planned after the primary studies have already been performed, there are some initiatives underway to plan the meta-analyses prospectively. For example, a consortium of hospitals may plan to perform a series of studies with the goal of incorporating all of these studies into a meta-analysis. In this case, the goal might be to ensure good power for the summary effect, rather than for the individual studies. In this situation, the meta-analyst may have direct influence over the sample sizes of the individual studies and the number of studies (or hospitals). We have seen in this chapter that power considerations depend on the intended meta-analysis model. In particular, for a fixed-effect meta-analysis only the total sample size across studies is important, whereas for a random-effects meta-analysis the option of using five hospitals with 1000 patients each (for a total of 5000 patients) versus ten hospitals with 500 patients each (for the same total) can yield substantially different values for power.

A power analysis should be performed when the review is being planned, and not after the review has been completed. Researchers sometimes conduct a power analysis after the fact, and report that *Power was low, and therefore the absence of a significant effect is not informative*. While this is correct, it is preferable to address the same question by simply reporting the observed effect size with its confidence interval. For example, *The effect size is 0.4 with a confidence interval of −0.10 to +0.90* is much more informative than the statement that *Power was low*. The statement of effect size with confidence intervals not only makes it clear that we cannot rule out a clinically important effect, but also gives a range for what this effect might be (here, as low as −0.10 and as high as +0.90).

PLANNING FOR PRECISION RATHER THAN FOR POWER

A power analysis can focus directly on power (the likelihood of a test giving a statistically significant result) or may focus on precision (the likelihood that a confidence interval will be a specific width). The two approaches are closely related, although the latter is more straightforward. As we shall see below, estimating precision is an early step on the way towards estimating power. We shall define precision formally as one divided by the variance.

POWER ANALYSIS IN PRIMARY STUDIES

The formulas for power analysis are very similar for meta-analysis and for primary studies. Before turning to meta-analysis we review some key issues in power analysis for primary studies, to provide a context.

The statistical significance computed *after* the data are collected is a function of three elements: the true effect size, the precision with which it is estimated (strongly dependent on sample size) and the criterion used for statistical significance (alpha). A study is more likely to be statistically significant if the effect size is large, the precision is high or criterion for statistical significance is liberal (i.e. alpha is large).

Power, which is simply a prediction about statistical significance, is determined by the same three elements in the same way.

This parallel is obvious in the formulas for significance and for power. Consider a significance test based on a test statistic, Z. The observed value is computed as

$$Z = \frac{M}{\sqrt{V_M}}, \tag{29.4}$$

where M is an estimate of effect size *from the data* and V_M its variance. This Z value is evaluated with reference to the standard normal distribution, with a two-tailed p-value of

$$p = 2[1 - \Phi(|Z|)]. \tag{29.5}$$

In power analysis we consider the distribution of Z, not under the null hypothesis, but under specific alternatives. We will use a parameter lambda (λ) to represent an alternative true value of Z, defined as

$$\lambda = \frac{\delta}{\sqrt{V_\delta}}, \tag{29.6}$$

where δ is the true effect size, and V_δ its variance.

Note: we are using V_δ for both the true variance in (the Z equation) and λ in (the lambda equation). Strictly, these are different and might be notated differently. However, in meta-analysis we do not usually distinguish between the two (we assume the estimated variances are known) so we will not in this chapter.

The power of a study is the probability of observing values of Z that are statistically significant when the true mean of Z is λ. For a two-tailed test,

$$\text{Power} = (1 - \Phi(c_\alpha - \lambda)) + \Phi(-c_\alpha - \lambda), \tag{29.7}$$

where c_α is the critical value of Z associated with significance level α (thus, for $\alpha = 0.05$, $c_\alpha = 1.96$).

The actual computation of power for a given effect size (δ), precision ($1/V_\delta$), and α is usually straightforward. In power analysis the challenge is to identify a plausible range of values for each of these factors in order to determine values for the power of the study in realistic circumstances. The same formulas are used for sample size calculations, in which the power, effect size and α are fixed, and the required value of V_δ is computed. From V_δ, a sample size to meet these criteria can be computed. In the following discussion we focus mainly on the investigation of power rather than the computation of sample size.

Finding a range of values for the effect size

The effect size used to compute power is defined as the true (population) effect size. However, since we don't actually know the population effect size we must select a number to serve that function. In a sample size calculation, we use the smallest effect size that it would be important to detect, and this depends entirely on the context of the study. For example, if we are looking at a treatment to reduce risk of death we might decide that even a small effect is important. By contrast, if we are looking at treatment to reduce the risk of flu, we might decide that only a relatively large effect is worth detecting.

In power analysis, we must pick plausible values for the effect size, and usually a range of values is investigated. This range should be based on substantive or clinical importance, and where possible should be informed by available data. For example, if we are working with a class of drugs that typically yields a 10–15% reduction in events, then we should probably use an effect size that falls in (or near) this range. Prior studies or a pilot study can help to identify a plausible range, and researchers may also fall back on the use of conventions, such as Cohen's proposals for small, medium and large effects in social science research (Cohen, 1987).

Finding a range of values for the precision

The major determinant of precision is sample size. The range of possible sample sizes will be determined by practical constraints, which will vary substantially from one study to the next. For a primary experimental study, a pilot study may provide information about the potential sample size by showing how many people can be enrolled over a given period of time.

Other determinants of precision depend on the type of data being collected. For example, for continuous outcomes, precision depends on the inherent variability across individuals, expressed using the standard deviation.

Finding a range of values for significance level (α)

In any significance test we need to balance the risk of a type I error (the true effect is zero but we reject the null) and a type II error (the true effect is not zero but we fail to reject the null). As we move the criterion for significance (alpha) toward zero we reduce the risk of a type I error but increase risk of a type II error.

There is a common convention that alpha should be set at 0.05 (or 5%) and power at 80%, which makes sense if the damage associated with a type I error is four times as severe as that associated with a type II error (with power at 80%, the risk of a type II error is 20%, which is four times the risk of a type I error). In fact, though, it would be better to adjust these risks as appropriate for a given study. For example, if a positive result will be seen as definitive and result in an immediate change in clinical practice, we would want to protect against a type I error and would therefore use a conservative value of alpha (say, 0.01). On the other hand, if a significant result will lead to other trials to replicate the effect, while a nonsignificant result will discourage further research of the treatment, we might be more concerned with a type II error. In this case we might use a more liberal value of alpha (say 0.10) as a mechanism to increase power.

Illustrative example

Suppose that we plan to investigate the impact of a drug to reduce pain from migraine headaches. Patients will be allocated at random to either treatment or placebo, and assessed after two hours on a 100-point scale. The standard deviation of scores on this scale is 10. We plan to perform this study in a hospital's migraine clinic, where we can enroll about 10 patients a month, and we wish to use a significance level of $\alpha = 0.05$. Suppose it is proposed that the study runs for five months. During this period we can recruit 25 patients per group. Patients report that a difference of 2 to 4 points on this scale (corresponding to a standardized mean difference of 0.2 or 0.4) would represent a meaningful effect to them, and this effect is consistent with data from previous studies.

The effect size index is d with two independent groups, and so we compute the variance using (4.20),

$$V_d = \frac{n_1 + n_2}{n_1 \times n_2} + \frac{d^2}{2(n_1 + n_2)} . \tag{29.8}$$

For our sample size of 25 and effect size of 0.3, we can estimate this variance as

$$V_d = \frac{25 + 25}{25 \times 25} + \frac{0.30^2}{2(25 + 25)} = 0.0809 .$$

The parameter λ is given by

$$\lambda = \frac{0.30}{\sqrt{0.0809}} = 1.0547 .$$

The Z-value required for significance with alpha (2-tailed) of 0.05 is

$$c_\alpha = \Phi(1 - 0.05/2) = 1.96.$$

In Excel $=$NORMSINV$(1 - 0.05/2) = $ returns 1.96, and finally,

$$\text{Power} = 1 - \Phi(1.96 - 1.0547) + \Phi(-1.96 - 1.0547) = 0.1840.$$

In Excel, $=$1-NORMSDIST$(1.96 - 1.0547) + $ NORMSDIST$(-1.96 - 1.0547) = 0.1840$.

In words, the power to detect an effect size of 0.30 is 0.184, or 18.4%. This is obviously much lower than the values of 80% or 90% that are typically desirable in a randomized trial. By applying the same formula while varying the effect size (0.20, 0.30, 0.40) and sample size (from 10 to 300 per group) we can create a graph that displays the power of the study under different scenarios.

Figure 29.1 shows power as a function of sample size for $\delta = 0.40, 0.30$, and 0.20, assuming alpha, two-tailed, is set at 0.05. Reading left to right at 0.90 on the Y axis, to yield power of 90% for a large, medium or small effect we would need a sample size of around 140, 240, or more than 300 per group. We might then decide to enroll 240 patients per group, which will allow us to complete the study in 48 months. Reading from top to bottom at 240 on the X axis, the study will have power of about

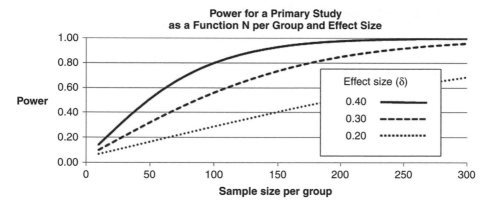

Figure 29.1 Power for a primary study as a function of n and δ.

99% to detect the larger effect of 0.40, 90% to detect the moderate effect of 0.30, and 60% to detect the smaller effect of 0.20.

With this as prologue we can turn to meta-analysis and consider how the process is analogous to that for the primary study, and how it differs.

POWER ANALYSIS FOR META-ANALYSIS

Power analysis for a main effect

The logic of power analysis for meta-analysis is very similar to the logic of power analysis for primary studies. Again, we could either investigate how power is likely to depend on plausible values of the effect size, precision and alpha, or we could compute a precision for a given effect size, alpha and power. In meta-analysis, the precision reflects both the sample sizes of the studies *and* the number of studies. When using power analysis to compute the precision, we therefore need to consider both aspects of sample size. There are differences in the implications of precision of sample sizes, depending on whether we adopt a fixed-effect or random-effects model for the meta-analysis.

For power analysis, plausible values for the effect size and precision are needed. Alpha should be chosen to reflect the potential impact of a type I error. The effect sizes should be based on substantive issues ('What effect size would it be important to detect?'). Both the effect size and the precision could be informed by a pilot study. In a primary study this might mean actually performing the study on a small scale to get a sense of the likely effect size as well as the number of persons who might be recruited. In the meta-analysis this might mean locating and coding a subset of the literature to get a sense of the effect sizes, of the sample sizes within studies, and also of the number of studies that meet the inclusion criteria.

In this chapter, we assume that every study has the same precision (in the notation of Part 3, V_{Y_i} is the same in every study). For a discussion of power analysis when the V_{Y_i} are not equal, see Hedges and Pigott (2001).

Power for main effect using fixed-effect model

The formulas for significance and for power have the same structure as they did for primary studies. Concretely, the test of significance for the main effect in a fixed-effect meta-analysis is based on a test statistic Z, computed as

$$Z = \frac{M}{\sqrt{V_M}}, \tag{29.9}$$

but M and V_M are now the effect size and variance of the *summary effect* observed in the synthesis rather than for a single study. Recall that V_M is calculated as one divided by the sum of the weights awarded to the individual studies, where the weights are inverse-variances. If all studies had the same variance, say V_Y, then V_M is equivalent to V_Y/k, where k is the number of studies.

As before, Z is evaluated with reference to the standard normal distribution which yields the corresponding p-value. For a two-tailed test,

$$p = 2[1 - (\Phi(|Z|))]. \tag{29.10}$$

Similarly, power analysis is again based on lambda (λ), defined as

$$\lambda = \frac{\delta}{\sqrt{V_\delta}}, \tag{29.11}$$

but now δ and V_δ are the (hypothesized) *true* effect size and its variance for the summary effect. As before, the power formula for a two-tailed test is

$$\text{Power} = 1 - \Phi(c_\alpha - \lambda) + \Phi(-c_\alpha - \lambda). \tag{29.12}$$

Illustrative example

Above, we presented the power analysis for a primary study to assess the impact of a treatment for migraine headaches. For a single study with $n = 25$ per group, assuming an effect size of 0.30, we computed the variance as 0.0809, lambda as 1.0547, and power as 0.18.

Suppose that we are planning a meta-analysis to address the same question and instead of a single study with $n = 25$ per group, we have ten studies where each has this sample size. Since the variance of a single study is

$$\frac{25 + 25}{25 \times 25} + \frac{0.30^2}{2(25 + 25)} = 0.0809,$$

the variance of the summary effect is

$$V_M = \frac{0.0809}{10} = 0.00809.$$

Then, lambda is

$$\lambda = \frac{0.30}{\sqrt{0.00809}} = 3.3354,$$

$$C_\alpha = \Phi(1 - 0.05/2) = 1.96,$$

and

$$Power = 1 - \Phi(1.96 - 3.3354) + \Phi(-1.96 - 3.3354) = 0.9155.$$

In Excel, =NORMSINV$(1 - 0.05/2)$ returns 1.96, and
= 1-NORMSDIST$(1.96 - 3.3354)$ + NORMSDIST$(-1.96 - 3.3354)$ returns 0.9155.

In other words, while the formula for power is identical to the formula for a primary study, the variance is reduced by a factor of k (the number of studies), which yields a k-fold increase in lambda and an increase in power.

We can apply the formula while varying the effect size and the number of studies to graph power as a function of effect size and number of studies. In Figure 29.2 we assume an n of 25 per group within each study, alpha (2-tailed) of 0.05 and a fixed-effect model. The graph shows power for an effect size (δ) of 0.4, 0.3, 0.2, and the number of studies varies from 1 to 25.

Reading from left to right, to ensure power of 90% for an effect size of 0.40, 0.30 or 0.20 we would need 6 studies, 10 studies, or 22 studies. Suppose that it becomes clear from a pilot study that there are likely to be at least 20 studies that meet the inclusion criteria. At that point, the researchers might decide to proceed as planned. Based on this number, and reading the graph from top to bottom, if the true effect is 0.40 or 0.30 power will exceed 99%, and if the true effect is 0.20, power will approach 90%.

By contrast, if it seemed that there would be only 5 or 10 studies that met the inclusion criteria the reviewers might wish to obtain a more accurate estimate of the number (the difference between 5 and 10 is important). Alternatively, there may be

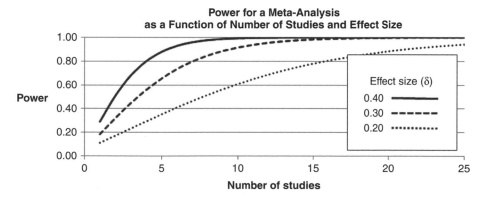

Figure 29.2 Power for a meta-analysis as a function of number studies and δ.

reasonable ways of modifying the research question to increase the number of relevant studies.

Power for main effect using random-effects model

The formulas for significance and for power under the random-effects model have the same structure as those for a fixed effect meta-analysis. Using the notation introduced in Chapter 12 where an asterisk (*) indicates that a statistic is based on random-effects variance, the test of significance for the main effect is still based on a test statistic (for example) Z^*, computed as

$$Z^* = \frac{M^*}{\sqrt{V_{M^*}}} , \tag{29.13}$$

but M^* and V_{M^*} are now the estimated mean effect size and its variance using random-effects weights. As before, Z^* is evaluated with reference to the standard normal distribution which yields the corresponding p-value. For a two-tailed test,

$$p^* = 2[1 - (\Phi(|Z^*|))] . \tag{29.14}$$

Similarly, power analysis is still based on lambda (λ^*), defined as

$$\lambda^* = \frac{\delta^*}{\sqrt{V_{\delta^*}}} , \tag{29.15}$$

but now δ^* and V_{δ^*} are the true mean effect size and its variance for the summary effect. The variance incorporates variance within studies and variance between studies. Consider the simple situation in which each study has the same within-study variance, say V_Y. Then the variance may be written as

$$V_\delta^* = \frac{V_Y + \tau^2}{k} , \tag{29.16}$$

Plausible values of the within-study variance, V_Y, might be obtained using the same procedures as those used for the fixed-effect model. Plausible values of the between-studies variance, τ^2, might be obtained using data from the pilot study, by computing the effect sizes for the studies gathered as part of the pilot and looking at how much these effects actually vary from study to study. Alternatively, the between-studies variance in a previous, similar, meta-analysis might be suitable. Finally, Hedges and Pigott propose a convention that can be used to represent small, medium, and large degrees of heterogeneity. This convention is to set τ^2 equal to 0.33, 0.67, or 1.0 times the within-study variance, so that the total variance $V_{\delta^*} = 1.33V_Y/k$, $1.67V_Y/k$, or $2.00V_Y/k$

As before, the critical value of alpha is given by

$$C_\alpha = \Phi(1 - \alpha/2) , \tag{29.17}$$

and power for a two-tailed test is then given by

$$\text{Power} = 1 - \Phi(C_\alpha - \lambda^*) + \Phi(-C_\alpha - \lambda^*). \tag{29.18}$$

In practice, the effect size is likely to be the same under the random-effects model as it had been under the fixed–effect model. However, the variance will always be larger under the random-effects model as compared with the fixed-effect model (see Chapter 13).

Illustrative example

The example above for the fixed-effect model can be used here as well if we assume that the true effect size varies from study to study, and the random-effects model is therefore appropriate. Again, we assume an effect size of d = 0.30 and 10 studies with 25 patients per group. The within-study variance for one study is computed as

$$V_Y = \frac{25 + 25}{25 \times 25} + \frac{0.30^2}{2(25 + 25)} = 0.0809.$$

If we assume a moderate degree of between-study heterogeneity and apply the convention, the variance of the summary effect is computed as

$$V_\delta^* = \frac{1.667 \times 0.0809}{10} = 0.0135.$$

The parameter λ^* is computed as

$$\lambda^* = \frac{0.30}{\sqrt{0.0135}} = 2.5836.$$

The critical value of alpha is given by

$$C_\alpha = \Phi(1 - 0.05/2) = 1.96.$$

In Excel, =NORMSINV(1−0.05/2) returns 1.96.

Power is then given by

$$\text{Power} = 1 - \Phi(1.96 - 2.5836) + \Phi(-1.96 - 2.5836) = 0.7336.$$

This computation can be done in EXCEL as
=1-NORMSDIST(1.96−2.5836) + NORMSDIST(−1.96−2.5836).

As before, we can create a graph that shows power under a series of assumptions. Figure 29.3 is based on the middle effect size of $\delta = 0.30$, and shows how power will vary if the dispersion is small, medium, or large. We could create a similar graph for an effect size (δ) of 0.20 or of 0.40.

Reading from left to right, if the between-studies dispersion is small, moderate, or large, then we would need about 12, 15, or 20 studies to get power of 90%. Assume that the pilot study shows that we can locate at least 15 studies. Reading from top to bottom at 15 on the X-axis, we see that if dispersion is small, medium or large,

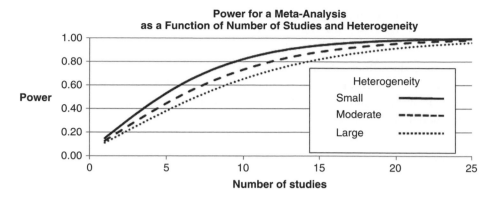

Figure 29.3 Power for a meta-analysis as a function of number studies and heterogeneity.

power would be around 0.95, 0.92 or 0.90. Of course, power will be lower for an effect size of 0.20 and higher for an effect size of 0.40.

Notes about random effects

Under the random-effects model the variance of each study (and of the summary effect) includes two components, the variance within studies and the variance between studies. The practical impact is that power will depend both on the total sample size and also the number of studies. If there is substantial study-to-study dispersion, then the only way to yield good power is to include a large number of studies (which reduces this element of the variance). If the number of studies is small, then power could remain low even if the total sample size across studies reaches into the tens of thousands or even higher.

It is important to understand that the fixed-effect model and random-effects model address different hypotheses, and that they use different estimates of the variance because they make different assumptions about the nature of the distribution of effects across studies, as explained in Chapter 13. Researchers sometimes remark that power is lower under the random-effects model than for the fixed-effect model. While this statement may be true, it misses the larger point: it is not meaningful to compare power for fixed- and random-effects analyses since the two values of power are not addressing the same question.

POWER ANALYSIS FOR A TEST OF HOMOGENEITY

Many meta-analyses include a test of homogeneity, which asks whether or not the between-studies dispersion is more than would be expected by chance. The test of significance is discussed in Chapter 16, and is based on Q, the sum of the squared deviations of each study's effect size estimate (Y_i) from the summary effect (M), with each deviation weighted by the inverse of that study's variance. Concretely,

$$Q = \sum_{i=1}^{k} W_i (Y_i - M)^2 . \tag{29.19}$$

Q is then evaluated with reference to the chi-squared distribution with $k-1$ degrees of freedom. Power for this test depends on three factors. The larger the ratio of between-studies to within-studies variance, the larger the number of studies, and the more liberal the criterion for significance, the higher the power. We can compute power under two alternative scenarios. In the first scenario we do not assume any meta-analytic model (such as fixed-effect or random-effects) for the true effects in the different studies. In the second scenario we assume a random-effects model for these true effects. In both scenarios we assume that the within-study variance V_{Y_i} is the same in each study. For a discussion of power analysis when the V_{Y_i} are not equal, see Hedges and Pigott (2001).

Power for a test of homogeneity in the absence of a meta-analytic model

Researchers who apply the fixed-effect model sometimes test the dispersion for significance. Technically, if the fixed-effect model of homogeneity is true, there is no dispersion, since the model asserts that the between-studies variance is zero. However, it is possible to perform this test (and to compute power) in the absence of a meta-analytic model (a model in which the effect sizes are taken to be fixed, but not necessarily equal).

The expected value of the test statistic (Q), is equal to $df + \lambda$, where the non-centrality parameter λ is computed as

$$\lambda = df \times \left(\frac{\tau^2}{V_Y} \right) . \tag{29.20}$$

In this formula df is $k-1$ (k being the number of studies). Here τ^2 and V_Y are the between-studies variance and the within-studies variance respectively, but power depends only the ratio of these two values (rather than their absolute values).

Power is then given by

$$\text{Power} = 1 - F(C_\alpha | k - 1; \lambda), \tag{29.21}$$

where

$$F(X | df ; \lambda)$$

is the cumulative distribution function of a noncentral chi-square with df degrees of freedom and noncentrality parameter λ, and where C_α is the $100(1-\alpha)$ percent point of the central chi-squared distribution.

To approximate this value in Excel we can proceed as follows. First, the function =CHIINV(*alpha,df*) returns the alpha critical value C_α. Then,

$$a = 1 + \frac{\lambda}{df + \lambda} \,, \tag{29.22}$$

$$b = df + \frac{\lambda^2}{df + 2\lambda} \,, \quad \text{and} \tag{29.23}$$

$$X = \frac{C_\alpha}{a} \,. \tag{29.24}$$

Finally, the expression =1-GAMMADIST($X,b/2,2$,TRUE) returns the value of power.

Illustrative example

Suppose that we are planning a meta-analysis with six studies, and we want to compute power to test for a large amount of dispersion (in which $\tau^2 = V_Y$) with alpha set at 0.05. Then,

$$\lambda = 5\left(\frac{1}{1}\right) = 5 \,.$$

(Note that we don't need to know the actual variances, only the ratio of τ^2 to V_Y. Using the conventions, this ratio is 1.000., 0.667, or 0.333 for large, moderate, and small dispersion.)

In Excel, the chi-squared critical value corresponding to α of 0.05 for 5 df is given by the function =CHIINV(0.05,5), which returns 11.0705. The intermediate values a and b are computed as

$$a = 1 + \frac{5}{5 + 5} = 1.5 \quad \text{and}$$

$$b = 5 + \frac{5^2}{5 + 2 \times 5} = 6.6667 \,.$$

Finally, power is given by the Excel function =1-GAMMADIST(11.0705/1.5, 6.6667/2, 2, TRUE), which returns 0.3553.

Note that we assumed a large amount of dispersion, and the number of studies is typical for many meta-analyses, yet power is quite low. In this example we would need 26 studies to boost power into the 80% range.

Power for a test of homogeneity under the random-effects model

Power of the test is slightly different if we impose a random-effects model on the effects across the studies. The formulas are the same as those for the test in the absence of a meta-analytic model except for the final step. Now, we use instead an Excel expression of the form =CHIDIST(x, df) to return power, where

$$X = \frac{C_\alpha}{1 + \dfrac{\tau^2}{V_Y}}. \tag{29.25}$$

In this example, $= \text{CHIDIST}(11.0705/(1 + 1/1), 5)$ returns 0.3541, or 35.4%.

In this chapter we have presented the logic of power analysis for systematic reviews, and presented formulas for tests of the main effect and for tests of homogeneity. Hedges and Pigott (2004) discuss power for tests of subgroup analyses, and for meta-regression.

SUMMARY POINTS

- The process of power analysis for a meta-analysis closely parallels the issues of power analysis for a primary study.
- Under the fixed-effect model, the 'sample size' factor is driven by the number of subjects accumulated across studies. Power for a meta-analysis of ten studies with 100 persons each is the same as power for one study with 1000 persons (provided the effect size is constant). Therefore, a fixed-effect analyses with a decent number of studies and/or some large studies, will often have good power to detect any nontrivial effect size.
- Under the random-effects model power depends not only on the total number of subjects but also on the number of studies. Even if the effect size is large and the cumulative number of subjects is large, if there are only a few studies and the variance between-studies is substantial, power could be very low.
- The absence of statistical significance should never be interpreted as evidence that an effect is absent. This is important to keep in mind since power to detect heterogeneity in effect sizes, and power to detect the relationship between subgroup membership and effect size, or between covariate values and effect size, is often quite low.

Further reading

Borenstein, M. (1994). The case for confidence intervals in controlled clinical trials. *Controlled Clinical Trials*, Oct; 15(5): 411–28.

Borenstein, M. (1997). Hypothesis testing and effect size estimation in clinical trials. *Annals of Allergy, Asthma and Immunology*, Jan; 78(1), 5–16(12).

Cohen J. Statistical Power Analysis for the Behavioral Sciences (2nd ed) 1987. Lawrence Erlbaum Associates, Hillsdale NJ.

Hedges L.V. and Pigott T.D. (2001). The power of statistical tests in meta-analysis, *Psychological Methods*, 6, 203–17.

Hedges L.V. and Pigott T.D., (2004). The power of statistical tests for moderators in meta-analysis, *Psychological Methods*, 9, 426–45.

Sutton, A.J., Cooper, N.J., Jones, D.R., Abrams, K.A., Lambert, P., Thompson, J.R. (2007). Evidence based sample size calculations for the future trials based on results of current meta-analysis. *Statistics in Medicine* 26, 2479–2500.

Sutton, A.J., Donegan, S., Takwoingi, Y., Garner, P., Gamble, C., Donald, A. (in press) An encouraging assessment of methods to inform priorities for updating systematic reviews. *Journal of Epidemiology*.

CHAPTER 30

Publication Bias

INTRODUCTION

While a meta-analysis will yield a mathematically accurate synthesis of the studies included in the analysis, if these studies are a biased sample of all relevant studies, then the mean effect computed by the meta-analysis will reflect this bias. Several lines of evidence show that studies that report relatively high effect sizes are more likely to be published than studies that report lower effect sizes. Since published studies are more likely to find their way into a meta-analysis, any bias in the literature is likely to be reflected in the meta-analysis as well. This issue is generally known as publication bias.

The problem of publication bias is not unique to systematic reviews. It affects the researcher who writes a narrative review and even the clinician who is searching a database for primary papers. Nevertheless, it has received more attention with regard to systematic reviews and meta-analyses, possibly because these are promoted as being more accurate than other approaches to synthesizing research.

In this chapter we first discuss the reasons for publication bias and the evidence that it exists. Then we discuss a series of methods that have been developed to assess

Introduction to Meta-Analysis   M. Borenstein, L. V. Hedges, J. P. T. Higgins, H. R. Rothstein
© 2009, John Wiley & Sons, Ltd

the likely impact of bias in any given meta-analysis. At the end of the chapter we present an illustrative example.

THE PROBLEM OF MISSING STUDIES

When planning a systematic review we develop a set of inclusion criteria that govern the types of studies that we want to include. Ideally, we would be able to locate all studies that meet our criteria, but in the real world this is rarely possible. Even with the advent of (and perhaps partly due to an over-reliance on) electronic searching, it is likely that some studies which meet our criteria will escape our search and not be included in the analysis.

If the missing studies are a *random* subset of all relevant studies, the failure to include these studies will result in less information, wider confidence intervals, and less powerful tests, but will have no systematic impact on the effect size. However, if the missing studies are *systematically* different than the ones we were able to locate, then our sample will be biased. The specific concern is that studies that report relatively large effects for a given question are more likely to be published than studies that report smaller effects for the same question. This leads to a bias in the published literature, which then carries over to a meta-analysis that draws on this literature.

Studies with significant results are more likely to be published

Several lines of research (reviewed by Dickersin, 2005) have established that studies with statistically significant results are more likely to find their way into the published literature than studies that report results that are not statistically significant. And, for any given sample size the result is more likely to be statistically significant if the effect size is larger. It follows that if there is a population of studies that looked at the magnitude of a relationship, and the observed effects are distributed over a range of values (as they always are), the studies with effects toward the higher end of that range are more likely to be statistically significant and therefore to be published. This tendency has the potential to produce very large biases in the magnitude of the relationships, particularly if studies have relatively small sample sizes (see, Hedges, 1984; 1989).

A particularly enlightening line of research was to identify groups of studies as they were initiated, and then follow them prospectively over a period of years to see which were published and which were not. This approach was taken by Easterbrook, Berlin, Gopalan, & Matthews (1991), Dickersin, Min, & Meinert (1992), Dickersin & Min (1993a), among others. Nonsignificant studies were less likely to be published than significant studies (61–86% as likely), and when published were subject to longer delay prior to publication. Similar studies have demonstrated that researchers selectively report their findings in the reports they do publish, sometimes even changing what is labeled *a priori* as the main hypothesis (Chan *et al.*, 2004).

Published studies are more likely to be included in a meta-analysis

If persons performing a systematic review were able to locate studies that had been published in the grey literature (any literature produced in electronic or print format that is not controlled by commercial publishers, such as technical reports and similar sources), then the fact that the studies with higher effects are more likely to be published in the more mainstream publications would not be a problem for meta-analysis. In fact, though, this is not usually the case.

While a systematic review *should* include a thorough search for all relevant studies, the actual amount of grey/unpublished literature included, and the types, varies considerably across meta-analyses. When Rothstein (2006) reviewed the 95 meta-analytic reviews published in *Psychological Bulletin* between 1995 and 2005 to see whether they included unpublished or *grey* research, she found that 23 of the 95 clearly did not include any unpublished data. Clarke and Clarke (2000) studied the references from healthcare protocols and reviews published in The Cochrane Library in 1999, and found that about 92% of references to studies included in reviews were to journal articles. Of the remaining 8%, about 4% were to conference proceedings, about 2% were to unpublished material (for example personal communication, *in press* documents and data on file), and slightly over 1% were to books or book chapters. In a similar vein, Mallet, Hopewell, & Clarke (2002) looked at the sources of grey literature included in the first 1000 Cochrane systematic reviews, and found that nearly half of them did not include any data from grey or unpublished sources. Since the meta-analyses published in the Cochrane Database have been shown to retrieve a higher proportion of studies than those published in many journals, these estimates probably understate the extent of the problem.

Some have suggested that it is legitimate to exclude studies that have not been published in peer-reviewed journals because these studies tend to be of lower quality. For example, in their systematic review, Weisz *et al.* (1995) wrote 'We included only published psychotherapy outcome studies, relying on the journal review process as one step of quality control' (p. 452). However, it is not obvious that journal review assures high quality, nor that it is the *only* mechanism that can do so. For one thing, not all researchers aim to publish their research in academic journals. For example, researchers working for government agencies, independent think-tanks or consulting firms generally focus on producing reports, not journal articles. Similarly, a thesis or dissertation may be of high quality, but is unlikely to be submitted for publication in an academic journal if the individual who produced it is not pursuing an academic career. And of course, peer review may be biased, unreliable, or of uneven quality. Overall, then, publication status cannot be used as a proxy for quality; and in our opinion should not be used as a basis for inclusion or exclusion of studies.

Other sources of bias

Other factors that can lead to an upward bias in effect size and are included under the umbrella of publication bias are the following. Language bias (English-language databases and journals are more likely to be searched, which leads to an over-sampling of statistically significant studies) (Egger *et al.*, 1997; Jüni *et al.*, 2002); availability bias (selective inclusion of studies that are easily accessible to the researcher); cost bias (selective inclusion of studies that are available free or at low cost); familiarity bias (selective inclusion of studies only from one's own discipline); duplication bias (studies with statistically significant results are more likely to be published more than once (Tramer *et al.*, 1997)) and citation bias (whereby studies with statistically significant results are more likely to be cited by others and therefore easier to identify (Gøtzsche, 1997; Ravnskov, 1992)).

METHODS FOR ADDRESSING BIAS

In sum, it is possible that the studies in a meta-analysis may overestimate the true effect size because they are based on a biased sample of the target population of studies. But how do we deal with this concern? The only true test for publication bias is to compare effects in the published studies formally with effects in the unpublished studies. This requires access to the unpublished studies, and if we had that we would no longer be concerned. Nevertheless, the best approach would be for the reviewer to perform a truly comprehensive search of the literature, in hopes of minimizing the bias. In fact, there is evidence that this approach is somewhat effective. Cochrane reviews tend to include more studies and to report a smaller effect size than similar reviews published in medical journals. Serious efforts to find unpublished, and *difficult to find* studies, typical of Cochrane reviews, may therefore reduce some of the effects of publication bias.

Despite the increased resources that are needed to locate and retrieve data from sources such as dissertations, theses, conference papers, government and technical reports and the like, it is generally indefensible to conduct a synthesis that categorically excludes these types of research reports. Potential benefits and costs of grey literature searches must be balanced against each other. Readers who would like more guidance in the process of literature searching and information retrieval may wish to consult Hopewell, Mallett and Clarke (2005), Reed and Baxter (2009), Rothstein and Hopewell (2009), or Wade, Turner, Rothstein and Lavenberg (2006).

Since we cannot be certain that we have avoided bias, researchers have developed methods intended to assess its potential impact on any given meta-analysis. These methods address the following questions:

- Is there evidence of any bias?
- Is it possible that the entire effect is an artifact of bias?
- How much of an impact might the bias have?

We shall illustrate these methods as they apply to a meta-analysis on passive smoking and lung cancer.

ILLUSTRATIVE EXAMPLE

Hackshaw *et al.* (1997) published a meta-analysis with data from 37 studies that reported on the relationship between so-called second-hand (passive) smoking and lung cancer. The paper reported that exposure to second-hand smoke increased the risk of lung cancer in the nonsmoking spouse by about 20%. Questions were raised about the possibility that studies with larger effects were more likely to have been published (and included in the analysis) than those with smaller (or nil) effects, and that the conclusion was therefore suspect.

THE MODEL

In order to gauge the impact of publication bias we need a model that tells us which studies are likely to be missing. The model that is generally used (and the one we follow here) makes the following assumptions: (a) Large studies are likely to be published regardless of statistical significance because these involve large commitments of time and resources. (b) Moderately sized studies are at risk for being lost, but with a moderate sample size even modest effects will be significant, and so only some studies are lost here. (c) Small studies are at greatest risk for being lost. Because of the small sample size, only the largest effects are likely to be significant, with the small and moderate effects likely to be unpublished.

The combined result of these three items is that we expect the bias to increase as the sample size goes down, and the methods described below are all based on this model. Other, more sophisticated methods have been developed for estimating the number of missing studies and/or adjusting the observed effect to account for bias. These have rarely been used in actual research because they are difficult to implement and also because they require the user to make some relatively sophisticated assumptions and choices.

Before proceeding with the example we call the reader's attention to an important caveat. The procedures that we describe here look for a relationship between sample size and effect size, and if such a relationship is found, it is attributed to the existence of missing studies. While this is *one possible reason* that the effect size is larger in the smaller studies, it is also possible that the effect size *really is larger* in the smaller studies. We mention this caveat here to provide a context for the discussion that follows, and return to it near the end of the chapter, in the section entitled *small-study effects*.

GETTING A SENSE OF THE DATA

A good place to start in assessing the potential for bias is to get a sense of the data, and the forest plot can be used for this purpose. Figure 30.1 is a forest plot of the studies in the passive smoking meta-analysis. In this example, an increase in risk is indicated by a risk ratio greater than 1.0. The overwhelming majority of studies show an increased risk for second-hand smoke, and the last row in the spreadsheet

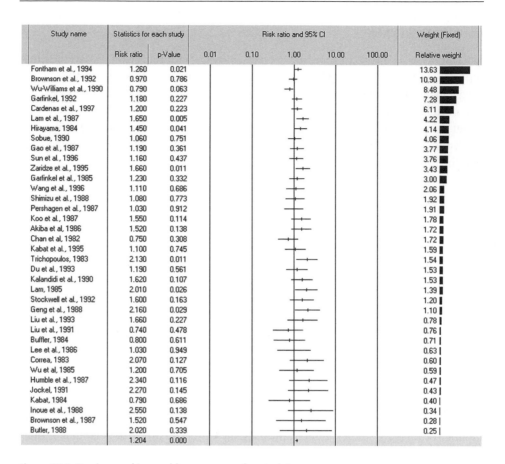

Study name	Statistics for each study		Risk ratio and 95% CI					Weight (Fixed)
	Risk ratio	p-Value	0.01	0.10	1.00	10.00	100.00	Relative weight
Fontham et al., 1994	1.260	0.021						13.63
Brownson et al., 1992	0.970	0.786						10.90
Wu-Williams et al., 1990	0.790	0.063						8.48
Garfinkel, 1992	1.180	0.227						7.28
Cardenas et al., 1997	1.200	0.223						6.11
Lam et al., 1987	1.650	0.005						4.22
Hirayama, 1984	1.450	0.041						4.14
Sobue, 1990	1.060	0.751						4.06
Gao et al., 1987	1.190	0.361						3.77
Sun et al., 1996	1.160	0.437						3.76
Zaridze et al., 1995	1.660	0.011						3.43
Garfinkel et al., 1985	1.230	0.332						3.00
Wang et al., 1996	1.110	0.686						2.06
Shimizu et al., 1988	1.080	0.773						1.92
Pershagen et al., 1987	1.030	0.912						1.91
Koo et al., 1987	1.550	0.114						1.78
Akiba et al, 1986	1.520	0.138						1.72
Chan et al, 1982	0.750	0.308						1.72
Kabat et al., 1995	1.100	0.745						1.59
Trichopoulos, 1983	2.130	0.011						1.54
Du et al., 1993	1.190	0.561						1.53
Kalandidi et al., 1990	1.620	0.107						1.53
Lam, 1985	2.010	0.026						1.39
Stockwell et al., 1992	1.600	0.163						1.20
Geng et al., 1988	2.160	0.029						1.10
Liu et al., 1993	1.660	0.227						0.78
Liu et al., 1991	0.740	0.478						0.76
Buffler, 1984	0.800	0.611						0.71
Lee et al., 1986	1.030	0.949						0.63
Correa, 1983	2.070	0.127						0.60
Wu et al, 1985	1.200	0.705						0.59
Humble et al., 1987	2.340	0.116						0.47
Jockel, 1991	2.270	0.145						0.43
Kabat, 1984	0.790	0.686						0.40
Inoue et al., 1988	2.550	0.138						0.34
Brownson et al., 1987	1.520	0.547						0.28
Butler, 1988	2.020	0.339						0.25
	1.204	0.000						

Figure 30.1 Passive smoking and lung cancer – forest plot.

shows the summary data for the fixed-effect model. The risk ratio is 1.204 and the 95% confidence interval is 1.120 to 1.295.

The studies have been plotted from most precise to least precise, so that larger studies appear toward the top and smaller studies appear toward the bottom. This has no impact on the summary effect, but it allows us to see the relationship between sample size and effect size. As we move toward the bottom of the plot the effects shift toward the right, which is what the model would predict if bias is present.

If the analysis includes some studies from peer-reviewed journals and others from the grey literature, we can also group by source and see if the grey papers (which may be representative of any missing studies) tend to have smaller effects than the others.

The funnel plot

Another mechanism for displaying the relationship between study size and effect size is the funnel plot.

Traditionally, the funnel plot was plotted with effect size on the X axis and the sample size or variance on the Y axis. Large studies appear toward the top of the graph and generally cluster around the mean effect size. Smaller studies appear toward the bottom of the graph, and (since smaller studies have more sampling error variation in effect sizes) tend to be spread across a broad range of values. This pattern resembles a funnel, hence the plot's name (Light and Pillemer, 1984; Light *et al.*, 1994).

The use of the standard error (rather than sample size or variance) on the Y axis has the advantage of spreading out the points on the *bottom half* of the scale, where the smaller studies are plotted. This could make it easier to identify asymmetry. This affects the display only, and has no impact on the statistics, and this is the route we follow here (Figure 30.2).

IS THERE EVIDENCE OF ANY BIAS?

In the *absence* of publication bias, the studies will be distributed symmetrically about the mean effect size, since the sampling error is random. In the *presence* of publication bias the studies are expected to follow the model, with symmetry at the top, a few studies missing in the middle, and more studies missing near the bottom. If the direction of the effect is toward the right (as in our example), then near the bottom of the plot we expect a gap on the left, where the nonsignificant studies would have been if we had been able to locate them.

In the running example (Figure 30.2) the risk ratio (in log units) is at the bottom and the standard error is on the Y axis (which has been reversed, so low values are at

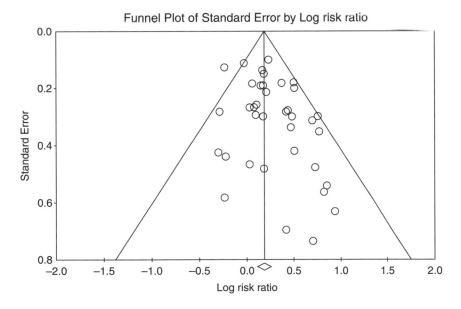

Figure 30.2 Passive smoking and lung cancer – funnel plot.

the top). The subjective impression does support the presence of asymmetry. Toward the bottom of the graph most studies appear toward the right (indicating more risk), which is consistent with the possibility that some studies are missing from the left.

First, we ask if there is evidence of *any* bias. Because the interpretation of a funnel plot is largely subjective, several tests have been proposed to quantify or test the relationship between sample size and effect size. Two early proposals are in common use (Begg and Mazumdar, 1994, Egger *et al.*, 1997); a comprehensive review appears in Chapter 10 of Higgins and Green (2008).

While these tests provide useful information, several caveats are in order. First, the tests (like the funnel plot) may yield a very different picture depending on the index used in the analysis (risk difference versus risk ratio, for example). Second, this approach makes sense only if there is a reasonable amount of dispersion in the sample sizes and a reasonable number of studies. Third, even when these criteria are met, the tests tend to have lower power. Therefore, the absence of a significant correlation or regression cannot be taken as evidence of symmetry.

In any event, even if we could somehow solve these problems, the question addressed by the tests (is there evidence of *any* bias) is of limited import. A more interesting question would be *How much bias is there, and what is its impact on our conclusions?*

IS THE ENTIRE EFFECT AN ARTIFACT OF BIAS?

The next question one might ask is whether or not the observed overall effect is robust. In other words, can we be confident that the effect is not solely an artifact of bias?

Rosenthal's *Fail-safe N*

An early approach to dealing with publication bias was Rosenthal's *Fail-safe N*. Suppose a meta-analysis reports a significant *p*-value based on *k* studies. We are concerned that studies with smaller effects are missing, and if we were to retrieve all the missing studies and include them in the analysis, the *p*-value for the summary effect would no longer be significant. Rosenthal (1979) suggested that we actually compute how many missing studies we would need to retrieve and incorporate in the analysis before the *p*-value became nonsignificant. For purposes of this exercise we would assume that the mean effect in the missing studies was zero. If it should emerge that we needed only a few studies (say, five or ten) to 'nullify' the effect, then we would be concerned that the true effect was indeed zero. However, if it turned out that we needed a large number of studies (say, 20,000) to nullify the effect, there would be less reason for concern.

Rosenthal referred to this as a *File drawer* analysis (file drawers being the presumed location of the missing studies), and Harris Cooper suggested that the number of missing studies needed to nullify the effect should be called the *Fail-safe N* (Rosenthal, 1979; Begg and Mazumdar, 1994).

While Rosenthal's work was critical in focusing attention on publication bias, this approach is of limited utility for a number of reasons. First, it focuses on the question of statistical significance rather than substantive significance. That is, it asks how many hidden studies are required to make the effect not statistically significant, rather than how many hidden studies are required to reduce the effect to the point that it is not of substantive importance. Second, the formula assumes that the mean effect size in the hidden studies is zero, when in fact it could be negative (which would require fewer studies to nullify the effect) or positive but low. Finally, the *Fail-safe N* is based on significance tests that combine *p*-values across studies, as was common at the time that Rosenthal suggested the method. Today, the common practice is to compute a summary effect, and then compute the *p*-value for this effect. The *p*-values computed using the different approaches actually test different null hypotheses, and are not the same. For these reasons this approach is not generally appropriate for analyses that focus on effect sizes. We have addressed it at relative length only because the method is well known and because of its important historical role.

That said, for the passive smoking review the *Fail-safe N* is 398, suggesting that there would need to be nearly 400 studies with a mean risk ratio of 1.0 added to the analysis, before the cumulative effect would become statistically nonsignificant.

Orwin's *Fail-safe N*

As noted, two problems with Rosenthal's approach are that it focuses on statistical significance rather than substantive significance, and that it assumes that the mean effect size in the missing studies is zero. Orwin (1983) proposed a variant on the Rosenthal formula that addresses both of these issues. First, Orwin's method allows the researcher to determine how many missing studies would bring the overall effect to a specified level other than zero. The researcher could therefore select a value that would represent the smallest effect deemed to be of substantive importance, and ask how many missing studies it would take to bring the summary effect below this point. Second, it allows the researcher to specify the mean effect in the missing studies as some value other than zero. This would allow the researcher to model a series of other distributions for the missing studies (Becker, 2005; Begg and Mazumdar, 1994).

In the running example, Orwin's *Fail-safe N* is 103, suggesting that there would need to be over 100 studies with a mean risk ratio of 1.0 added to the analysis before the cumulative effect would become trivial (defined as a risk ratio of 1.05).

HOW MUCH OF AN IMPACT MIGHT THE BIAS HAVE?

The approaches outlined above ask whether bias has had *any* impact on the observed effect (those based on the funnel plot), or whether it might be *entirely* responsible for the observed effect (*Fail-safe N*). As compared with these extreme positions, a third approach attempts to estimate how much impact the bias had, and to estimate what the effect size would have been in the absence of bias. The hope is to classify each meta-analysis into one of three broad groups, as follows.

- The impact of bias is probably trivial. If all relevant studies were included the effect size would probably remain largely unchanged.
- The impact of bias is probably modest. If all relevant studies were included the effect size might shift but the key finding (that the effect is, or is not, of substantive importance) would probably remain unchanged.
- The impact of bias may be substantial. If all relevant studies were included, the key finding (that the effect size is, or is not, of substantive importance) could change.

Duval and Tweedie's *Trim and Fill*

As discussed above, the key idea behind the funnel plot is that publication bias may be expected to lead to asymmetry. If there are more small studies on the right than on the left, our concern is that there may be studies missing from the left. (In the running example we expect suppression of studies on the left, but in other cases we would expect suppression on the right. The algorithm requires the reviewer to specify the expected direction.)

Trim and Fill uses an iterative procedure to remove the most extreme small studies from the positive side of the funnel plot, re-computing the effect size at each iteration until the funnel plot is symmetric about the (new) effect size. In theory, this will yield an unbiased estimate of the effect size. While this *trimming* yields the adjusted effect size, it also reduces the variance of the effects, yielding a too narrow confidence interval. Therefore, the algorithm then adds the original studies back into the analysis, and imputes a mirror image for each. This *fill* has no impact on the point estimate but serves to correct the variance (Duval and Tweedie, 2000a, 2000b).

A major advantage of this approach is that it addresses an important question, *What is our best estimate of the unbiased effect size?* Another nice feature of this approach is that it lends itself to an intuitive visual display. The computer programs that incorporate *Trim and Fill* are able to create a funnel plot that includes both the observed studies and the imputed studies, so the researcher can see how the effect size shifts when the imputed studies are included. If this shift is trivial, then one can have more confidence that the reported effect is valid. A problem with this method is that it depends strongly on the assumptions of the model for why studies are missing, and the algorithm for detecting asymmetry can be influenced by one or two aberrant studies.

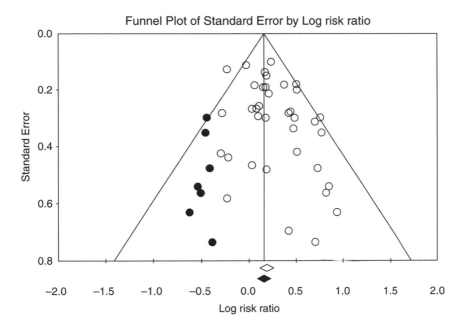

Figure 30.3 Passive smoking and lung cancer – funnel plot with imputed studies.

We can re-display the funnel plot, taking into account the *Trim and Fill* adjustment. In Figure 30.3, the observed studies are shown as open circles, and the observed point estimate in log units is shown as an open diamond at 0.185 (0.113, 0.258), corresponding to a risk ratio of 1.204 (1.120, 1.295). The seven imputed studies are shown as filled circles, and the imputed point estimate in log units is shown as a filled diamond at 0.156 (0.085, 0.227), corresponding to a risk ratio of 1.169 (1.089, 1.254). The 'adjusted' point estimate suggests a lower risk than the original analysis. Perhaps the key point, though, is that the adjusted estimate is fairly close to the original – in this context, a risk ratio of 1.17 has the same substantive implications as a risk ratio of 1.20.

Restricting analysis to the larger studies

If publication bias operates primarily on smaller studies, then restricting the analysis to large studies, which might be expected to be published irrespective of their results, would in theory overcome any problems. The question then arises as to what threshold defines a *large* study. We are unable to offer general guidance on this question. A potentially useful strategy is to illustrate all possible thresholds by drawing a cumulative meta-analysis.

A cumulative meta-analysis is a meta-analysis run first with one study, then repeated with a second study added, then a third, and so on. Similarly, in a cumulative forest plot, the first row shows the effect based on one study, the second row shows the cumulative effect based on two studies, and so on. We discuss cumulative meta-analysis in more detail in Chapter 42.

To examine the effect of different thresholds for study size, the studies are sorted in the sequence of largest to smallest (or of most precise to least precise), and a cumulative meta-analysis performed with the addition of each study. If the point estimate has stabilized with the inclusion of the larger studies and does not shift with the addition of smaller studies, then there is no reason to assume that the inclusion of smaller studies had injected a bias (i.e. since it is the smaller studies in which study selection is likely to be greatest). On the other hand, if the point estimate does shift when the smaller studies are added, then there is at least a *prima facie* case for bias, and one would want to investigate the reason for the shift.

This approach also provides an estimate of the effect size based solely on the larger studies. And, even more so than *Trim and Fill*, this approach is entirely transparent: We compute the effect based on the larger studies and then determine if and how the

Study name	Cumulative statistics		Cumulative risk ratio (95% CI)			Weight (Fixed)
	Point	p-Value	0.50	1.00	2.00	Relative weight
Fontham et al., 1994	1.260	0.021				13.63
Brownson et al., 1992	1.122	0.124				24.53
Wu-Williams et al.,	1.025	0.699				33.01
Garfinkel, 1992	1.052	0.388				40.29
Cardenas et al., 1997	1.070	0.213				46.40
Lam et al., 1987	1.109	0.046				50.62
Hirayama, 1984	1.132	0.013				54.75
Sobue, 1990	1.127	0.013				58.81
Gao et al., 1987	1.131	0.009				62.58
Sun et al., 1996	1.132	0.006				66.34
Zaridze et al., 1995	1.154	0.001				69.76
Garfinkel et al., 1985	1.157	0.001				72.77
Wang et al., 1996	1.155	0.001				74.83
Shimizu et al., 1988	1.154	0.001				76.75
Pershagen et al., 1987	1.150	0.001				78.66
Koo et al., 1987	1.158	0.000				80.44
Akiba et al, 1986	1.165	0.000				82.15
Chan et al, 1982	1.154	0.000				83.87
Kabat et al., 1995	1.153	0.000				85.46
Trichopoulos, 1983	1.166	0.000				87.00
Du et al., 1993	1.166	0.000				88.53
Kalandidi et al., 1990	1.173	0.000				90.05
Lam, 1985	1.182	0.000				91.45
Stockwell et al., 1992	1.187	0.000				92.65
Geng et al., 1988	1.195	0.000				93.75
Liu et al., 1993	1.199	0.000				94.53
Liu et al., 1991	1.194	0.000				95.29
Buffler, 1984	1.190	0.000				96.00
Lee et al., 1986	1.189	0.000				96.63
Correa, 1983	1.193	0.000				97.23
Wu et al, 1985	1.193	0.000				97.82
Humble et al., 1987	1.197	0.000				98.29
Jockel, 1991	1.201	0.000				98.72
Kabat, 1984	1.199	0.000				99.12
Inoue et al., 1988	1.202	0.000				99.46
Brownson et al., 1987	1.202	0.000				99.75
Butler, 1988	1.204	0.000				100.00
	1.204	0.000				

Figure 30.4 Passive smoking and lung cancer – cumulative forest plot.

effect shifts with the addition of the smaller studies (a clear distinction between larger and smaller studies will not usually exist, but is not needed).

Figure 30.4 shows a cumulative forest plot of the data. Note the difference between the cumulative plot and the standard version shown earlier. Here, the first row is a 'meta' analysis based only on the Fontham *et al.* study. The second row is a meta-analysis based on two studies (Fontham *et al.* and Brownson *et al.*), and so on. The last study to be added is Butler (1988), and so the point estimate and confidence interval shown on the line labeled 'Butler' are identical to that shown for the summary effect on the line labeled 'Fixed'. Note that the scale on this plot is 0.50 to 2.00.

The studies have been sorted from the most precise to the least precise (roughly corresponding to largest to smallest). With the 18 largest studies in the analysis, starting at the top (inclusive of Chan and Fung, 1982) the cumulative relative risk is 1.15. With the addition of another 19 (smaller) studies, the point estimate shifts to the right, and the relative risk is 1.20. As such, our estimate of the relative risk has increased. However, the key point is that even if we had limited the analysis to the 18 larger studies, the relative risk would have been 1.15 (with 95% confidence interval of 1.07, 1.25) and the clinical implications probably would have been the same.

Note also that the analysis that incorporates all 37 studies assigns 83% of its weight to the first 18 (see the bar graph in the right-hand column). In other words, if small studies *are* introducing a bias, we are protected to some extent by the fact that small studies are given less weight. Recall, however, that random-effects meta-analyses award relatively more weight to smaller studies than fixed-effect meta-analyses, so a cumulative meta-analysis based on a random-effects model may not reveal such protection.

A major advantage of this approach is that it provides an estimate of the unbiased effect size (under the strong assumptions of the model) and lends itself to an intuitive visual display. Unlike *Trim and Fill*, this approach will not be thrown by one or two aberrant studies.

SUMMARY OF THE FINDINGS FOR THE ILLUSTRATIVE EXAMPLE

The various statistical procedures approach the problem of bias from a number of directions. One would not expect the results of the different procedures to 'match' each other since the procedures ask different questions. Rather, the goal should be to synthesize the different pieces of information provided by the various procedures.

Getting a sense of the data

There are a substantial number of studies in this analysis. While the vast majority show an increased risk, only a few are statistically significant. This suggests that the mechanism of publication bias based on statistical significance was not a powerful one in this case.

Is there evidence of bias?

The funnel plot is noticeably asymmetric, with a majority of the smaller studies clustering to the right of the mean. This visual impression is confirmed by Egger's test which yields a statistically significant p-value. The rank correlation test did not yield a significant p-value, but this could be due to the low power of the test. As a whole the smaller studies did tend to report a higher association between passive smoking and lung cancer than did the larger studies.

Is it possible that the observed relationship is entirely an artifact of bias?

Rosenthal's *Fail-safe N* is 398, suggesting that there would need to be nearly 400 studies with a mean risk ratio of 1.0 added to the analysis, before the cumulative effect would become statistically nonsignificant. Similarly, Orwin's *Fail-safe N* is 103, suggesting that there would need to be over 100 studies with a mean risk ratio of 1.0 added to the analysis before the cumulative effect would become trivial (defined as a risk ratio of 1.05). Given that the authors of the meta-analysis were able to identify only 37 studies that looked at the relationship of passive smoking and lung cancer, it is unlikely that nearly 400 studies, or even 103 studies, were missed. While we may have overstated the risk caused by second-hand smoke, it is unlikely that the actual risk is zero.

What impact might the bias have on the risk ratio?

The complete meta-analysis showed that passive smoking was associated with a 20% increase in risk of lung cancer. By contrast, the meta-analysis based on the larger studies reported an increased risk of 16%. Similarly, the *Trim and Fill* method suggested that if we removed the asymmetric studies, the increased risk would be imputed as 15%.

Earlier, we suggested that the goal of a publication bias analysis should be to classify the results into one of three categories (a) where the impact of bias is trivial, (b) where the impact is not trivial but the major finding is still valid, and (c) where the major finding might be called into question. This meta-analysis seems to fall squarely within category *b*. There *is* evidence of larger effects in the smaller studies, which is consistent with our model for publication bias. However, there is no reason to doubt the validity of the core finding, that passive smoking is associated with a clinically important increase in the risk of lung cancer.

SOME IMPORTANT CAVEATS

Most of the approaches discussed in this chapter look for evidence that the effect sizes are larger in the smaller studies, and interpret this as reflecting publication bias. This relationship between effect size and sample size lies at the core of the forest plot, as well as the correlation and regression tests. It also drives the algorithm for *Trim and Fill* and the logic of restricting the analysis to the larger studies.

Therefore, it is important to be aware that these procedures are subject to a number of caveats. They may yield a very different picture depending on the index used in the analysis (e.g. risk difference versus risk ratio). The procedures can easily miss real dispersion. They have the potential to work only if there is a reasonable amount of dispersion in the sample sizes and also a reasonable number of studies. Even when these conditions are met, the tests (correlation and regression) tend to have lower power. Therefore, our failure to find evidence of asymmetry should not lead to a false sense of assurance.

SMALL-STUDY EFFECTS

Equally important, when there is clear evidence of asymmetry, we cannot assume that this reflects publication bias. The effect size *may* be larger in small studies because we retrieved a biased sample of the smaller studies, but it is also possible that the effect size really is larger in smaller studies for entirely unrelated reasons.

For example, the small studies may have been performed using patients who were quite ill, and therefore more likely to benefit from the drug (as is sometimes the case in early trials of a new compound). Or, the small studies may have been performed with better (or worse) quality control than the larger ones. Sterne *et al.* (2001) use the term *small-study effect* to describe a pattern where the effect is larger in small studies, and to highlight the fact that the mechanism for this effect is not known.

Adjustments for publication bias should always be made with this caveat in mind. For example, we should report 'If the asymmetry is due to bias, our analyses suggest that the adjusted effect would fall in the range of ...' rather than asserting 'the asymmetry is due to bias, and therefore the true effect falls in the range of ...'

CONCLUDING REMARKS

It is almost always important to include an assessment of publication bias in relation to a meta-analysis. It will either assure the reviewer that the results are robust, or alert them that the results are suspect. This is important to ensure the integrity of the individual meta-analysis. It is also important to ensure the integrity of the field. When a meta-analysis ignores the potential for bias and is later found to be incorrect, the perception is fostered that meta-analyses cannot be trusted.

SUMMARY POINTS

- Publication bias exists when the studies included in the analysis differ system-atically from all studies that should have been included. Typically, studies with larger than average effects are more likely to be published, and this can lead to an upward bias in the summary effect.
- Methods have been developed to assess the likely impact of publication bias on any given meta-analysis. Using these methods we report that if we adjusted the

---

CONTINUED

effect to remove the bias, (a) the resulting effect would be essentially unchanged, or (b) the effect might change but the basic conclusion, that the treatment works (or not) would not be changed, or (c) the basic conclusion would be called into question.

• Methods developed to address publication bias require us to make many assumptions, including the assumption that the pattern of results is due to bias, and that this bias follows a certain model.

• Publication bias is a problem for meta-analysis, but also a problem for narrative reviews or for persons performing any search of the literature.

Further reading

Chalmers, T.C., Frank, C.S., & Reitman, D. (1990). Minimizing the three states of publication bias. *JAMA* 263: 1392–1395.

Dickersin, K., Chan, S., Cha.mers,T.C., Sacks, H.S., & Smith, H. (1987) Publication bias in clinical trials. *Controlled Clinical Trials* 8: 348–353.

Dickersin, K,. Min, Y.L., & Meinert, C.L. (1992). Factors influencing publication of research results: Follow-up of applications submitted to two institutional review boards. *JAMA* 267: 374–378.

Hedges, L.V. (1984) Estimation of effect size under nonrandom sampling: The effects of censoring studies yielding statistically insignificant mean differences. *Journal of Educational Statistics*, 9, 61–85.

Hedges, L.V. (1989) Estimating the normal mean and variance under a selection model. In Gleser, L, Perlman, M.D., Press, S.J., Sampson, A.R. *Contributions to Probability and Statistics: Essays in Honor of Ingram Olkin* (pp. 447–458). NY: Springer Verlag.

Hunt, M.M. (1999) *The New Know-Nothings: The Political Foes of the Scientific Study of Human Nature*. New Brunswick, NJ, Transacation.

International Committee of Medical Journal Editors. *Uniform Requirements for Manuscripts Submitted to Biomedical Journals: Writing and Editing for Biomedical Publication*. Updated October 2007. Available at http://www.icmje.org/#clin_trials.

Ioannidis, J.P. (2007). Why most published research findings are false: author's reply to Goodman and Greenland. *PLoS Med* 4: e215.

Lau, J., Ioannidis, J.P., Terrin, N., Schmid, C.H., & Olkin, I. (2006). The case of the misleading funnel plot. *BMJ* 333: 597–600.

Rosenthal, R. (1979). The 'File drawer problem' and tolerance for null results. *Psychol Bull* 86: 638–641.

Rothstein, H.R., Sutton, A.J., & Borenstein, M. (2005). *Publication Bias in Meta-analysis: Prevention, Assessment and Adjustments*. Chichester, UK, John Wiley & Sons, Ltd.

Sterne, J.A., Egger, M. & Smith, G. D. (2001). Systematic reviews in healthcare: investigating and dealing with publication and other biases in meta-analysis. *Bmj* 323: 101–105.

Sterne, J.A., Egger, M. (2001). Funnel plots for detecting bias in meta-analysis: guidelines on choice of axis. *J Clin Epidemiol* 54: 1046–1055.

Sutton A.J., Duval S.J., Tweedie, R.L., Abrams, K.R., & Jones, D.R. (2000). Empirical assessment of effect of publication bias on meta-analyses. *BMJ* 320: 1574–1577.

PART 7

Issues Related to Effect Size

CHAPTER 31

Overview

The focus of this volume has been almost exclusively on meta-analysis of effect sizes (though some other approaches will be addressed in Chapter 36). We compute an effect size for each study, and it is these values that form the core of the analysis. We use them to assess dispersion across studies, to compute a summary effect, to compare effects across subgroups, and so on. In this part we offer some context for this approach.

Readers who are accustomed to working with significance tests and p-values in primary studies may wonder why we don't synthesize these p-values. This is addressed in Chapter 32.

Some may wonder why we compute an effect size for each study, rather than simply aggregating the summary data (for example, summing all the cell counts for a series of 2×2 tables) and then computing an effect size for the final table. This is addressed in Chapter 33.

In this volume we have worked primarily with measures that assess the impact of treatments or the relationship between variables, but the same idea can be extended to other kinds of measures as well. In Chapter 34 we provide an overview of some other applications, such as estimating prevalence. We also outline some other approaches to meta-analysis, such as the use of individual participant data, and of Bayesian meta-analysis.

Introduction to Meta-Analysis   M. Borenstein, L. V. Hedges, J. P. T. Higgins, H. R. Rothstein
© 2009, John Wiley & Sons, Ltd

CHAPTER 32

Effect Sizes Rather than *p*-Values

Introduction
Relationship between *p*-values and effect sizes
The distinction is important
The *p*-value is often misinterpreted
Narrative reviews vs. meta-analyses

INTRODUCTION

A central theme in this volume is the fact that we usually prefer to work with effect sizes, rather than *p*-values. Readers who are accustomed to working with significance tests and *p*-values in primary studies may wonder why we don't synthesize these *p*-values. The reason reflects a fundamental issue that applies both to primary studies and to meta-analysis, and is the subject of this chapter. Since narrative reviews typically work with *p*-values while meta-analyses typically work with effect sizes, the distinction between effect sizes and *p*-values also reflects a difference between narrative reviews and meta-analysis, and we address this as well.

Note that meta-analysis methods are available for working with *p*-values, and we will describe these in Chapter 36.

RELATIONSHIP BETWEEN *p*-VALUES AND EFFECT SIZES

There are two general approaches to data analysis, both in primary studies and in meta-analysis. One is significance testing, where the researcher poses the null hypothesis (for example, that the treatment effect is zero) and then attempts to disprove that hypothesis. The other is effect-size estimation, where the researcher estimates the magnitude of the effect size. Both approaches start with the same values but express them in different ways.

Introduction to Meta-Analysis   M. Borenstein, L. V. Hedges, J. P. T. Higgins, H. R. Rothstein
© 2009, John Wiley & Sons, Ltd

Suppose a study of independent groups reports a standardized mean difference of 0.50 with a standard error of 0.20. To perform a significance test we compute

$$Z = \frac{d}{SE_d},$$ (32.1)

and then compare the observed Z-value to the Z-value required for statistical significance. In this example

$$Z = \frac{0.50}{0.20} = 2.5000.$$

We then compare the observed Z-value of 2.50 with the Z-value of 1.96 (corresponding to the two-tailed alpha of 0.05) and conclude that the effect is statistically significant.

The complementary approach is to report the effect size (which reflects the magnitude of the effect) and its confidence interval (which reflects the precision of the estimate). In this example the effect size is $d = 0.50$. The confidence interval is given by

$$LL_d = d - 1.96 \times SE_d$$ (32.2)

and

$$UL_d = d + 1.96 \times SE_d$$ (32.3)

where 1.96 corresponds to the two-tailed 0.05 significance value. Concretely, the lower limit and upper limit for d are

$$LL_d = 0.50 - 1.96 \times 0.20 = 0.1080$$

and

$$UL_d = 0.50 + 1.96 \times 0.20 = 0.8920.$$

The two approaches are consistent with each other in that the p-value for a test of the null will fall under 0.05 if and only if the 95% confidence interval for the effect size excludes the null value. We can see this in Figure 32.1. The top line reflects the effect size approach, with a line representing the confidence interval extending from the effect size toward the null. The bottom line reflects the significance testing

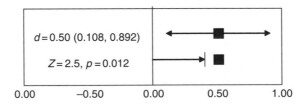

Figure 32.1 Estimating the effect size versus testing the null hypothesis.

approach, with a line representing the nonsignificance region extending from the null toward the effect size. The line is the same length in either case ($Z \times SE_d$), which means that the top line will include the null if and only if the bottom line includes the effect size.

Note. There may be small differences in the length of the line but the difference is generally trivial.

THE DISTINCTION IS IMPORTANT

Since the two approaches are consistent with each other, the decision to use one or the other is largely a matter of choice. However, it is an important choice, because by focusing on different questions (the viability of the null versus the magnitude of the effect) the two approaches shift the attention of the researcher in important ways. While researchers in many fields tend to favor significance tests, there are good reasons to focus on effect sizes instead.

First, the effect size is what we need to decide on a course of action. If a clinician or patient needs to make a decision about whether or not to employ a treatment, they want to know if the treatment reduces the risk of death by 5% or 10% or 20%, and this is the information carried by the effect size. Similarly, if we are thinking of implementing an intervention to increase the test scores of students, or to reduce the number of incarcerations among at-risk juveniles, or to increase the survival time for patients with pancreatic cancer, the question we ask is about the magnitude of the effect. The p-value tells us *only* that the effect may be (or is probably not) zero.

Second, the p-value is often misinterpreted. Because researchers *care about* the effect size, they tend to take whatever information they have and press it into service as an indicator of effect size. A statistically significant p-value is assumed to reflect a clinically important effect, and a nonsignificant p-value is assumed to reflect a trivial (or zero) effect. However, these interpretations are not necessarily correct. The problem with using the p-value as a surrogate for effect size is that the p-value incorporates information about both the size of the effect and also the size of the sample (or the precision with which the effect is estimated). While a significant p-value *may* reflect a large effect size, it could also reflect a small effect size that had been measured in a large study. Similarly, while a nonsignificant p-value *may* reflect a small effect size, it could also reflect a large effect size that had been measured in a small study.

For example, Figure 32.2 is a plot of two studies. Study A has a p-value of 0.119 while Study B has a p-value of < 0.001, which might suggest that the effect is stronger in Study B. In fact, the effect size is the same (0.50) in both studies. The difference in p-values reflects a difference in sample size (40 in Study A versus 200 in Study B), not a difference in effect size.

By contrast, when we work with the effect size we focus on the question of interest, which is to estimate the magnitude of the effect. We report the effect size as 0.50, and (as a separate matter) the precision (-0.129 to 1.129 for Study A, and

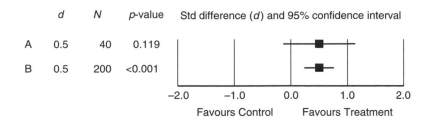

Figure 32.2 The *p*-value is a poor surrogate for effect size.

0.219 to 0.781 for Study *B*). Additionally, this approach avoids the mistakes outlined in the previous paragraph. Because we work with the effect sizes directly we
avoid the problem of interpreting nonsignificant *p*-values to indicate the absence of
an effect (or of interpreting significant *p*-values to indicate a large effect).

THE *p*-VALUE IS OFTEN MISINTERPRETED

While we would argue that researchers should shift their focus to effect sizes even
when working entirely with primary studies, the shift *is absolutely critical* when our
goal is to synthesize data from multiple studies. A narrative reviewer who works
with *p*-values (or with reports that were based on *p*-values) and uses these as the
basis for a synthesis, is facing an impossible task. Where people tend to misinterpret
a single *p*-value, the problem is much worse when they need to compare a series of
p-values. Consider the following three examples.

Suppose we are told that four studies reported *p*-values of 0.28, 0.28, 0.28, and
0.003. A reviewer working with these *p*-values might assume that the effect was
larger in the last study. The studies are shown in Figure 32.3. The effect size is the
same in all the studies, and the *p*-values differ only because the sample size was
larger in the last study.

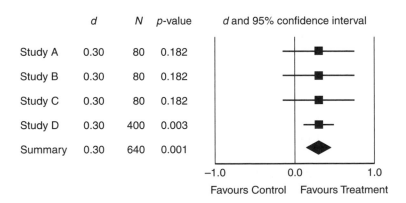

Figure 32.3 Studies where *p*-values differ but effect size is the same.

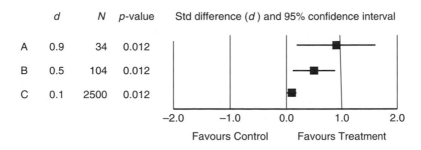

Figure 32.4 Studies where *p*-values are the same but effect sizes differ.

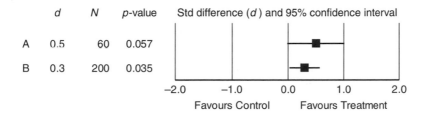

Figure 32.5 Studies where the more significant *p*-value corresponds to weaker effect size.

Suppose we are told that three studies each reported a *p*-value of 0.012. Many would assume that the treatment effect is consistent across studies. The studies are shown in Figure 32.4. Study *A* has a large effect (and poor precision), Study *B* has a moderate effect (and modest precision), while Study *C* has a small effect (and excellent precision).

Suppose we are told that studies *A* and *B* reported *p*-values of 0.057, and 0.035. Many would assume that the effect size was higher in Study *B*. The studies are shown in Figure 32.5, and it turns out that the effect was *weaker* in study *B*.

NARRATIVE REVIEWS VS. META-ANALYSES

The narrative review typically works with *p*-values (or with conclusions that are based on *p*-values), and therefore lends itself to these kinds of mistakes. *p*-values that differ are assumed to reflect different effect sizes but may not (Figure 32.3), *p*-values that are the same are assumed to reflect similar effect sizes but may not (Figure 32.4), and a more significant *p*-value is assumed to reflect a larger effect size when it may actually be based on a smaller effect size (Figure 32.5). By contrast, the meta-analysis works with effect sizes. As such it not only focuses on the question of interest (what is the size of the effect) but allows us to compare the effect size from study to study.

There is an additional difference between meta-analysis and narrative reviews. Where the narrative review treats each item of information as discrete (and the synthesis takes place in the reviewer's head), meta-analysis incorporates all of the effect sizes in a single statistical analysis. Even if the p-value did move in tandem with the effect size (for example, if all studies in the analysis had the same sample size), the narrative review provides no mechanism for assessing the dispersion in effect size from one study to the next. By contrast, meta-analysis usually works directly with the effect size (which is separated from the sample size), and uses established statistical techniques to isolate and quantify the true dispersion.

SUMMARY POINTS

- To synthesize data from a series of studies we need to work with the effect size rather than the p-value from each study and we need to incorporate all of the effect sizes in a single analysis, rather than working with discrete results from the separate studies.
- The narrative review fails on both counts. It works with the p-values from the primary studies (either directly, or because most studies basc their results section and discussion on the p-values). And, it tries to perform a synthesis working with a series of discrete results.
- By contrast, meta-analysis has developed methods to meet these two goals. It works with the effect sizes, and incorporates all of these in a single analysis.

CHAPTER 33

Simpson's Paradox

Introduction
Circumcision and risk of HIV infection
An example of the paradox

INTRODUCTION

To compute the summary effect in a meta-analysis we compute an effect size for each study and then combine these effect sizes, rather than pooling the data directly. For example, if we start with 2×2 tables we compute an odds ratio for each table and then combine these odds ratios. We *do not* pool the cell counts across tables to create a pooled 2×2 table and then compute the odds ratio for this table.

This approach allows us to study the dispersion of effects before proceeding to the summary effect. For a random-effects model this approach also allows us to incorporate the between-studies dispersion into the weights.

There is one additional reason for using this approach, and that reason is the subject of this chapter. The reason is to ensure that each effect size is based on the comparison of a group with *its own* control group, and thus avoid a problem known as Simpson's paradox. In some cases, particularly when we are working with observational studies, this is a critically important feature.

To illustrate this point we present a review published by Van Howe (1999) which concluded that circumcision is associated with increased risk of HIV. Matthias Egger presented a critique of this review at the Cochrane Colloquium in Cape Town in 1999, and (with O'Farrell), also published a commentary in the *International Journal of STD and AIDS* (O'Farrell and Egger, 2000). What follows draws heavily on this work.

CIRCUMCISION AND RISK OF HIV INFECTION

Van Howe (1999) published a review article in the *International Journal of STD and AIDS* that looked at the relationship between circumcision and HIV infection in Africa. The article was based on data from 33 studies, which Van Howe classified into one of three groups based on the populations studied. The *High-risk* populations included

Table 33.1 HIV as function of circumcision (by subgroup).

Sample	Studies	N	Prevalence HIV
High risk	15	13,238	25%
Partner	7	13,515	11%
Random	11	17,267	9%
Total	33	44,020	

long-distance truck drivers and patients recruited at STD clinics. The *Partner* studies looked at HIV infection in men whose partner was HIV positive. The *Random population* surveys did not target specific groups. The prevalence of HIV in the men in these three groups was 25%, 11% and 9%, respectively (see Table 33.1).

The data for all 33 studies are shown in Table 33.2. An odds ratio less than 1.0 means that circumcision is associated with *higher* risk of HIV, and an odds ratio greater than 1.0 means that circumcision is associated with *lower* risk of HIV.

In the first study, Bwayo(a), the risk of HIV is 52% (92/178) for noncircumcised versus 21% (160/772) for circumcised, yielding an odds ratio of 4.09 (lower risk for circumcised), and so on for the remaining studies. Of the 33 studies, 8 associated circumcision with higher risk (an odds ratio of less than 1.0), and 25 with lower risk (an odds ratio greater than 1.0).

The same data are shown graphically in Figure 33.1.

Study name	Statistics for each study			HIV / Total		Odds ratio and 95% CI				
	Odds ratio	Z-Value	p-Value	Non-Circ	Circumcized	0.01	0.10	1.00	10.00	100.00
Bwayo (a)	4.092	8.084	0.000	92 / 178	160 / 772					
Bwayo (b)	2.585	3.015	0.003	22 / 68	37 / 237					
Kreiss	2.168	2.696	0.007	59 / 77	254 / 422					
Hira	2.430	1.946	0.052	418 / 590	10 / 20					
Cameron	10.230	4.713	0.000	18 / 79	6 / 214					
Pepin	2.225	1.449	0.147	5 / 47	13 / 256					
Greenblatt	3.339	2.336	0.019	11 / 39	8 / 76					
Diallo	3.402	5.273	0.000	38 / 84	212 / 1085					
Simonsen	2.683	2.791	0.005	17 / 87	21 / 253					
Tyndall	4.587	8.269	0.000	85 / 178	105 / 632					
Nasio	4.668	8.421	0.000	86 / 164	137 / 717					
Mehendal	1.634	2.755	0.006	837 / 4248	38 / 291					
Bollinger	2.905	1.019	0.308	50 / 291	1 / 15					
Chiasson	1.749	1.747	0.081	36 / 833	14 / 556					
Sassan	2.219	2.894	0.004	75 / 93	415 / 636					
Hunter	2.973	6.034	0.000	43 / 373	165 / 3930					
Carael	1.134	0.469	0.639	90 / 195	34 / 79					
Chao	0.282	-8.919	0.000	442 / 5286	75 / 307					
Moss	2.125	1.519	0.129	24 / 40	12 / 29					
Allen	1.103	0.776	0.438	275 / 887	132 / 456					
Sedlin	1.492	1.131	0.258	32 / 58	33 / 73					
Konde-Luc	2.136	1.780	0.075	153 / 1669	6 / 133					
Barongo	0.620	-2.272	0.023	55 / 1411	42 / 684					
Grosskurth	0.577	-3.554	0.000	158 / 4762	61 / 1087					
Van de	0.890	-0.243	0.808	46 / 270	6 / 32					
Seed	1.526	2.324	0.020	171 / 593	51 / 243					
Malamba	2.179	2.646	0.008	111 / 225	21 / 68					
Quigley	0.936	-0.320	0.749	101 / 373	48 / 169					
Urassa 1	0.615	-2.316	0.021	56 / 1357	42 / 642					
Urassa 2	0.685	-1.810	0.070	105 / 2145	32 / 458					
Urassa 3	1.023	0.075	0.940	38 / 347	19 / 177					
Urassa 4	2.005	3.996	0.000	112 / 828	54 / 746					
Urassa 5	0.784	-1.204	0.229	101 / 466	48 / 184					

Figure 33.1 HIV as function of circumcision – by study.

AN EXAMPLE OF THE PARADOX

Van Howe summed the counts in each cell across the 33 studies (see the line labeled *Total* in Table 33.2) to yield Table 33.3. Using this table he computed the risk of HIV as 14% (3962/28341) for noncircumcised versus 15% (2312/15679) for circumcised, and the odds ratio as 0.94 (95% confidence interval 0.89 to 0.99) with *p*-value under 0.05. Van Howe concludes that 'When the raw data are combined, a

Table 33.2 HIV as function of circumcision – by study.

Study name	Noncircumcised		Circumcised		Prevalence		Odds Ratio
	HIV+	Total	HIV+	Total	Noncircumcised	Circumcised	
High risk							
Bwayo (a)	92	178	160	772	0.52	0.21	4.09
Bwayo (b)	22	68	37	237	0.32	0.16	2.59
Kreiss	59	77	254	422	0.77	0.60	2.17
Hira	418	590	10	20	0.71	0.50	2.43
Cameron	18	79	6	214	0.23	0.03	10.23
Pepin	5	47	13	256	0.11	0.05	2.23
Greenblatt	11	39	8	76	0.28	0.11	3.34
Diallo	38	84	212	1085	0.45	0.20	3.40
Simonsen	17	87	21	253	0.20	0.08	2.68
Tyndall	85	178	105	632	0.48	0.17	4.59
Nasio	86	164	137	717	0.52	0.19	4.67
Mehendal	837	4248	38	291	0.20	0.13	1.63
Bollinger	50	291	1	15	0.17	0.07	2.90
Chiasson	36	833	14	556	0.04	0.03	1.75
Sassan	75	93	415	636	0.81	0.65	2.22
Partner							
Hunter	43	373	165	3930	0.12	0.04	2.97
Carael	90	195	34	79	0.46	0.43	1.13
Chao	442	5286	75	307	0.08	0.24	0.28
Moss	24	40	12	29	0.60	0.41	2.13
Allen	275	887	132	456	0.31	0.29	1.10
Sedlin	32	58	33	73	0.55	0.45	1.49
Konde-Luc	153	1669	6	133	0.09	0.05	2.14
Random population							
Barongo	55	1411	42	684	0.04	0.06	0.62
Grosskurth	158	4762	61	1087	0.03	0.06	0.58
Van de Perre	46	270	6	32	0.17	0.19	0.89
Seed	171	593	51	243	0.29	0.21	1.53
Malamba	111	225	21	68	0.49	0.31	2.18
Quigley	101	373	48	169	0.27	0.28	0.94
Urassa 1	56	1357	42	642	0.04	0.07	0.61
Urassa 2	105	2145	32	458	0.05	0.07	0.69
Urassa 3	38	347	19	177	0.11	0.11	1.02
Urassa 4	112	828	54	746	0.14	0.07	2.00
Urassa 5	101	466	48	184	0.22	0.26	0.78
Total	3962	28341	2312	15679	0.14	0.15	0.94

Table 33.3 HIV as a function of circumcision – full population.

	HIV Positive	HIV Negative	Total	% HIV
Noncircumcised	3962	24379	28341	14%
Circumcised	2312	13367	15679	15%

man with a circumcised penis is at *greater risk* of acquiring and transmitting HIV than a man with a non-circumcised penis.'

This conclusion seems to be at odds with the full table of data, where the preponderance of studies (25 of the 33) had odds ratios greater than 1.0, meaning that circumcision was associated with *lower risk* of HIV. This anomaly is also evident on the plot, where 25 studies line up on the right-side of 1.0, with only 8 on the left. Also, the 8 studies on the left are not large enough to have pulled the effect so far to the left. Therefore, it seems counter-intuitive that the summary effect should fall to the left.

In fact, this intuition is correct. When the data are analyzed using standard meta-analysis techniques, circumcision is associated with a *lower risk* of HIV. Under the random-effects model the odds ratio is 1.67 with a 95% confidence interval of 1.25 to 2.24, Z of 3.42 and p-value of 0.001. The fixed-effect model is not appropriate here since the effects are clearly heterogeneous ($Q = 419$, $df = 32$, $p<0.0001$) but the fixed-effect model would lead to the same conclusion with an odds ratio of 1.40, 95% confidence interval of 1.29 to 1.51, $Z = 8.43$, and a p-value of <0.0001. These findings are consistent with the visual impression of the data, and contradict Van Howe's conclusions.

The reason that Van Howe reported a *higher risk* for circumcision is that rather than compute an effect size for each study and then pool these effects, he pooled the 2×2 tables for each study and then used the combined table to compute the odds ratio. The reason that this matters is as follows.

Recall that the 33 studies included three kinds of populations, *High risk*, *Partners*, and *Random*, with prevalence rates of 25%, 11% and 9%, respectively. It turns out that a disproportionate number of the circumcised patients were from the *High risk* studies. Among circumcised persons 39% came from the *high risk* studies while only 29% came from the *Random* studies. Among the noncircumcised, by contrast, 25% came from the high risk studies while 45% came from the *Random* studies. The proportion of noncircumcised and circumcised subjects drawn from each kind of study is shown in Table 33.4.

Table 33.4 HIV as a function of circumcision – by risk group.

	High Risk	Partner	Random
Noncircumcised	25%	30%	45%
Circumcised	39%	32%	29%

Table 33.5 HIV as a function of circumcision/risk group – full population.

	HIV Positive	HIV Negative	Total	% HIV
Noncircumcised, low HIV prevalence population	3962	24379	28341	14%
Circumcised, high HIV prevalence population	2312	13367	15679	15%

In this light, the labels in Table 33.3 might better reflect the facts if we modified them as shown in Table 33.5. Rather than *Noncircumcised* versus *Circumcised*, the rows are labeled *Noncircumcised low HIV prevalence population* versus *Circumcised, high HIV prevalence population*.

In sum, the problem with Van Howe's analysis is that by summing the raw data he introduced confounding. That is, the noncircumcised men cannot legitimately be compared with the circumcised population because they differ in other ways. The increased risk of HIV that appeared to be associated with circumcision was also associated with an array of high-risk behaviors (and more likely due to those than to the circumcision). By contrast, when we compute an effect size for each study we control for these confounds (at least to the extent possible when working with observational studies).

Egger also showed what happens if we compute the odds ratio *within* each of the three groups that Van Howe had delineated. Within the high risk group, circumcision is associated with a decreased risk (by about two-thirds) of HIV. Within each of the other two groups of studies the relationship between circumcision and HIV (if any) is small (see Figure 33.2).

Egger used this pattern of effects to formulate several hypotheses about the mechanisms by which circumcision might have an impact on the risk of HIV infection, and suggested that these be tested in future studies. This is an elegant and appropriate use of meta-analysis, to direct the formulation and conduct of future studies.

Egger also noted that given the heterogeneity of effects it would be a mistake to draw any conclusions from the analysis at this point. As Egger said in concluding his presentation at Capetown, 'I am not suggesting that you all run right out and get circumcised.'

The problem addressed in this chapter has been known to statisticians for a long time, and is generally called Simpson's paradox. The term paradox refers to the fact that one group can do better in *every one* of the included studies, but still do worse when the raw data are pooled. The problem is not limited to studies that use proportions, but can exist also in studies that use means or other indices. The problem exists only when the base rate (or mean) varies from study to study *and* the proportion of participants from each group varies as well. For this reason, the problem is generally limited to observational studies, although it can exist in randomized trials when allocation ratios vary from study to study.

For readers who choose to savor these papers in the original, note that the Van Howe paper seems to include a number of typographical errors which we corrected for this

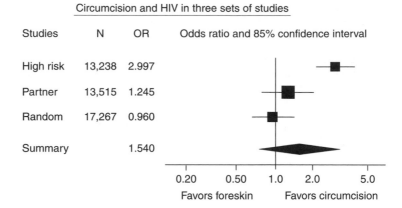

Figure 33.2 HIV as function of circumcision – in three sets of studies.

chapter (in particular, the Van Howe abstract reverses the direction of the odds ratio from the one used in the body of paper). Note also that Egger raises many questions about Van Howe's methodology in addition to the ones outlined here.

SUMMARY POINTS

- In a meta-analysis we compute an effect size for each study and combine these effect sizes, rather than combining the summary data and then computing an effect size for the combined data.
- This allows us to determine whether or not the effects are consistent across studies.
- This also ensures that each study serves as its own control, which minimizes the potential impact of confounders.
- If we were to pool data across studies and then compute the effect size from the pooled data, we may get the wrong answer, due to Simpson's paradox.

Further reading

Chudnovsky, A & Niederberger, C.S. (2007). The foreskin dilemma: To cut or not to cut. *J Androl* 28: 5–7.

O'Farrell, N., & Egger, M. (2000). Circumcision in men and the prevention of HIV infection: a 'meta-analysis' revisited. *Int J STD AIDS*, 11, 137–142.

Siegfried, N., Muller, M., Volmink, J., *et al*. (2003). Male circumcision for prevention of heterosexual acquisition of HIV in men. Cochrane Database of Systematic Reviews Issue 3. Art. No.: CD003362. DOI: 10.1002/14651858.CD003362.

Siegfried, N., Muller, M., Deeks, J., *et al*. (2005) HIV and male circumcision-a systematic review with assessment of the quality of studies. *Lancet Infect Dis* 5:165–173.

Van Howe, R.S. (1999). Circumcision and HIV infection: review of the literature and meta-analysis. *Int J STD AIDS*, 10(1), 8–16.

Van Howe R.S., Cold, C.J., Storms, M.R., *et al.* (2000). Male circumcision and HIV prevention. *BMJ* 321: 1467–1468; author reply 1469.

Van Howe R.S., Svobodo, J.S., & Hodges, M. (2005). HIV infection and circumcision: cutting through the hyperbole, *Journal of the Royal Society for the Promotion of Health*, 125: 259–265.

CHAPTER 34

Generality of the Basic Inverse-Variance Method

Introduction
Other effect sizes
Other methods for estimating effect sizes
Individual participant data meta-analyses
Bayesian approaches

INTRODUCTION

The basic idea of meta-analysis is to compute an effect size from each of several studies, and to calculate a weighted average of these effect size estimates. We have shown how the weights can reflect either a fixed-effect assumption or a random-effects assumption. We have also seen how we can examine differences in effect sizes across studies, using subgroup analyses and meta-regression.

In all of our examples so far, we have applied these methods to *comparative studies* or studies of *association*. For example, we might compare the outcomes of people randomized to different treatments in a clinical trial by looking at the difference in means or the ratio of risks. Or, we could use the same techniques to compare the scores in two existing groups, such as males and females.

Precisely the same approach to meta-analysis can be used to work with other kinds of studies and other kinds of data. We will use the term *point estimate* as a more generic term than effect size estimate, to reflect the fact that we are not necessarily looking at the effect of one thing on another. The only requirements for meta-analysis to be possible are that

- The point estimate can be expressed as a single number.
- We can compute a variance for the point estimate.

Introduction to Meta-Analysis   M. Borenstein, L. V. Hedges, J. P. T. Higgins, H. R. Rothstein
© 2009, John Wiley & Sons, Ltd

OTHER EFFECT SIZES

We now provide some examples of situations in which these requirements are met and where meta-analysis can therefore be used to combine findings across studies. We do not attempt to provide detailed methodology for any of these. Rather, our aim is to provide a flavor of the range of applications for the basic methods. Many of the relevant formulas are provided in the companion volume, *Computing Effect Sizes for Meta-Analysis* (Borenstein, Hedges, Higgins and Rothstein, 2009, John Wiley & Sons, Ltd).

Single descriptive statistics

A meta-analysis can be used to combine single descriptive statistics. For example, a sample of continuous measures might be summarized simply by its mean, and a meta-analysis might be performed to synthesize means across samples (or studies).

Similarly, a sample of binary outcomes might be summarized simply by the proportion of successes, the risk of an event, or the prevalence of a condition. For example, a meta-analysis was used to assess the prevalence of food allergies in the general population (Rona *et al.*, 2007). Prevalence was estimated from each study, along with its variance, and combined in a meta-analysis using standard techniques. However, as is often the case for single-group studies, very substantial heterogeneity was observed. For instance, while the average prevalence of self-reported milk allergy was a little over 3% in a meta-analysis, with a tight 95% confidence interval from around 2.5% to 4%, the results from the individual studies ranged from 1.2% to 17%.

Physical constants

Meta-analysis methods have a long history in the field of physics. For example, Raymond Birge published a paper on methods for combining estimates of physical constants from different experiments in 1932. In 1941, he summarized numerous attempts that had been made to measure the speed of light in a vacuum, and calculated weighted averages of their findings (Birge, 1941). A similar approach has been used for other important constants. These are essentially meta-analyses of the multiple experiments, although the term meta-analysis was not introduced until 1976.

Two-group studies with other types of data

Although we have described in some detail different indices for comparing two groups when the outcomes are continuous or binary, we should make it clear that other types of data may be encountered. Three particular different types of data are as follows.

Ordinal data arise when each individual is assigned to one of *three or more* categories, and these categories have a logical ordering. For example, the symptoms of a condition after a period of treatment might be assessed as 'mild', 'moderate' or 'severe'. A single effect size can be computed from studies with ordinal data for use in meta-analysis. For example, under assumptions of a proportional odds model, an odds ratio is available (this is not computed in the same way as in Chapter 5).

Time-to-event (survival) data are used when we know how long each person was followed, and the outcome (either the event occurred or the follow-up period ended). Typically we compute a hazard ratio to reflect the treatment effect in each study and use meta-analysis to synthesize these hazard ratios across studies.

Rate data arise when the data includes both a period of observation and the number of times a specific event occurs during this period. This type of data is used to determine whether the incidence of a (repeatable) event is lower in one group than the other. In particular, it allows for individuals to have more than one event.

Methods are available for comparing two groups when any of these types of data are encountered. As noted above, the sorts of indices that are most commonly encountered are odds ratios for ordinal data, hazard ratios for time-to-event data and rate ratios for rate data. The meta-analysis would proceed in the same way, in each of these particular cases working in the logarithmic scale because the indices are ratios rather than differences.

Three-group studies

We provide one example of how basic meta-analysis methods have been applied to studies with three groups, in the field of genetic epidemiology. There is considerable interest in understanding how our genetic make-up affects our risk of developing diseases such as cancer and cardiovascular disease. Many studies are therefore investigating these relationships by measuring genetic variants and looking at the association between these variants and disease. Most genetic variants have two versions, called alleles. Crudely put, one of these alleles may usually be considered the *normal* variant, with the other having arisen as a mutation at some point during human evolution. For each genetic variant, we receive one copy from our father and one from our mother. We therefore end up with one of three possible combinations: two normal alleles, two mutant alleles or one normal allele and one mutant allele.

A simple genetic association study divides individuals into three groups according to their genetic variants, and cross-tabulates these groups against disease status. For example, one study by Lacasaña-Navarro and colleagues (2006) measured a specific variant in the methylenetetrahydrofolate reductase (MTHFR) gene, and compared the distributions of people having different combinations of alleles with their gastric cancer status. The two alleles for this specific variant (at position 677 in the gene) are termed 677C and 677T. The results are shown in Table 34.1.

Table 34.1 Simple example of a genetic association study.

Genotype	Interpretation	Cases	Controls	Total
677C, 677C	normal, normal	56	144	200
677C, 677T	normal, mutation	85	179	264
677T, 677T	mutation, mutation	60	104	164
Total		201	427	628

There are several ways in which this study can be included in a basic meta-analysis. However, comparisons among three groups cannot be reduced to a single number without making assumptions or ignoring some of the information. A published meta-analysis by Boccia (2008) and colleagues created a 2×2 table by excluding the middle (normal, mutation) group. Thus, they compared people with two mutation alleles with people with two normal alleles. This simple approach imposes no assumptions about the way in which the genetic variants determine risk, but does not make use of all of the data. To use all of the data in a standard meta-analysis, we have to make assumptions. Three common assumptions are

- A *dominant* genetic model, in which we assume that at least one mutation is sufficient to alter risk of disease (and it does not matter whether one or two mutation alleles is present)
- A *recessive* model, in which we assume both mutation alleles are required to alter risk of disease (and having one is no different from having none)
- An *additive* model, in which we assume there is a similar change in risk for each additional mutation allele

To perform a meta-analysis assuming a dominant or a recessive model, the 3×2 table from each study is collapsed into a 2×2 table from each study, by combining either the second two rows (for a dominant model) or the first two rows (recessive model) in the table above. To perform an additive model, alternative methods need to be used for each study such as logistic regression. In every case, however, a log odds ratio and its variance is obtained for each study, and the meta-analysis proceeds in exactly the same way as we have described earlier in the book.

Regression coefficients

A final example of the broad range of types of study amenable to meta-analysis is the combination of regression coefficients, or beta weights. This is the synthesis of results from several regression analyses, and should not to be confused with meta-regression. For example, Sirmans and colleagues (2006) were interested in the relationship between house price and various characteristics of the house such as its square footage, age, number of bedrooms and presence of a swimming pool. Tackling each of these separately, they compiled studies that have looked at the relationship (e.g. between square footage and house price) and obtained regression coefficients to characterize the relationship. These could then be combined in a meta-analysis, using the variances of the coefficients in the weights.

However, the main aim of these authors was not simply to obtain an overall regression coefficient, but to examine whether the regression coefficients depend on other study-level characteristics, such as the location and timing of the study, and whether or not the regression analysis controlled for other house characteristics (e.g. number of bedrooms). The primary analysis is therefore a meta-regression of regression coefficients.

OTHER METHODS FOR ESTIMATING EFFECT SIZES

In the previous section we discussed how the basic meta-analysis method of computing inverse-variance weighted averages can be applied to diverse types of studies and to diverse types of data. In a fixed-effect meta-analysis, the weighted average provides a summary estimate of a common effect size. In a random-effects meta-analysis, the weighted average (using revised weights) provides an estimate of the mean effect size across studies. In a random-effects meta-analysis we also compute an estimate of the standard deviation of effect sizes across studies.

The inverse-variance weighted average approach is not the only way to perform a meta-analysis. Both fixed-effect meta-analyses and random-effects meta-analyses can be undertaken using a variety of other statistical methods. The need to consider other methods typically arises either to refine the analysis of data within a study, or to refine the analysis of variation across studies (or, quite frequently, for both).

Refined methods tailored to the type of data within a study

First, we may wish to analyze the data *within a study* using methods specific to the type of data we have. For instance, if we have 2×2 tables from binary data, the methods we have described involve the computation of an effect size for each study (such as a log odds ratio or a risk difference) and its variance. For most purposes this is appropriate, but when studies are small, or when events are rare, other methods can have better statistical properties. To understand why this might be, note that the basic inverse-variance method assumes that the variance from each study is truly the variance of that study's effect size estimate. However, in reality the variance is only an estimate of the true variance. For large studies, the estimate is close to the true variance and the assumption is not problematic. For small studies, the variance may not be well estimated.

Methods based directly on 2×2 tables for binary data do not require us to estimate the variance. Some examples are the Mantel-Haenszel method and the one-step method commonly referred to as the Peto method. We discuss these methods in Chapter 37.

Another situation in which we might prefer to analyse a study using methods specific to the type of data is when we have the original data from each study, often referred to as *individual participant data*. We could compute a standardized mean difference, or an odds ratio, or some other effect size, from these data and perform an inverse-variance meta-analysis. However, we might alternatively wish to perform the meta-analysis directly on the complete original dataset. We discuss the potential advantages of this approach in the next section.

Refined methods for analysing between-study variation

The second reason for considering other methods for meta-analysis is that we may wish to combine results *across studies* using more sophisticated statistical techniques. In particular, in random-effects meta-analysis, we estimate the between-study standard deviation, τ. When the number of studies is small, this can be estimated with considerable error, as we describe in Chapters 17 and 40. Methods are available that allow uncertainty in τ to be taken into account. One such possibility is a Bayesian approach to the meta-analysis, which we discuss at the end of this chapter. A further consideration in the random-effects inverse-variance method is the assumption that the true effects in different studies follow a normal distribution. It is usually very difficult to assess whether this assumption is reasonable. Methods are available that assume other distributions, and even methods that allow the data to determine the shape of the distribution. These are advanced methods that so far have mostly been considered only by statistical methods researchers.

INDIVIDUAL PARTICIPANT DATA META-ANALYSES

When the meta-analyst has access to all of the original data from each study, the meta-analysis may be referred to as an *individual participant data* (or *individual patient data*) meta-analysis. This usually involves collaboration with the authors of the original studies included in the meta-analysis. There are many advantages to individual participant data (IPD) meta-analysis over literature-based meta-analysis (or summary data meta-analysis), which are summarized by Stewart and Tierney (2002). These include

- Being able to perform consistent data checking and (if necessary) data cleaning
- Having available a complete and up-to-date dataset on which to base analyses
- Being able to perform a wide variety of statistical analyses in the same way in every study
- Being able to examine the effects of participant-level covariates
- Further benefits of having direct contact with study authors, for example in collating descriptive information about the studies, interpreting results and identifying further studies.

With access to individual participant data, the range of possible analysis methods is substantial. Methods can be broadly categorized as methods that analyze each study separately and then combine effect sizes using standard meta-analysis techniques, and (on the other hand) methods that analyze all of the data in one go.

Applying standard meta-analysis methods to individual participant data

A common approach is to analyze each study in a consistent way and to perform an inverse-variance meta-analysis on the resulting effect size estimates and their variances. For example, a mean difference could be computed from each study, and these combined using the standard methods.

Having access to IPD, however, allows for consistent, and even complex, analyses of the data from each study. For instance, a problem sometimes encountered in summary data meta-analysis is that studies provide effect size estimates that are adjusted for different sets of covariates. For example, one study might adjust for age and sex; and another might adjust for age, sex and smoking behavior. With access to the raw data, the meta-analyst can adjust for the same covariates in every study.

Another common limitation of summary data is that studies present basic results in such different ways that a common effect size cannot readily be computed for each study. This is particularly the case for time-to-event data. Because a pair of observations is collected on each individual (the length of observation and whether the event occurs at the end of this period), time-to-event data cannot conveniently be reduced to simple summaries such as a 2×2 table. Thus, only results of *analyses* tend to be presented, which may differ across studies. Many of the existing IPD meta-analyses in the medical area address time-to-event outcomes, since a common method of analysis can be applied to each study prior to the meta-analysis.

Analyzing individual patient data in a single analysis

Given IPD for a series of primary studies, any method that could be used to analyze the individual studies can be used to analyze the complete data set. The key principle underlying the analysis of an IPD dataset is that the individual identities of the studies are respected. In this way we avoid the problem of Simpson's paradox discussed in Chapter 33. In statistical terminology, we say that the analysis is stratified by study. This is often achieved in practice by including a dummy covariate for each study.

An advantage of analyzing all IPD together (rather than analyzing each study separately and then synthesizing the effect sizes) is that information may be borrowed from one study to another. For example, suppose we are interested in whether the effect of a weight-loss intervention depends on age, and we have several small trials of the intervention, each performed in a similar population with mixed ages. We cannot use meta-regression for such a question because age is a participant-level rather than a study-level covariate (the mean age will be roughly the same for every study). If we have IPD from the trials, including each participant's age, then we can obtain a powerful analysis of the effect of age on intervention by analyzing all of the data at once, providing we stratify by study. We can decide to borrow information from one study to another to further increase the power. For example, we could assume that the standard deviation for weight losses is the same in every study.

In fact, every one of the meta-analysis models we have discussed up to this point in the book can be performed in a single analysis of IPD, by making different assumptions in the statistical model. However, some of the random-effects models are difficult to implement. Therefore, the simpler approach of analyzing each study individually, and then synthesizing the effect sizes in a meta-analysis, remains the most popular in practice.

BAYESIAN APPROACHES

The methods we describe in this book are classical, or frequentist, methods for statistics. They revolve around estimating unknown parameters along with confidence intervals, and performing statistical tests in order to determine the extent to which the results are compatible with a null hypothesis (the p-value).

An alternative approach to statistics is the Bayesian approach. This stems from a different philosophy of probability, and in particular from an interpretation of probability as an uncertainty (or a belief) rather than a frequency. Bayesian statistics attaches probability distributions to the parameters of interest. The main parameters of interest in a meta-analysis are the overall mean effect size and, in a random-effects meta-analysis, the standard deviation (τ) of true effect sizes across studies. We might, for example, represent our uncertainty about an overall mean log odds ratio by attaching a normal distribution centered on our *best guess* and with tails describing how confident we are about it.

A Bayesian analysis starts by attaching a prior probability distribution to each unknown quantity. This describes *a priori* uncertainty (or belief) about the quantity before seeing the data. In many cases, the prior distribution is used to express ignorance (e.g. as a flat distribution). The Bayesian analysis itself combines the prior distribution with the data, turning it into a posterior probability distribution for the unknown quantity. When the prior distribution represents prior ignorance, the posterior distribution is simply a summary of what the data tell us about the quantity. Thus a Bayesian analysis can be viewed as a generalization of the classical method, with the flexibility to include prior information in a formal way if desired.

Instead of producing confidence intervals, Bayesian analyses produce *credible intervals* (sometimes called probability intervals, and not to be confused with the credibility interval described in Chapter 38). A 95% credible interval from a Bayesian analysis is a summary of the posterior distribution, such that the probability is equal to 95% that the true quantity is within the interval. This is a particularly intuitive way to express uncertainty, and is one of the most appealing aspects of a Bayesian analysis.

We can make further statements about the unknown quantity after a Bayesian analysis. In particular, we can state the probability that the quantity lies in any specified range. For instance, we can state the probability that the quantity is smaller than (or bigger than) zero. This is a bit like a *p*-value, but is a more direct statement since it does not require a null hypothesis for its interpretation.

The controversial aspect of Bayesian meta-analysis is the source of the prior distribution. In practice, several different prior distributions are often compared. If very different prior distributions all lead to the same posterior distribution, then we can conclude that the data are sufficiently convincing to overwhelm any *a priori* belief, and the analysis might be considered robust. However, if the prior is influential, then this usually means that there are insufficient data, and both a Bayesian and a classical meta-analysis ought to be interpreted with some caution.

The combination of prior distribution and data to produce the posterior distribution is computationally very demanding. This is partly why Bayesian methods have only become prominent in recent years. Flexible software is now available for performing Bayesian analyses, particularly the WinBUGS software. In fact, this software is so flexible that very complicated meta-analysis models can be fitted even more easily than in a classical framework. We therefore expect to see more meta-analyses undertaken using Bayesian methods, and for the models they implement to become more and more complex.

SUMMARY POINTS

- The basic inverse-variance approach to meta-analysis can be applied to a very large class of problems. All we need is a point estimate and its variance from each study.
- Meta-analyses that use the raw data from every included study are often called individual patient data meta-analyses, at least in the medical area. These offer unrivalled flexibility in methods.
- Bayesian methods are based on different philosophical approach to statistics. Results of Bayesian analyses have an appealing interpretation, and they readily allow more complex models to be fitted to meta-analysis datasets, but they require specialized software and require specification of a prior distribution for each parameter.

Further reading

Stewart, L.A. & Tierney, J.F. (2002). To IPD or not to IPD? Advantages and disadvantages of systematic reviews using individual patient data. *Evaluation and the Health Professions* 25: 76–97.

Sutton, A.J. & Abrams, K.R. (2001). Bayesian methods in meta-analysis and evidence synthesis. *Statistical Methods in Medical Research* 10: 277–303.

PART 8

Further Methods

CHAPTER 35

Overview

Thus far, we have concentrated on a specific approach to meta-analysis, based on obtaining an estimate of effect size, along with its variance, from each study. These effect estimates are combined across studies using a weighted average, with inverse variances as weights. In this Part we consider some alternate approaches.

In Chapter 36 we discuss methods based on combining *p*-values, rather than effect sizes, and also a method based on direction of effect in each study (ignoring the magnitude of the effect). We explain how these methods work, outline their limitations, and discuss when it may be appropriate to apply them.

In Chapter 37 we discuss further methods for dichotomous (binary) outcome data. These include the *Mantel-Haenszel* methods and a 'one-step' method known widely as the *Peto* method.

Finally, in Chapter 38 we discuss further methods for correlational data, detailing in particular a method due to Hunter and Schmidt known to many as *psychometric meta-analysis*.

Introduction to Meta-Analysis   M. Borenstein, L. V. Hedges, J. P. T. Higgins, H. R. Rothstein
© 2009, John Wiley & Sons, Ltd

CHAPTER 36

Meta-Analysis Methods Based on Direction and p-Values

Introduction
Vote counting
The sign test
Combining p-values

INTRODUCTION

In this volume we have concentrated almost exclusively on meta-analysis of *effect sizes*. This reflects current practice, as the overwhelming majority of meta-analyses published over the past two decades *are* meta-analyses of effect sizes. A meta-analysis of effect sizes addresses the magnitude of the effect, which is what we care about. By contrast, a meta-analysis of p-values tells us only that the effect is probably not zero.

Nevertheless, there are cases where a meta-analysis of effect sizes is not possible, and in those cases the only option may be to test a null hypothesis. In this chapter we outline a few options for this goal and explain where these might be used.

VOTE COUNTING

Vote counting is the process of counting the number of studies that are statistically significant and the number that are not, and then choosing the winner. This approach is discussed in Chapter 28 where we explain why it has no validity whatsoever. We mention it here only to be sure that it is not confused with the sign test (below) which is a valid approach.

THE SIGN TEST

In a sign test, we count the number of studies with findings in one direction and compare this with the number of studies with findings in the other direction,

Introduction to Meta-Analysis   M. Borenstein, L. V. Hedges, J. P. T. Higgins, H. R. Rothstein
© 2009, John Wiley & Sons, Ltd

irrespective of whether the findings were statistically significant. The sign test takes into account *neither* the actual effect magnitudes observed in the studies *nor* the amount of evidence within each study (for example, the sample sizes). As such it has very limited value. However, it might be considered in any of the following cases.

- When no numerical data are provided from the studies, but directions of effect are provided
- When the numerical data are of such different types that they cannot be combined statistically
- When the studies are so diverse in their populations or other characteristics that a pooled effect size is meaningless, but the studies are still addressing a question sufficiently similar that the direction of the effect is meaningful.

If a treatment is truly ineffective, we would expect half of the studies to lie on each side of the no-effect line. We can test this formally by comparing the number of studies in one direction versus the null value of 50%.

For example, in the streptokinase meta-analysis (Chapter 2), 25 out of 33 studies favored the treatment (i.e. had a point estimate of the risk ratio less than 1.0), and 8 studies favored the control (i.e. had a point estimate of the risk ratio greater than 1.0). The two-sided p-value for the sign test is 0.00455 (in Excel, the function = 2*BINOM-DIST(8,33,0.5,TRUE) returns 0.00455). Or, the one-sided p-value for the sign test is 0.0023 (the function =BINOMDIST(8,33,0.5,TRUE) returns 0.0023). Note that in Excel we need to enter the *smaller* of the two numbers and the total (here, 8 and 33).

COMBINING p-VALUES

Another option when we don't want to work with effect sizes is to work directly with the p-values from each test, to yield an overall p-value. Unlike the sign test or the p-value for a summary effect size, both of which test the null that the *mean effect* across studies is zero (or 1.0 for a ratio), the tests based on combining p-values tests the null that the effect size is zero *in all studies*. In other words, if we combine p-values and obtain a significant effect, we would conclude that the effect is real *in at least one* of the included studies.

In deciding which approach to use (a meta-analysis of effect sizes or of p-values), the fact that some (or all) studies reported p-values (and not an effect size) should not be a factor. This is because starting with the p-value and some additional information (such as the sample size) we can usually back-compute the effect size and its variance, and then perform a meta-analysis of the effect sizes.

Rather, the approach of combining p-values may be considered under the following conditions.

- If we want to test the null that the effect is zero *in all the studies*. This might be the case, for example, if each study looked for a different serious side effect for a drug, and we want to know if there is evidence that *any* of the side effects is present. We assume here that the separate tests have adequate power.

- When we have the *p*-values but not the sample sizes from each study (and therefore cannot back-compute the effect size)
- When the studies are so diverse in their populations or other characteristics that a pooled effect size is meaningless, but it *is* meaningful to ask if any of the effects is nonzero.

The last two of these points are the same as those we listed for the sign test, but here we have more information from each study (the *p*-value as well as the direction of effect). Since the null hypothesis is different for the sign test (a nonzero effect on average) than for the test of combined *p*-values (a nonzero effect in at least one study), we would select the test that matches our null hypothesis.

We describe two methods for performing meta-analyses of *p*-values. For both methods it is critical that the starting point for the analysis is a set of exact one-tailed (or one-sided) *p*-values. This means that an effect in one direction yields a *p*-value in the range of 0.0 to < 0.5, while an effect in the other direction yields a *p*-value in the range of > 0.5 to 1.0. A study where the effect was identical in both groups would have a *p*-value of exactly 0.50.

If we start with a two-tailed *p*-value, we convert this to a one-tailed *p*-value as follows. If the effect is in the expected direction, then

$$p_1 = \frac{p_2}{2} . \tag{36.1}$$

If the effect is in the other direction, then

$$p_1 = 1 - \left(\frac{p_2}{2}\right) . \tag{36.2}$$

One-tailed *p*-values contain information about the direction of effect, whereas two-tailed *p*-values do not. For instance, consider the studies in Figure 36.1. The first two studies (*A* and *B*) have the same two-sided *p*-value, but have effects in opposite directions: the first favors control but the second favors treatment. The one-tailed *p*-value reflects this.

The same is true for studies *C* and *D*. We include these extra studies in the schematic as a reminder that the methods we describe for combining *p*-values treat studies *A* and C in exactly the same way, and treat studies *B* and *D* in exactly the same way. In other words, they do not distinguish between a *p*-value arising from a large effect in a small study and the same *p*-value arising from a smaller effect in a larger study.

As was true when we were working with effect sizes (and using a *p*-value to compute the effect size) we need to start with the actual *p*-value. If we are told only that the *p*-value falls under 0.05 (for example) we may elect to work with 0.05 or to omit the study from the analysis. Using 0.05 when the actual value could be much lower than 0.05 will lower the chances of a type I error if the null is true, but increase the chances of a type II error if the null is false.

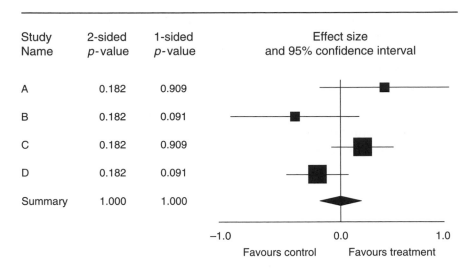

Study Name	2-sided p-value	1-sided p-value	Effect size and 95% confidence interval
A	0.182	0.909	
B	0.182	0.091	
C	0.182	0.909	
D	0.182	0.091	
Summary	1.000	1.000	

Figure 36.1 Effect size in four fictional studies.

The first test based on p-values is known as Fisher's method. We calculate

$$X^2 = -2 \sum_{i=1}^{k} \ln(p_i) \,, \tag{36.3}$$

that is, minus 2 times the sum of the logged p-values, where p_i is the one-sided p-value from study (i) and k is the number of studies. Under the null hypothesis of no effect in every study, X^2 will follow a central chi-squared distribution with degrees of freedom equal to $2 \times k$, so we can report a p-value for the aggregated evidence across studies.

The second method is known as Stouffer's method. We calculate a standard normal deviate, Z_i, from each one-sided p-value (this standard normal deviate is often calculated directly from the effect size and its standard error rather than via the p-value), and calculate

$$Z_{Stouffer} = \frac{\sum_{i=1}^{k} Z_i}{\sqrt{k}} \,, \tag{36.4}$$

where k is again the number of studies. Under the null hypothesis of no effect in every study, $Z_{Stouffer}$ will follow a standard normal distribution, so we can report a p-value for the aggregated evidence across studies.

Table 36.1 Streptokinase data – calculations for meta-analyses of *p*-values.

Study	Risk ratio	Lower limit	Upper limit	Z	Two-tailed *p*-value	One-tailed *p*-value	Log(one-tailed *p*-value)
Fletcher	0.229	0.030	1.750	−1.420	0.155	0.078	−2.554
Dewar	0.571	0.196	1.665	−1.026	0.305	0.152	−1.881
European 1	1.349	0.743	2.451	0.984	0.325	0.837	−0.177
European 2	0.703	0.534	0.925	−2.519	0.012	0.006	−5.134
Heikinheimo	1.223	0.669	2.237	0.654	0.513	0.743	−0.296
Italian	1.011	0.551	1.853	0.034	0.973	0.513	−0.667
Australian 1	0.779	0.478	1.268	−1.005	0.315	0.157	−1.849
Frankfurt 2	0.457	0.252	0.828	−2.581	0.010	0.005	−5.315
NHLBI SMIT	2.377	0.649	8.709	1.307	0.191	0.904	−0.100
Frank	0.964	0.332	2.801	−0.068	0.946	0.473	−0.749
Valere	1.048	0.481	2.282	0.117	0.907	0.547	−0.604
Klein	2.571	0.339	19.481	0.914	0.361	0.820	−0.199
UK-Collab	0.922	0.609	1.394	−0.386	0.699	0.350	−1.051
Austrian	0.608	0.417	0.886	−2.590	0.010	0.005	−5.338
Australian 2	0.702	0.443	1.110	−1.514	0.130	0.065	−2.734
Lasierra	0.282	0.034	2.340	−1.172	0.241	0.121	−2.116
N Ger Collab	1.161	0.840	1.604	0.905	0.366	0.817	−0.202
Witchitz	0.813	0.263	2.506	−0.361	0.718	0.359	−1.025
European 3	0.612	0.356	1.050	−1.782	0.075	0.037	−3.286
ISAM	0.880	0.619	1.250	−0.713	0.476	0.238	−1.436
GISSI-1	0.827	0.749	0.914	−3.738	0.000	0.000	−9.286
Olson	0.429	0.041	4.439	−0.710	0.477	0.239	−1.432
Baroffio	0.079	0.005	1.350	−1.752	0.080	0.040	−3.222
Schreiber	0.333	0.038	2.925	−0.991	0.322	0.161	−1.828
Cribier	1.095	0.073	16.427	0.066	0.948	0.526	−0.642
Sainsous	0.500	0.132	1.887	−1.023	0.306	0.153	−1.876
Durand	0.621	0.151	2.555	−0.660	0.510	0.255	−1.367
White	0.174	0.040	0.761	−2.323	0.020	0.010	−4.596
Bassand	0.604	0.188	1.944	−0.845	0.398	0.199	−1.614
Vlay	0.462	0.048	4.461	−0.668	0.504	0.252	−1.378
Kennedy	0.654	0.322	1.331	−1.171	0.241	0.121	−2.114
ISIS-2	0.769	0.704	0.839	−5.869	0.000	0.000	−19.940
Wisenberg	0.244	0.051	1.164	−1.770	0.077	0.038	−3.260
Sum				−33.677			−89.268

We will again use the streptokinase example to illustrate these methods (but note that we are testing a different null hypothesis than we had earlier). Table 36.1 presents risk ratios and their 95% confidence intervals for the 33 studies. The Z statistics are obtained as

$$Z_i = \frac{\ln(RR_i)}{\left(\ln(\text{Upper limit}_i) - \ln(\text{Lower limit})\right)/(2 \times 1.96)}, \quad (36.5)$$

or

$$Z_i = \frac{\ln(RR_i)}{SE_{\ln(RR_i)}} , \qquad (36.6)$$

where the numerator is the log risk ratio and the denominator is the standard error of the log risk ratio. The one-tailed p-values are obtained by comparing the Z values with a standard normal distribution. In Excel, the function $=$NORMSDIST(Z) can be used. For example, $=$NORMSDIST(-1.420) returns 0.078 for the Fletcher study. The sum of the Z values is -33.677, and the sum of the logs of the one-sided p-values is -89.268.

For Fisher's method, we compute

$$X^2 = -2 \times -89.268 = 178.5360.$$

The overall p-value across studies is obtained by comparing this with a chi-squared distribution with 66 degrees of freedom. In Excel, the function $=$CHIDIST($178.54,66$) returns a very small p-value ($p = 2.6 \times 10^{-12}$).

For Stouffer's method, we compute

$$Z_{Stouffer} = \frac{-33.677}{\sqrt{33}} = -5.862.$$

The overall p-value across studies is obtained by comparing this with a standard normal distribution. In Excel, the function $=$NORMSDIST(-5.862) returns a very small p-value ($p = 2.3 \times 10^{-9}$).

Both methods provide strong evidence of the benefit of streptokinase in at least one study.

SUMMARY POINTS

- A meta-analysis of effect sizes is generally the preferred approach since it addresses the issue of interest (*What is the magnitude of the effect?*) rather than the null hypothesis (*Is the effect size zero?*). However, when this approach is not possible, we may consider an approach that tests the null.
- The sign test addresses the null hypothesis that the mean effect across all studies is zero. It can be used when we know the direction (but not the magnitude) of the effects, or when the studies are so different that it does not make sense to combine effect sizes.
- Tests to combine p-values address the null hypothesis that the effect in all studies is zero.

CHAPTER 37

Further Methods for Dichotomous Data

Introduction
Mantel-Haenszel method
One-Step (Peto) formula for odds ratio

INTRODUCTION

In this chapter we present two methods, the Mantel-Haenszel method and the one-step method (also known as the Peto method) for performing a meta-analysis on odds ratios. For both methods we assume the data from each study are presented in the form of a 2×2 table with cells labeled as in Table 37.1.

MANTEL-HAENSZEL METHOD

Widely familiar to epidemiologists, although perhaps less familiar to others, the Mantel-Haenszel (*MH*) method is unusual in being a weighted average of odds ratios rather than of log odds ratios. If we use Y_i to denote the odds ratio in study i, then Y_i is computed as

$$Y_i = \frac{A_i D_i}{B_i C_i}.$$ (37.1)

Table 37.1 Nomenclature for 2×2 table of events by treatment.

	Events	Non-Events	
Treated	*A*	*B*	n_1
Control	*C*	*D*	n_2

Introduction to Meta-Analysis   M. Borenstein, L. V. Hedges, J. P. T. Higgins, H. R. Rothstein
© 2009, John Wiley & Sons, Ltd

In the Mantel-Haenszel method, the weight assigned to each study is

$$W_i = \frac{B_i C_i}{n_i},$$

(37.2)

where

$$n_i = A_i + B_i + C_i + D_i,$$

(37.3)

and the weighted mean is then computed as

$$OR_{MH} = \frac{\sum_{i=1}^{k} W_i Y_i}{\sum_{i=1}^{k} W_i}.$$

(37.4)

This is the sum of the products (effect size multiplied by weight) divided by the sum of the weights. This formula is identical to the one for inverse-variance, but the weights (W) have been defined differently and the effect size (Y) is in raw units rather than log units.

While the odds ratio itself is computed in raw units, the variance is computed in log units. Therefore we need to transform the odds ratio into log units to compute the Z-score and confidence intervals. The natural log of the *MH* odds ratio is simply

$$lnOR_{MH} = \ln(OR_{MH}).$$

(37.5)

Recall that in the inverse variance formula the variance of the summary effect was defined as the reciprocal of the sum of the weights. This is not the case here. Rather, the *MH* approach calls for us to accumulate separate values, which will be summed across studies and then used to compute the variance of the summary effect.

For each study (*i*),

$$R_i = \frac{A_i D_i}{n_i},$$

(37.6)

$$S_i = \frac{B_i C_i}{n_i},$$

(37.7)

$$E_i = \frac{(A_i + D_i) A_i D_i}{n_i^2},$$

(37.8)

$$F_i = \frac{(A_i + D_i) B_i C_i}{n_i^2},$$

(37.9)

$$G_i = \frac{(B_i + C_i) A_i D_i}{n_i^2},$$

(37.10)

and

$$H_i = \frac{(B_i + C_i) B_i C_i}{n_i^2}.$$

(37.11)

Then the variance of the summary effect, in log units, is

$$V_{InOR_{MH}} = 0.5 \left(\frac{\sum_{i=1}^{k} E_i}{\left(\sum_{i=1}^{k} R_i\right)^2} + \frac{\sum_{i=1}^{k} F_i + \sum_{i=1}^{k} G_i}{\sum_{i=1}^{k} R_i \times \sum_{i=1}^{k} S_i} + \frac{\sum_{i=1}^{k} H_i}{\left(\sum_{i=1}^{k} S_i\right)^2} \right) \quad (37.12)$$

and

$$SE_{lnOR_{MH}} = \sqrt{V_{lnOR_{MH}}}. \quad (37.13)$$

The 95% confidence interval for the summary effect in log units would be computed as

$$LL_{lnOR_{MH}} = lnOR_{MH} - 1.96 \times SE_{lnOR_{MH}} \quad (37.14)$$

and

$$UL_{lnOR_{MH}} = lnOR + 1.96 \times SE_{lnOR_{MH}}. \quad (37.15)$$

The Z-value is given by

$$Z = \frac{lnOR_{MH}}{SE_{lnOR_{MH}}}. \quad (37.16)$$

For a one-tailed test the p-value is given by

$$p = 1 - \Phi(\pm|Z|), \quad (37.17)$$

where we choose '+' if the difference is in the expected direction and '−' otherwise. Or, for a two-tailed test by

$$p = 2[1 - (\Phi(\pm|Z|))]. \quad (37.18)$$

Table 37.2 Mantel-Haenszel – odds ratio.

| | Cell Counts | | | | | Compute Odds Ratio | | |
	A	B	C	D	N	Odds Ratio	Weight	OR*WT
Saint	12	53	16	49	130	0.6934	6.5231	4.5231
Kelly	8	32	10	30	80	0.7500	4.0000	3.0000
Pilbeam	14	66	19	61	160	0.6810	7.8375	5.3375
Lane	25	375	80	320	800	0.2667	37.5000	10.0000
Wright	8	32	11	29	80	0.6591	4.4000	2.9000
Day	16	49	18	47	130	0.8526	6.7846	5.7846
Sum							67.0452	31.5452

Table 37.3 Mantel-Haenszel – variance of summary effect.

	Cell Counts					Compute Variance of Combined effect					
	A	B	C	D	N	R	S	E	F	G	H
Saint	12	53	16	49	130	4.5231	6.5231	2.1224	3.0608	2.4007	3.4622
Kelly	8	32	10	30	80	3.0000	4.0000	1.4250	1.9000	1.5750	2.1000
Pilbeam	14	66	19	61	160	5.3375	7.8375	2.5020	3.6738	2.8355	4.1637
Lane	25	375	80	320	800	10.0000	37.5000	4.3125	16.1719	5.6875	21.3281
Wright	8	32	11	29	80	2.9000	4.4000	1.3413	2.0350	1.5588	2.3650
Day	16	49	18	47	130	5.7846	6.7846	2.8033	3.2879	2.9813	3.4967
Sum						31.5452	67.0452	14.5064	30.1295	17.0388	36.9157

We present a worked example for Dataset 2, which was originally presented in Chapter 18 and served as an example for the inverse-variance method.

From the results in Table 37.2, the Mantel-Haenszel summary odds ratio is computed as

$$OR_{MH} = \frac{31.5452}{67.0452} = 0.4705,$$

and the log odds ratio is

$$lnOR_{MH} = \ln(0.4705) = -0.7539.$$

The confidence interval for the summary effect is calculated in log units as follows (see Table 37.3).

For the first study (Saint), for example,

$$R = \frac{(12)(49)}{130} = 4.5231,$$

$$S = \frac{(53)(16)}{130} = 6.5231,$$

$$E = \frac{(12 + 49)(12)(49)}{130^2} = 2.1224,$$

$$F = \frac{(12 + 49)(53)(16)}{130^2} = 3.0608,$$

$$G = \frac{(53 + 16)(12)(49)}{130^2} = 2.4007,$$

and

$$H = \frac{(53 + 16)(53)(16)}{130^2} = 3.4622.$$

The variance of the log odds ratio is given by

$$V_{lnOR_{MH}} = 0.5 \times \left(\frac{14.5064}{31.5452^2} + \frac{30.1295 + 17.0388}{31.5452 \times 67.0452} + \frac{36.9157}{67.0452^2} \right) = 0.0225,$$

so

$$SE_{lnOR_{MH}} = \sqrt{0.0225} = 0.1502,$$

$$LL_{lnOR_{MH}} = -0.7539 - 1.96 \times 0.1502 = -1.0482,$$

$$UL_{lnOR_{MH}} = -0.7539 + 1.96 \times 0.1502 = -0.45951,$$

and

$$Z = \frac{-0.7539}{0.1502} = -5.0211.$$

For a one-tailed test p is given by

$$p = 1 - \Phi(+5.0211) = 0.00000026,$$

which, in Excel is $=(1\text{-}(\text{NORMSDIST}(\text{ABS}(Z))))$. Or, for a two-tailed test, p is given by

$$p = 2[1 - (\Phi(|-5.0211|))] = 0.00000051$$

which, in Excel is $=(1\text{-}(\text{NORMSDIST}(\text{ABS}(Z))))^*2$.

Finally, we would convert the values back to raw units for display, using

$$OR_{MII} = 0.4705,$$

$$LL_{OR_{MH}} = \exp(-1.0482) = 0.3506,$$

and

$$UL_{OR_{MH}} = \exp(0.4596) = 0.6315.$$

The Z-value and p-value are the same as for the log values.

The Mantel-Haenszel method was developed for combining odds ratios across 2×2 tables. It has since been extended by others to combine risk ratios or risk differences across 2×2 tables. Similar formulas are available for these, although we do not present them since they provide little insight into the pooling mechanism and they can readily be implemented in meta-analysis software (see Chapter 44).

The Mantel-Haenszel method is based on the fixed-effect model, where the weight assigned to each study is based on that study alone and not on the variance across studies.

ONE-STEP (PETO) FORMULA FOR ODDS RATIO

The one-step method for computing the summary odds ratio works on the log odds ratio scale, and is a variant of the basic inverse-variance approach. However, this method uses a different formula than the one presented earlier for both the odds ratio and its variance. The one-step method is sometimes called the Peto method.

The log odds ratio in study (i) is estimated using

$$Y_i = \frac{O_i - E_i}{I_i},\tag{37.19}$$

where the observed count, O_i is given by

$$O_i = A_i,\tag{37.20}$$

and the expected count, E_i, is given by

$$E_i = \frac{(A_i + B_i) \times (A_i + C_i)}{n_i},\tag{37.21}$$

where

$$n_i = A_i + B_i + C_i + D_i,\tag{37.22}$$

and

$$I_i = \frac{(A_i + B_i) \times (C_i + D_i) \times (A_i + C_i) \times (B_i + D_i)}{n_i^2 \times (n_i - 1)}.\tag{37.23}$$

The variance of the log odds ratio estimate for a single study is

$$V_{Y_i} = \frac{1}{I_i},\tag{37.24}$$

where the weight given to the study is its inverse-variance given by

$$W_i = \frac{1}{V_{Y_i}}.\tag{37.25}$$

Note that the weight is just I_i. The meta-analysis is given by the weighted average of the log odds ratio estimates

$$lnOR_{onestep} = \frac{\displaystyle\sum_{i=1}^{k} W_i Y_i}{\displaystyle\sum_{i=1}^{k} W_i}\tag{37.26}$$

with variance given by

$$V_{lnOR_{onestep}} = \frac{1}{\sum\limits_{i=1}^{k} W_i}. \tag{37.27}$$

An alternative way of writing these results is

$$lnOR_{onestep} = \frac{\sum\limits_{i=1}^{k}(O_i - E_i)}{\sum\limits_{i=1}^{k} I_i}, \tag{37.28}$$

with variance given by

$$V_{lnOR_{onestep}} = \frac{1}{\sum\limits_{i=1}^{k} I_i}. \tag{37.29}$$

The standard error (in log units) is

$$SE_{lnOR_{onestep}} = \sqrt{V_{lnOR_{onestep}}}. \tag{37.30}$$

The 95% confidence interval for the summary effect in log units would be computed as follows.

$$LL_{lnOR_{onestep}} = lnOR_{onestep} - 1.96 \times SE_{lnOR_{onestep}} \tag{37.31}$$

and

$$UL_{lnOR_{onestep}} = lnOR_{onestep} + 1.96 \times SE_{lnOR_{onestep}}. \tag{37.32}$$

The Z-value is given by

$$Z = \frac{lnOR_{onestep}}{SE_{lnOR_{onestep}}}. \tag{37.33}$$

The p-value for a one-tailed test given by

$$p = 1 - \Phi(\pm|Z|), \tag{37.34}$$

where we choose '+' if the difference is in the expected direction and '−' otherwise. Or, for a two-tailed test as

$$p = 2[1 - (\Phi(|Z|))]. \tag{37.35}$$

In Excel, the two-tailed p-value is given by =(1-(NORMSDIST(ABS(Z))))*2.

In Table 37.4 we apply these formulas to Dataset 2 (see Table 14.4). Then, using sums computed in Table 37.4, we compute

Table 37.4 One-step – odds ratio and variance.

	A	B	C	D	N	O	E	O–E	I	Y	W	WY
Saint	12	53	16	49	130	12	14	−2	5.5349	−0.3613	5.5349	−2.0000
Kelly	8	32	10	30	80	8	9	−1	3.5316	−0.2832	3.5316	−1.0000
Pilbeam	14	66	19	61	160	14	16.5	−2.5	6.5896	−0.3794	6.5896	−2.5000
Lane	25	375	80	320	800	25	52.5	−27.5	22.8332	−1.2044	22.8332	−27.5000
Wright	8	32	11	29	80	8	9.5	−1.5	3.6677	−0.4090	3.6677	−1.5000
Day	16	49	18	47	130	16	17	−1	6.3256	−0.1581	6.3256	−1.0000
Sum											48.4827	−35.5000

$$lnOR_{onestep} = \frac{-35.5000}{48.4827} = -0.7322,$$

$$V_{lnOR_{onestep}} = \frac{1}{48.4827} = 0.0206,$$

$$SE_{lnOR_{onestep}} = \sqrt{0.0206} = 0.1436,$$

$$LL_{lnOR_{onestep}} = -0.7322 - 1.96 \times 0.1436 = -1.0137,$$

$$UL_{lnOR_{onestep}} = -0.7322 + 1.96 \times 0.1436 = -0.4507,$$

$$Z = \frac{-0.7322}{0.1436} = -5.098,$$

$$p = 1 - \Phi(-5.098) = 0.00000017,$$

and

$$p = 2[1 - (\Phi(|-5.098|))] = 0.00000034.$$

Finally, we would convert the values back to raw units for display, using

$$OR_{onestep} = \exp(-0.7322) = 0.481,$$

$$LL_{OR_{onestep}} = \exp(-1.0137) = 0.363,$$

and

$$UL_{OR_{onestep}} = \exp(-0.4507) = 0.637,$$

In the one-step approach, like the basic approach, all analyses are carried out on the log of the odds ratio. We compute a weighted mean of the log values, and then exponentiate this value to report the summary effect.

When one or more of the cells in the 2×2 table is empty (that is, a value of zero), the basic inverse-variance formula cannot work with zero, and the typical approach is to add the value 0.5 (or some other value) to all four cells. However, both the Mantel-Haenszel method and the one-step approach are able to work with a value of zero, and so no adjustment is needed.

The one-step approach follows the same logic as the basic scheme, in that it uses inverse-variance weights at all points in the analysis, and differs from the *basic* approach only in that it uses a slightly different way of computing the log odds ratio and its variance. As such, the one-step approach can be extended to the random-effects model. In practice, though, this is rarely done.

SUMMARY POINTS

- The Mantel-Haenszel method for combining odds ratios is an alternative to the fixed-effect inverse variance method.
- The one-step (Peto) method for combining odds ratios is an inverse-variance method, but uses an alternate approach to computing the odds ratio and variance in each study. This method offers some advantages when some studies have empty cells.

CHAPTER 38

Psychometric Meta-Analysis

INTRODUCTION

Most meta-analyses aim to summarize the results obtained in studies that were carried out with an implicit assumption that those results are the *best available* estimates of effect. However, any study has methodological flaws that affect its results. If we were able to *correct* estimates for these flaws, it would be preferable to perform a meta-analysis of these corrected results. Then we can address what the study results *would have been* if all of the studies had been free of methodological imperfections (including finite sample size) and to estimate parameters describing the effects in these methodologically perfect studies.

Unfortunately it is typically difficult, if not impossible, to know the specific impact of these methodological flaws. A growing literature addresses attempts to determine the likely biases using theoretical considerations or information from other studies and other meta-analyses. One approach to meta-analysis has focused since its inception almost exclusively on developing ways to adjust estimates of effect for methodological limitations of the studies. This is the field of psychometric meta-analysis (also called validity generalization or Hunter-Schmidt meta-analysis). This field has also adopted a somewhat different (though closely related) set of methods for combining results in meta-analysis than those that have been discussed previously. This chapter provides an overview of two issues. One is the approach to adjusting estimates of effect (known as artifact correction), which will be of interest to nearly anyone thinking about using meta-analysis. The other is the methods that are commonly used to combine results in the field of psychometric meta-analysis, which will be of interest primarily to researchers who use correlations as their effect size measure.

Psychometric meta-analysis

Methodological flaws in research studies affect study results in ways that might be thought of as artifacts of the study design. Much of the work on psychometric meta-analysis has focused on the case of studies that use continuous outcome measures and use effect size measures involving standardization (such as correlation coefficients or standardized mean differences). Since the measuring instruments are subject to measurement error (imperfect reliability), they produce effect size estimates that are made smaller (attenuated) by this measurement error. If the samples in some studies are selected in ways that do not contain the full range of variation on either independent or dependent variables, effect size estimates are reduced (or attenuated) due to this restriction of range. The dichotomization of variables that are inherently continuous in order to form binary categories produces effect size estimates that are attenuated by the reduction in variance that results from the (artificial) dichotomization. A more complete list of methodological problems that can have an impact on observed effects may be found in Hunter and Schmidt (2004). Psychometric meta-analysts rightly argue that what researchers really would like to know about is the relationship between the constructs (or variables) in a study that are *not* artifacts of study design. Therefore the answers to scientific questions are best provided by estimating the results that would have been observed had each study been free of methodological imperfections. This is what psychometric meta-analysis would call the *true values*.

Psychometric meta-analysis uses procedures based on psychometric principles (hence the name psychometric meta-analysis) to make corrections for attenuation due to measurement error and other artifacts at the level of the individual effect size estimate, before these effects are synthesized across the set of studies in the meta-analysis.

Many methodological artifacts have the effect of attenuating relationships among variables. Therefore, the average effect size corrected for the effects of artifacts (such as measurement unreliability or range restriction) will generally be larger than if the corrections were not made.

Our estimate of the *variation* in effects may also be different. The reason is that the impact of artifacts on effect sizes varies from study to study, and this increases the variability of the observed effect sizes. Consequently, the variation across studies in the effects corrected for artifacts (the variation that is of interest in psychometric meta-analyses) is typically less than that in the observed effects.

THE ATTENUATING EFFECTS OF ARTIFACTS

Psychometric meta-analyses usually represent the relationship between the observed (unadjusted) effect size and the *true* (adjusted) effect size via their ratio. In accordance with psychometric terminology, however, they use the term *attenuated* to refer to the observed effect, and the term *unattenuated* to refer to the adjusted effect. The ratio of the attenuated to the unattenuated effect describes the impact of the artifact on the effect size, and is called an *artifact multiplier* because the magnitude of the observed (attenuated) effect size is equal to the artifact multiplier times the unattenuated effect size. For example, if the effect size is a correlation coefficient (as it typically is in psychometric meta-analyses), and the artifact is measurement error (unreliability) in one of the two variables, then the ratio a of the attenuated correlation ρ to the unattenuated correlation ρ^u

$$a = \frac{\rho}{\rho^u} \qquad (38.1)$$

is the square root of the reliability coefficient of Y. (The reliability coefficient is an index used in psychometric theory and other areas to characterize the reproducibility of measurements.) Although a discussion of measurement theory in general, and reliability, in particular, are beyond the scope of this book, a sophisticated discussion of reliability can be found in Lord and Novick (1968) and an introductory discussion can be found in Crocker and Algina (1986). Other artifacts (such as restriction of the range of measurement for one or other variable) lead to different expressions for the artifact multiplier. Algebraic expressions for the artifact multipliers come from psychometric or statistical theory (see Hunter and Schmidt, 2004). While artifacts typically lead to attenuation (that is, $0 < a < 1$), this need not be so for all artifacts (e.g. in the case where the range of variables in the study population is greater than that in the reference population of interest).

If several artifacts influence an effect size parameter, we can compute an artifact multiplier for each. Then the combined effect of all of the artifacts can be expressed by a combined artifact multiplier that is the product of all of the individual artifact multipliers. This combined artifact multiplier can be used like any single artifact multiplier. The object of psychometric meta-analysis is to describe the distribution of the unattenuated effect size parameters (such as the ρ^u) given estimates of the observed (attenuated) effect size estimates (such as the r). It follows from (38.1) that the unattenuated correlation can be estimated from the observed correlation and the artifact multiplier as

$$r^u = \frac{r}{a} . \qquad (38.2)$$

Because the artifact multipliers are taken to be constants, it follows that the variance of r^u (call this V_r^u) is $1/a^2$ as large as the variance of r (call this V_r). That is,

$$V_r^u = \frac{V_r}{a^2} . \qquad (38.3)$$

Having obtained estimates of unattenuated correlations and their variances, we could implement any of the methods described in Parts 3 to 6. For instance, we could perform a fixed-effect or a random-effects meta-analysis using basic inverse-variance weighted averages, we could assess heterogeneity using a statistical test, or I^2, or by computing T^2, and could perform subgroup analyses and meta-regression to explore heterogeneity. The methods that are typically used in the psychometric meta-analysis field are somewhat different, however. In particular,

- Raw correlations are used as the effect size index instead of Fisher's Z-transformed correlations.
- Sample sizes are used as weights instead of inverse variances (which makes little difference for correlations, but which could yield very different results, were it applied to binary data).
- A different method is used to estimate τ^2.
- Heterogeneity is examined and reported in a different way.

META-ANALYSIS METHODS

We will describe first the methods used to perform a meta-analysis of the observed (attenuated) correlations, and then apply similar ideas to the unattenuated correlations. At this point we add subscripts (i) to refer to the different studies, and use k to denote the number of studies. The convention in psychometric meta-analysis is to use the sample sizes as weights for computing the mean correlation. This yields the mean

$$\bar{r} = \frac{\sum_{i=1}^{k} n_i r_i}{\sum_{i=1}^{k} n_i} . \tag{38.4}$$

To estimate the between-studies variance (τ^2) of the underlying attenuated correlation coefficients, we require a variance for the correlation from each study. We could use the usual variance estimate in (6.1). However, the convention in psychometric meta-analysis is to use the sample size weighted estimate of the mean effect size parameter to compute the sampling error variance, namely

$$V_{r_i} = \frac{[1 - (\bar{r})^2]^2}{n_i - 1} . \tag{38.5}$$

To compute the between-studies variance component of the observed (attenuated) effect size parameters we first compute the sample-size-weighted variance of the observed (attenuated) correlations

$$S^2 = \frac{\sum_{i=1}^{k} n_i (r_i - \bar{r})^2}{\sum_{i=1}^{k} n_i} . \tag{38.6}$$

Then the between-studies variance component of the observed (attenuated) effect size parameters is computed as the difference between S^2 and the sample-size-weighted average of the sampling error variances, namely

$$T^2 = S^2 - \frac{\sum\limits_{i=1}^{k} n_i V_{r_i}}{\sum\limits_{i=1}^{k} n_i} . \tag{38.7}$$

Note that the right hand side of this equation consists of two terms. The first term is a weighted variance of the observed correlations (with the ith correlation weighted by n_i) and the second term is a weighted average of the sampling error variances using the same weights. The between-studies variance estimate is the difference between an observed (weighted) variance and the (weighted) average of the sampling error variances. Thus the between-studies variance estimate can be seen as the observed variance *adjusting for* the sampling error variance.

A meta-analysis of unattenuated (artifact-corrected) correlation estimates follows a similar procedure with r_i^u replacing r_i and with revised weights. Recall that the artifact correction for the variance in each study is given by (38.3). The analogous correction to the sample size is to adjust it from n_i to $a_i^2 n_i$.

The mean unattenuated correlation is therefore

$$\bar{r}^u = \frac{\sum\limits_{i=1}^{k} n_i a_i^2 r_i^u}{\sum\limits_{i=1}^{k} n_i a_i^2} . \tag{38.8}$$

The weighted variance of the unattenuated correlations is

$$(S^u)^2 = \frac{\sum\limits_{i=1}^{k} n_i a_i^2 (r_i^u - \bar{r}^u)^2}{\sum\limits_{i=1}^{k} n_i a_i^2} . \tag{38.9}$$

Then the between-studies variance component of the unattenuated effect size parameters $(T^u)^2$ is computed as the difference between $(S^u)^2$ and the sample-size-weighted average of the sampling error variances of the unattenuated correlations, namely

$$(T^u)^2 = (S^u)^2 - \frac{\sum\limits_{i=1}^{k} n_i a_i^2 V_i^u}{\sum\limits_{i=1}^{k} n_i a_i^2} . \tag{38.10}$$

EXAMPLE OF PSYCHOMETRIC META-ANALYSIS

We now present a hypothetical example to illustrate the methods of psychometric meta-analysis. We will correct for only a single artifact, error of measurement (unreliability) in the dependent variable. In actual applications of psychometric meta-analysis, corrections for multiple artifacts (for example, error of measurement in both independent and dependent variables, and restriction of range in one or both variables) might be used.

Suppose that six studies were conducted to assess the validity of a pre-hire work sample test (independent variable) to predict the job performance (dependent variable) of dental hygienists six months after hire. The first two studies were conducted by a consortium of clinics run by schools of dentistry, and job performance was measured using a standard, professionally developed rating scale. The third and fourth studies were conducted in large multi-partner private dental practices, and job performance was measured using a home-grown rating scale developed by a group of the partners from the two practices. The fifth and sixth studies were done at clinics run by a nonprofit organization where dentists volunteered to work for free two weeks per year. Job performance was measured using a standardized work behavior assessment scale designed by the nonprofit organization.

The sample sizes (n), the observed (attenuated) correlations (r), and the criterion reliabilities are given in Table 38.1. We first perform a meta-analysis of the correlations as they were observed (the attenuated correlations). The calculations are provided in Table 38.2.

Table 38.1 Fictional data for psychometric meta-analysis.

Study	n	r	Criterion reliability
University 1	130	0.24	0.75
University 2	90	0.11	0.75
Private 1	30	0.05	0.60
Private 2	25	0.17	0.60
Volunteer 1	50	0.38	0.90
Volunteer 2	65	0.50	0.90

Table 38.2 Observed (attenuated) correlations.

Study	n_i	r_i	$n_i r_i$	$\bar{r}$	V_{r_i}	$n_i(r_i-\bar{r})^2$	$n_i V_{r_i}$
University 1	130	0.24	31.20	0.252179	0.0068	0.019283	0.88365
University 2	90	0.11	9.90	0.252179	0.0099	1.819338	0.88671
Private 1	30	0.05	1.50	0.252179	0.0302	1.226290	0.90709
Private 2	25	0.17	4.25	0.252179	0.0365	0.168835	0.91339
Volunteer 1	50	0.38	19.00	0.252179	0.0179	0.816910	0.89475
Volunteer 2	65	0.50	32.50	0.252179	0.0137	3.991991	0.89056
Total	390		98.35			8.042647	5.37615

We use the first three columns in Table 38.2 to compute the sum of n_i and the sum of $n_i r_i$. Then, the mean correlation is computed as

$$\bar{r} = \frac{\sum\limits_{i=1}^{6} n_i r_i}{\sum\limits_{i=1}^{6} n_i} = \frac{98.35}{390} = 0.2518,$$

which is inserted into column 4 in the table. Then, we complete the remaining columns in the table.

The variance of the correlation in study number i is

$$V_{r_i} = \frac{\left[1 - 0.25218^2\right]^2}{n_i - 1}$$

and these values are listed in Table 38.2.

The between-studies variance is computed as follows:

$$S^2 = \frac{8.0426}{390} = 0.0206 \quad \text{and}$$

$$T^2 = 0.0206 - \frac{5.3762}{390} = 0.0069.$$

Calculations for the unattenuated correlations appear in Table 38.3. The artifact multiplier for this particular example is the square root of the criterion reliability.

The mean unattenuated correlation is

$$\bar{r}^u = \frac{88.9048}{301.5} = 0.2949.$$

The between-studies variance is computed as

$$(S^u)^2 = \frac{6.6287}{301.5} = 0.0212$$

Table 38.3 Unattenuated correlations.

Study	n_i	a_i	r_i^u	$n_i a_i^2 r_i^u$	$V_{r_i}^u$	$n_i a_i^2$	$n_i a_i^2 (r_i^u - \bar{r}^u)^2$	$n_i a_i^2 V_{r_i}^u$
University 1	130	0.866	0.28	27.020	0.00906	97.500	0.030707	0.0068
University 2	90	0.866	0.13	8.574	0.01314	67.500	1.901896	0.0099
Private 1	30	0.775	0.06	1.162	0.05039	18.000	0.954894	0.0302
Private 2	25	0.775	0.22	3.292	0.06089	15.000	0.085290	0.0365
Volunteer 1	50	0.949	0.40	18.025	0.01988	45.000	0.502575	0.0179
Volunteer 2	65	0.949	0.53	30.832	0.01522	58.500	3.153359	0.0137
Total	390			88.905		301.500	6.628722	5.3762

and

$$(T^u)^2 = 0.0220 - \frac{5.3762}{301.5} = 0.0042.$$

The effect of the artifact of error of measurement in the criterion variable was to decrease the estimate of the average correlation from about 0.295 to about 0.252 or about 15%. In addition the artifact of error of measurement in the criterion variable increased the estimated variance of the unattenuated correlations compared to the observed (attenuated) correlations from about 0.0042 to about 0.0069 or about 64%. This example illustrates a common finding in psychometric meta-analyses: artifacts tend to reduce the magnitude of effects and increase their apparent variation in the sense that the unattenuated effect parameters are estimated to have a larger mean and smaller between-studies variance than the observed effects.

Explained variance in psychometric meta-analyses

It is conventional in psychometric meta-analyses to consider S^2 as the (estimated total) variance of the observed effect estimates and $(T^u)^2$ as the (estimated) variance of the true effects remaining after the artifacts effects have been removed. Thus

$$\frac{S^2 - (T^u)^2}{S^2} = 1 - \frac{(T^u)^2}{S^2} \tag{38.11}$$

is the proportion of variance in the observed (attenuated) effect estimates explained by artifacts.

Note that this definition is in the same spirit as the index I^2 in conventional meta-analysis, but I^2 focuses on unexplained, as opposed to explained variance. Thus

$$\frac{(T^u)^2}{S^2} \times 100\% \tag{38.12}$$

estimates a quantity similar to I^2 that reflects the percentage of the variance in the observed correlations that is *due to* the variance in the unattenuated correlation parameters.

In our example, the psychometric analysis would estimate the proportion of explained variance as

$$\frac{0.02062 - 0.0042}{0.0206} = 0.7987,$$

so that 79.9% of the total variance in the observed (attenuated) effect size estimates is explained by the artifacts of sampling error and measurement error in the criterion variable.

COMPARISON OF ARTIFACT CORRECTION WITH META-REGRESSION

In conventional meta-analysis, if criterion unreliability was hypothesized to influence effect size, it would be treated as a covariate. After the core meta-analysis was run, criterion unreliability would be regressed on effect size, to test whether it could explain some of the between-study variation in the (uncorrected) correlations. In this example, we conducted a random-effects meta-analysis on the (uncorrected) dental hygienist validity data. The overall mean effect was computed as 0.25, T^2 was computed 0.012, and I^2 was 44.481. We then performed a random-effects meta-regression (method of moments), regressing criterion unreliability on effect size. Results showed that the slope was significant with a p-value of 0.011. More to the point, T^2 was 0.00, meaning that all of the explainable variance was accounted for by differences in criterion reliability.

SOURCES OF INFORMATION ABOUT ARTIFACT VALUES

The most appropriate method of adjusting for the effects of artifacts is to correct each effect individually, using reliability and range restriction information that is provided in the study from which the effect is extracted. In most cases, however, this information is not available. This presents what is essentially a missing data problem. As in other cases of missing data, a variety of imputation techniques can be used to estimate the missing reliability and/or range restriction values. One technique that is recommended by the developers of psychometric meta- analysis is to create artifact distributions based on the information provided in the subset of studies that report the relevant data. In this case, the meta-analysis is conducted on the uncorrected effects and the average artifact value (e.g. reliability) from the artifact distribution is used to correct the average effect, while the standard deviation of the artifact values is used to correct the variance of the observed effects. The use of hypothetical distributions of artifacts in general, and in particular, the application of distributions created for meta-analyses of employment test validities to quite different research questions, has been criticized by many methodologists who are generally supportive of the psychometric meta-analysis framework. An alternative, when information about measurement reliability and range restriction is largely missing from the set of studies in the analysis, is to use the mean observed effect as the estimate of the population mean effect, and to remove the variance due to sampling error from the total observed variance, to produce an estimate of true variance in effects. Psychometric meta-analysis refers to this alternative as a *bare-bones* meta-analysis.

HOW HETEROGENEITY IS ASSESSED

When covariates are not hypothesized in advance of the meta-analysis

Psychometric meta-analyses do not usually use the chi-square test of homogeneity to test whether the observed variance is greater than the amount that would be expected due to sampling error. Instead, they have substituted the 75% decision rule, which proposes that if 75% or more of the total (observed) variance is due to artifacts, including sampling error, the researcher may conclude that, actually, all of the variance is artifactual, since there are several commonly operating artifacts for which no corrections can be made (such as transcriptional and coding errors, which are claimed to be ubiquitous), This rule was formulated for the original application of psychometric meta-analysis, the assessment of the consistency of employment test validities, and was tested through computer simulation of conditions typical of employment testing research. Its performance in other research areas remains unstudied, and it is not advisable to use this rule outside the area for which it was developed. Many users of psychometric meta analysis have objected to the 75% rule because it focuses on the percentage of true variance rather than on its magnitude, and may cause substantial remaining true variance to be ignored.

When there is an *a priori* hypothesis that a covariate may explain heterogeneity

In the cases of a hypothesized discrete covariate, the procedure followed by psychometric meta-analysis is to divide the studies into subgroups based on values of the hypothesized covariate. For example, if the hypothesis that the correlations will be higher for males than for females, studies of males will comprise one subgroup, and studies of females will comprise a second subgroup. Subgroup meta-analyses are conducted, and are declared to be different when the *true* means in each subgroup are different from each other, and the confidence intervals around each mean are largely non-overlapping.

For continuous covariates, the usual meta-regression procedures are followed, using correlations that are individually corrected for artifacts, and the corrected sampling error variances.

REPORTING IN PSYCHOMETRIC META-ANALYSIS

The findings of a psychometric meta-analysis focus on the value of three parameters: (1) the average percentage of the total (observed) variance of effects across studies that is explained by statistical and measurement artifacts, including sampling error; (2) the estimated mean true effect parameter; and (3) the estimated standard deviation of true effects. In a psychometric meta-analysis this last value represents the degree of dispersion across the true effects, that is, the degree of dispersion remaining after sampling error variance, and variance due to other artifacts, have been removed from the observed variance, It is used to form what psychometric meta-analysis refers to as the credibility interval. The credibility interval contains the distribution of true effects and is roughly analogous to the prediction interval discussed in Chapter 17. Typically, a psychometric meta-analysis results table presents the lower end of the 80 or 90% credibility interval, which is the estimated value of the effect above which 80 or 90% of true effects are expected to be found. The lower bound value of the credibility interval (because we care about the *minimum validity*) and the width of the interval are considered to be the most important results of the meta-analysis.

CONCLUDING REMARKS

The purpose of this chapter has been to explain the basic tenets of psychometric meta-analysis, and to explain how these differ from other methods of meta-analysis. A key characteristic of psychometric meta-analyses is the correction of individual study results for artifacts, so that we can estimate what the effect would be if there were no methodological limitations. This would be a desirable aim in any meta-analysis. Unfortunately methods are not established for many types of data, and even among supporters of psychometric meta-analysis, there is some disagreement about the specific operational procedures to be followed in making these corrections. Another characteristic of psychometric meta-analyses is the emphasis on credibility intervals rather than overall means. We have argued in Chapter 17 that analogous prediction intervals should be considered routinely for all meta-analyses.

Other differences are technical in nature. These include the way weights are assigned, the way between-studies variance is estimated, the use of correlation coefficients rather than Fisher's Z-transformed values, and the use of the average versus the individual effect in calculating the sampling error variance. The effects of these choices can be viewed entirely separately from other aspects of the procedures, and have been extensively examined through simulations, which suggest that the differences are likely to be trivial in many cases.

Finally, there are issues that remain the subject of disagreements among users of psychometric meta-analysis. These include the degree to which the assumptions needed to make the corrections are met in specific situations, the use of artifact distributions, the imputation of specific values for these distributions, and the use of the 75% rule to make decisions about the presence or absence of heterogeneity. These practices may be consequences of psychometric meta-analysis origins in test validity research, and may resolve themselves as relevant data accumulate from other research domains.

SUMMARY POINTS

- Psychometric meta-analysis attempts to correct for bias in study findings by adjusting for errors of measurement, restriction of range and other artifactual influences on effect sizes.
- Making these corrections typically produces effects that are higher in magnitude, and less variable across the set of studies in the meta-analysis, than would be the case if no corrections had been made.
- Psychometric meta-analysis emphasizes the distribution of true effects, rather than the overall mean effect. The inclusion of an estimate of the distribution of true effects should be adopted even by those who use conventional meta-analytic techniques.

Further Reading

Aguinis, H. (2001). Estimation of sampling variance of correlation in meta-analysis. *Personnel Psychology*, 54, 569–590.

Aguinis, H. & Pierce, C.A. (1998). Testing moderator variable hypotheses meta-analytically. *Journal of Management*, 24, 577–592.

Aguinis, H, Sturman, M., & Pierce, C.A. (2008). Comparison of three meta-analytic procedures for estimating moderating effects of categorical variables. *Organizational Research Methods* 11: 9–34.

Bobko, P. & Roth, P.L.(2008). Psychometric accuracy and (the continuing need for) quality thinking in meta-analysis. *Organizational Research Methods* 11: 114–126.

Crocker, L. & Algina, J. (1986). *Introduction to Classical and Modern Test Theory*. New York: Holt, Rinehart, & Winston.

Hunter, J.E. & Schmidt, F.L. (2004). *Methods of Meta-analysis: Correcting Error and Bias in Research Findings* (2nd ed.). Thousand Oaks, CA: Sage.

Lord, F.M. & Novick, M.R. (1968). *Statistical theories of mental test scores*. Reading, MA: Addison-Wesley.

Murphy, K.R. (2003). *Validity generalization: A critical review*. Mahwah, NJ: Lawrence Erlbaum.

Schmidt, F.L. & Hunter, J.E. (1977). Development of a general solution to the problem of validity generalization. *Journal of Applied Psychology*, 62, 529–540.

Meta-Analysis in Context

CHAPTER 39

OVERVIEW

Several chapters in this section address basic issues in meta-analysis. Chapter 40 addresses the basic question of when it makes sense to perform a meta-analysis, and Chapter 41 offers suggestions for how to report the results of a meta-analysis. The two share the theme that there is no single best way to perform (or report) a meta-analysis. Rather, there needs to be a match between the goals of a specific synthesis, the kinds of studies included, the methods applied, and the conclusions reported.

Chapter 42 describes a procedure called cumulative meta-analysis, which is a sequence of analyses performed with one study, then two, and so on, until all studies have been entered. This can be used to see how the body of evidence has shifted over time, or as a function of any moderator.

Chapter 43 is dedicated to criticisms of meta-analysis. There, we present a series of questions often raised by critics. We argue that some of the criticisms represent either a misunderstanding of the method, or poor applications of the method. Other criticisms represent problems that cannot easily be resolved, but we try to place these in context, by showing that these problems exist also in other kinds of reviews.

Introduction to Meta-Analysis   M. Borenstein, L. V. Hedges, J. P. T. Higgins, H. R. Rothstein
© 2009, John Wiley & Sons, Ltd

CHAPTER 40

When Does it Make Sense to Perform a Meta-Analysis?

Introduction
Are the studies similar enough to combine?
Can I combine studies with different designs?
How many studies are enough to carry out a meta-analysis?

INTRODUCTION

In the early days of meta-analysis (at least in its current incarnation) Robert Rosenthal was asked if it makes sense to perform a meta-analysis, given that the studies differ in various ways, and the analysis amounts to *combining apples and oranges*. Rosenthal answered that combining apples and oranges makes sense if your goal is to produce a fruit salad.

The goal of a meta-analysis is only rarely to synthesize data from a set of identical studies. Almost invariably, the goal is to broaden the base of studies in some way, expand the question, and study the pattern of answers. The question of whether it makes sense to perform a meta-analysis, and the question of what kinds of studies to include, must be asked and answered in the context of specific goals.

The ability to combine data from different studies to estimate the common effect (or mean effect), continues to be an important function of meta-analysis. However, it is not the only function. The goal of some syntheses will be to report the summary effect, but the goal of other syntheses will be to assess the dispersion as well as the mean effect, and the goal of others will be to focus on the dispersion exclusively.

For example, suppose that we are looking at the impact of a teaching intervention on student performance. Does it make sense to include studies that measured verbal skills and also studies that measured math skills? If our goal is to assess the impact on performance in general, then the answer is *Yes*. If our goal is to assess the impact on verbal skills alone, then the answer is *No*. Does it make sense to include studies that enrolled middle-school students and also studies that enrolled high-school students? Again, the answer depends on the question being asked.

In some cases, however, the decisions are less clear cut. For example, does it make sense to include both randomized trials and observational studies in the same analysis? What about quasi-experimental studies? Is it acceptable to include studies that used independent groups and also studies that used matched designs? The answers to these and other questions will need to be decided in the context of the research question being addressed. Our goal here is to outline the kinds of issues that may arise and provide a context for making these kinds of decisions.

ARE THE STUDIES SIMILAR ENOUGH TO COMBINE?

From a statistical perspective, there is no restriction on the similarity of studies based on the types of participants, interventions, or exposures. However, for the analysis to be meaningful, we need to pay careful consideration to the diversity of studies in these respects. For example, the research question might be *Does Drug A reduce the risk of heart attack as compared with a placebo; when used in a population of males, age 40–60 years, with no prior history of heart attack, and a cholesterol level of 250–300 on initial screening; where the dose was between 10– 15 mg per day; in studies that followed patients for at least a year, with a drop-out rate no higher than five percent, where the randomization and blinding met specific criteria; and where patients were under the care of a primary care physicians for the duration of the study?* In this case, the criteria for including studies in the analysis would be very narrow, and the goal of the analysis would be to yield a more precise estimate (and more powerful test) of the effect than would be possible with any single study. This kind of meta-analysis might be planned by a pharmaceutical company as part of the approval process, and this approach is entirely legitimate.

In most meta-analyses, however, the inclusion criteria will be broader than this. It is an important feature of a meta-analysis that it may (and usually must) address a broader question than those addressed by the primary studies it includes. Thus a certain amount of diversity among the studies is not only inevitable but also desirable. A good meta-analysis will anticipate this diversity and will interpret the findings with attention to the dispersion of results across studies. To modify the prior example by relaxing some of the criteria, a *pragmatic* review of the effects of Drug A versus placebo on the risk of heart attack might include both sexes, adults of any age with no prior history of heart attack, any cholesterol level; any dose of drug; in studies that followed patients for at least a year, with a drop-out rate no higher than twenty percent, where the randomization and blinding met specific criteria. The diversity of studies meeting these broader criteria may lead to heterogeneous results, and this heterogeneity needs to be recognized in the analysis and interpretation.

One approach to diversity is to apply the random-effects model and then address the diversity by reporting the expected range of true effects over the populations and interventions sampled. This could take the form of a prediction interval as explained in Chapter 17. This is appropriate if the effects fall over a small range, so that the substantive implications of the finding are the same across the range.

With sufficient data, we can also explore the diversity across studies. For example, we could investigate how the effect of a drug (as compared with a placebo) depends on the sex of a patient. Assume that these studies reported outcomes for males and females separately. We now have the ability to compute a summary effect in each of these subgroups and to determine whether (and how) the effect is related to sex. If the effect is similar in both groups, then we can report that the effect is robust, something that was not possible with the more narrow criteria. If the effect varies (say, the drug is effective for males but not for females) then the meta-analysis may have yielded important information that, again, was not possible when all studies adhered to the more narrow criteria. Note, however, that for many meta-analyses there is insufficient power to do this reliably. There may also be problems of confounding.

This basic approach, that we can define the inclusion criteria narrowly and focus on the summary effect, or define the inclusion criteria more broadly and explore the dispersion, holds true for any meta-analysis. This idea can play itself out in various ways, and we explore some of them here.

CAN I COMBINE STUDIES WITH DIFFERENT DESIGNS?

The appropriate types of study to include in a meta-analysis depend primarily on the type of question being addressed. For example, meta-analyses to evaluate the effect of an intervention will tend to seek randomized trials, in which interventions are assigned in an experimental fashion so that there are no important differences between those receiving and not receiving the intervention of interest. Meta-analyses to investigate the cause of a rare disease will tend to seek case-control studies, in which the past exposures of a collection of people with the disease are compared with those of a collection of people without the disease. Meta-analyses to examine the prevalence of a condition or a belief will tend to seek cross-sectional studies or surveys, in which a single group is examined and no within-study comparisons are made. And so on. Nevertheless, for any particular question there are typically several types of study that could yield a meaningful answer. A frequent question is whether studies with different designs can be combined in a meta-analysis.

Randomized trials versus observational studies

Some have argued that systematic reviews on the effects of interventions should be limited to randomized controlled trials, since these are protected from internal bias by design, and should exclude observational studies, since the effect sizes in these are almost invariably affected by confounders (and the confounders may vary from one study to the next). In our opinion, this distinction is somewhat arbitrary. It suggests that we would be better off with a set of poor quality randomized trials than with a set of high-quality observational studies (and leaves open the question of quasi-experimental studies). The key distinction should not be the design of the studies but the extent to which the studies are able to yield an unbiased estimate of the effect size in question.

For example, suppose we wish to evaluate the effects of going to a support group to give up smoking. We might locate five studies in which smokers were recruited and then randomly assigned to either of two conditions (invitation to a support group, or a control intervention). Because the trials use random assignment, differences between groups are attributed to differences in the effects of the interventions. If we include these trials in a meta-analysis, we are able to obtain a more precise estimate of the effect than we could from any single trial, and this effect can be attributed to the treatment. However, since trials cannot *impose* an intervention on people, the effect is of being *invited* to the support group rather than, necessarily, of attending the support group. Furthermore, the types of smokers who volunteer to be randomized into a trial may not be the types of smokers who might volunteer to join a support group.

Alternatively, suppose that we locate five studies that compared the outcomes of smokers who had voluntarily joined a support group with others who had not. Because these studies are observational, any differences allow us to draw conclusions about what proportions of people are likely to be smoking after joining a support group or not joining a support group, but do not allow us to attribute these differences to the treatment itself. For instance, those who enrolled for treatment are likely to have been more motivated to stop smoking. If we include these observational studies in a meta-analysis we are able to obtain a more precise estimate of the difference than we could from any single study, but the interpretation of this difference is subject to the same limitations as that of the primary studies.

Does it make sense to include both these randomized trials and these observational studies in the same meta-analysis? The two kinds of studies are asking different questions. The randomized trial asks if there is a relationship between treatment and outcome when we control for all other factors, while the observational study asks if there is a relationship when we do not control for these factors. Furthermore, the *treatment* is different, in that the randomized trial evaluates the effect of the invitation, and the observational study collects information based on actual participation in the support group.

It would probably not make sense to compute a summary value across both kinds of studies. The meta-analyst should first decide which question is of greater interest. Unfortunately neither would seem to address the fundamental question of whether participating in the support group increases the likelihood of stopping smoking. As is often the case, the researcher must decide between asking the sub-optimal question (about invitations) with minimal bias (through randomization) or the right question (about participation) with likely bias (using observational studies). Most would argue that randomized trials do ask highly relevant questions, allowing important conclusions to be drawn about causality even if they do not fully reflect the way intervention would be applied on a day to day basis. Thus the majority of meta-analyses of interventions are restricted to randomized trials, at least in health care, where randomized trials have long been the established method of evaluation. Of course, some important effects of interventions, such as long-term or rare outcomes (especially harms) often cannot be studied in randomized trials, so may need to be addressed using observational studies. We would generally recommend that randomized trials and observational studies be analyzed separately, though they might be put together if they do not disagree with each other and are believed to address a common question.

Studies that used independent groups, paired groups, clustered groups

Suppose that some of the studies compared means for treatment versus control using two independent groups, others compared means using paired groups and others used cluster-randomized trials. There is no technical problem with combining data from the three kinds of studies, but we need to assume that the studies are functionally similar in all other important respects. On the one hand, studies that used different designs may differ from each other in substantive ways as well. On the other hand, these differences may be no more important than the difference between (say) studies that enrolled subjects in cities and others that enrolled subjects in rural areas. If we are looking at the impact of a vaccination, then the biological function is probably the same in all three kinds of studies. If we are looking at the impact of an educational intervention, then we would probably want to test this assumption rather than take it on faith.

Can I combine studies that report results in different ways?

Meta-analysts frequently have to deal with results reported in different ways. Suppose we are looking at ways to increase the yield of grain, and are interested in whether a high dose of fertilizer works better than the standard dose. We might find studies that measure the impact of dose by randomizing different plots to receive one of the two doses, but which measure the outcome in different ways. Some studies might measure the average growth rate for the plants while others measure the yield after a certain number of weeks (and the timings might vary across studies). Some studies might measure the proportion of plants achieving a specific growth rate while others measure the time from application to production of a certain volume of grain. We might find further studies that apply a range of doses and examine the correlation between the dose and, for example, yield.

Even within studies investigating the same outcome, results can be reported in different ways. There are two types of variation here. First, different approaches to analysis could be used. For example, two studies might focus on the proportion of plants that fail under each dose of fertilizer, but one reports this as a ratio while another reports this as a difference in proportions. Second, even the same analysis can be reported using different statistics. For example, if several studies compare the mean yields between the two doses, some may report means with standard deviations, others means with a p-value, others differences in means with confidence intervals, and others F statistics from analysis of variance.

To what extent can all of these variations be combined in a meta-analysis? We address here only the statistical considerations, and assume that there is sound rationale for combining the different outcome measures in the analysis. Note that we have described binary outcomes (proportion of failing plants), continuous outcomes using different measurement scales (growth rate, yield), survival outcomes (time to fruit) and correlational data (dose-yield). The list of possibilities is longer, and we do not attempt a comprehensive summary of all options.

When studies are addressing the same outcome, measured in the same way, using the same approach to analysis, but presenting results in different ways, then the only obstacles to meta-analysis are practical. If sufficient information is available to estimate the effect size of interest, then a meta-analysis is possible. For instance, means with standard deviations, means with a p-value, and differences in means with a confidence interval can all be used to estimate the difference in mean yield (providing, in the first two situations, that the sample sizes are known). These three also allow calculation of a standardized difference in means, as does a suitable F statistic in combination with sample size. Detailed discussions of such conversions are provided in Borenstein *et al.* (2009).

When studies are addressing the same outcome, measured in the same way, but using different approaches to analysis, then the possibility of a meta-analysis depends on both statistical and practical considerations. One important point is that all studies in a meta-analysis must use essentially the same index of treatment effect. For example, we cannot combine a risk difference with a risk ratio. Rather, we would need to use the summary data to compute the same index for all studies.

There are some indices that are similar, if not exactly the same, and judgments are required as to whether it is acceptable to combine them. One example is odds ratios and risk ratios. When the event is rare, then these are approximately equal and can readily be combined. As the event gets more common the two diverge and should not be combined. Other indices that are similar to risk ratios are hazard ratios and rate ratios. Some people decide these are similar enough to combine; others do not. The judgment of the meta-analyst in the context of the aims of the meta-analysis will be required to make such decisions on a case by case basis.

When studies are addressing the same outcome measured in different ways, or different outcomes altogether, then the suitability of a meta-analysis depends mainly on substantive considerations. The researcher will have to decide whether a combined analysis would have a meaningful interpretation. If so, then the above statistical and practical considerations apply. A further consideration is how different scales used for different outcomes are to be dealt with. The standard approach for continuous outcome measures is to analyze each study as a standardized mean difference, so that all studies share a common metric.

There is a useful class of indices that are, perhaps surprisingly, combinable under some simple transformations. In particular, formulas are available to convert standardized mean differences, odds ratios and correlations to a common metric (see Chapter 7). These kinds of conversions require some assumptions about the underlying nature of the data, and violations of these assumptions can have an impact on the validity of the process. Also, we must remember that studies which used dichotomous data may be different in some substantive ways than studies which used continuous data, and studies measuring correlations may be different from those that compared two groups. As before, these are questions of degree rather than of qualitative differences among the studies.

HOW MANY STUDIES ARE ENOUGH TO CARRY OUT A META-ANALYSIS?

If we are working with a fixed-effect model, then it makes sense to perform a meta-analysis as soon as we have two studies, since a summary based on two or more studies yields a more precise estimate of the true effect than either study alone. Importantly, we are not concerned with dispersion in the observed effects because this is assumed to reflect nothing more than sampling error. There might be a concern that by reporting a summary effect we are implying a level of certainty that is not warranted. In fact, though, the summary effect is qualified by a confidence interval that describes the uncertainty of the estimate. Additionally, research shows that if we fail to provide this information researchers will impose their own synthesis on the data, which will invariably be less accurate and more idiosyncratic than the value than we compute using known formulas.

In most cases however, we should be working with the random-effects model, where the dispersion in effects is assumed to be real (at least in part). Unlike the fixed-effect analysis, where the estimate of the error is based on sampling theory (and therefore reliable), in a random-effects analysis, our estimate of the error may itself be unreliable. Specifically, when based on a small number of studies, the estimate of the between-studies variance (T^2), may be substantially in error. The standard error of the summary effect is based (in part) on this value, and therefore, if we present a summary effect with confidence interval, not only is the point estimate likely to be wrong but the confidence interval may provide a false sense of assurance.

A separate problem is that in a random-effects analysis, our understanding of the dispersion affects not only our estimate of the summary effect but also the thrust of the analysis. In other words, if the effect is consistent across studies we would report that the effect is robust. By contrast, if the effect varies substantially from study to study we would want to consider the impact of the dispersion. The problem is that when we have only a few studies to work with, we may not know what the dispersion actually looks like.

This suggests that if the number of studies is small enough it might be better not to summarize them statistically. However many statisticians would argue that, when faced with a series of studies, people have an almost irresistible tendency to draw some summary conclusions from them. Experience has shown that seemingly intuitive *ad hoc* summaries (such as vote counting, Chapter 28) are also often highly misleading. This suggests that a statistical summary with known, but perhaps poor, properties (such as high uncertainty) may be superior to inviting an *ad hoc* summary with unknown properties.

In sum, when the number of studies is small, there are no really good options. As a starting point we would suggest reporting the usual statistics and then explaining the limitations as clearly as possible. This helps preclude the kinds of ad hoc analyses mentioned in the previous paragraph, and is an accurate representation of what we can do with limited data.

SUMMARY POINTS

- The question of whether or not it makes sense to perform a meta-analysis is a question of matching the synthesis to the research question.
- If our goal is to report a summary effect, then the populations and interventions (and other variables) in the studies should match those in our target population. If our goal is to report on the dispersion of effects as a function of a covariate, then the synthesis must include the relevant studies and the analysis should focus on the differences in effects.
- Generally, we need to be aware of substantive differences among studies, but technical differences can be addressed in the analysis.
- A potentially serious problem exists when the synthesis is based on a small number of studies. Without sufficient numbers of studies we will have a problem estimating the between-studies variance, which has important implications for many aspects of the analysis.

Further Reading

Ioannidis, J.P.A., Patsopoulos, N.A., Rothstein, H.R. (2008). Reasons or excuses for avoiding meta-analysis in forest plots. *BMJ* 336: 1413–1415.

CHAPTER 41

Reporting the Results of a Meta-Analysis

Introduction
The computational model
Forest plots
Sensitivity analysis

INTRODUCTION

Most of the issues that one would address when reporting the results of a meta-analysis are similar to those for reporting the results of a primary study. There are some unique issues as well, and we address those here.

As we have throughout this volume, we deal here only with issues related to the meta-analysis, and not to the full systematic review. For a broader perspective, especially for reviews in medicine, see the *Cochrane Handbook for Systematic Reviews of Interventions* (Higgins and Green, 2008) and consider using some published Cochrane reviews as models for the full report.

Are the effects consistent?

A recurring theme in this volume has been that the goal of a meta-analysis is to synthesize the data, which is not necessarily the same as computing a single summary effect. Similarly, the issues discussed in the report should match those that are important to the synthesis.

- If the effect sizes are consistent, then the focus of the report is likely to be on the summary effect, and the fact that the effect size is robust, in that it does not vary across the range of studies included in the analysis.
- If the effect sizes vary modestly from study to study we may still report the summary effect size, but will want to pay attention also to the dispersion in effects. Usually, when we talk about whether or not the effects vary we are referring to substantive variation, so it would be helpful to report the range across

which the true effects vary. If there are sufficient studies in the analysis, we will be able to estimate this range with reasonable precision. If this is not possible, we should acknowledge this limitation. Similarly, it would be important to report I^2, the proportion of total variance attributed to variance in true effects. This helps to place the observed dispersion in context.

• If the effect sizes vary substantially, the report might focus on the variance, with the summary effect being of less (or even no) importance.

In all cases we need to be careful about the meaning of dispersion. We need to distinguish between the case where the effects are shown to be homogeneous (on the one hand) and the case where we simply fail to reject the hypothesis of homogeneity (on the other). Also, one measure of heterogeneity (I^2) tells us what proportion of the observed dispersion reflects differences in the true effect while another T^2 (or T) reflects the amount of heterogeneity on an absolute scale. While these measures tend to move in tandem, it is important to recognize that they are addressing two completely different aspects of heterogeneity, and it is important to use each appropriately in the report (see Chapter 17 on prediction intervals).

THE COMPUTATIONAL MODEL

A report should state the computational model used in the analysis and explain why this model was selected. A common mistake is to use the fixed-effect model on the basis that there is no evidence of heterogeneity. As explained in Chapter 13, the decision to use one model or the other should depend on the nature of the studies, and not on the significance of this test.

FOREST PLOTS

A recurring theme in this volume is the importance of interpreting statistics in context, and the forest plot helps to provide that context. The plot, as suggested by its appellation, allows the researcher to see both the forest and the trees (in the UK this would be the wood and the trees). We have used forest plots throughout this volume to illustrate various conceptual issues, precisely because the forest plot is an excellent vehicle for illustrating these issues. It can, and should, serve the same purpose in a report of a meta-analysis.

In the forest plot each study as well as the summary effect is depicted as a point estimate bounded by its confidence interval. It shows if the overall effect is based on many studies or a few, on studies that are precise or imprecise; whether the effects for all studies tend to line up, or whether they vary substantially from one study to the next. The plot puts a face on the statistics, helping to ensure that they will be interpreted properly, and highlighting anomalies, such as outliers, that require attention. The forest plot is a compelling piece of information and easy to understand, even for people who do not work with meta-analysis on a regular basis.

There are several variants of the forest plot that appear in the literature. Our goal here is to sensitize the reader to some of these variants, and point out the advantages and disadvantages of each.

Consider Figures 41.1 and 41.2, which represent the same set of studies. In both, the study is represented by a point which is bounded by the confidence interval for the effect size in that study. In Figure 41.1 the point is a vertical line, while in Figure 41.2 the point is a box, proportional (in area) to that study's weight in the analysis.

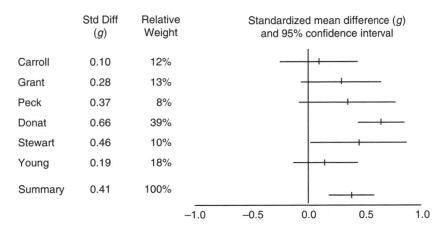

Figure 41.1 Forest plot using lines to represent the effect size.

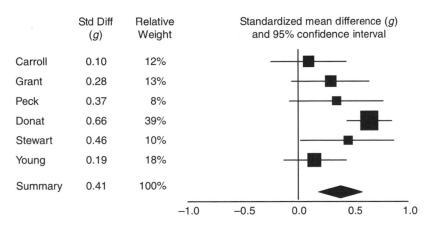

Figure 41.2 Forest plot using boxes to represent the effect size and relative weight.

Both plots use confidence intervals to track the precision, with a narrower interval reflecting better precision. What distinguishes between the two versions is the mechanism used to reflect the study's weight in the analysis, and the second version offers two advantages.

First, the boxes provide an important visual cue. In Figure 41.1 the only cue to the study weight is the width of the confidence interval, which requires careful attention and also is *inversely* proportional to the study weight. By contrast, in Figure 41.2 the studies with more weight are assigned *more* ink in the plot. The eye is naturally drawn to these studies, and we quickly get a sense of the relative impact of the different studies. In this example it is immediately apparent that the studies by Donat and by Young are dominant factors in the summary effect.

Second, the confidence interval (more precisely, the inverse of the squared standard error) is directly related to the weight only under the fixed-effect model. Under the random-effects model, the study weight is based also on the between-studies variance and may bear little relationship to the confidence interval.

The label *forest plot* also appears in the literature as *Forrest plot*. A paper in *BMJ* by Lewis and Clarke (2001) explains that this (incorrect) usage stems from a comment made by Richard Peto who, as a joke, attributed the plot's invention to breast cancer researcher Pat Forrest.

SENSITIVITY ANALYSIS

The issues addressed by a sensitivity analysis for a systematic review are similar to those that might be addressed by a sensitivity analysis for a primary study. That is, the focus is on the extent to which the results are (or are not) robust to assumptions and decisions that were made when carrying out the synthesis. The kinds of issues that need to be included in a sensitivity analysis will vary from one synthesis to the next. Our goal here is not to describe all of the possible sensitivity analyses that might be done in a meta-analysis, but to outline the kinds of issues that one might want to consider.

One kind of sensitivity analysis is concerned with the impact of decisions that lead to different data being used in the analysis. A common example of sensitivity analysis is to ask how results might have changed if different study inclusion rules had been used. This could be asked about studies classified on the basis of *a priori* criteria (for example, how would results have differed if we had included only randomized experiments instead of also including well designed quasi-experiments). It could also be asked about studies identified as outliers (studies whose effects differ very substantially from the others). Here the question is whether the conclusions reached might differ substantially if a single study or a few studies were omitted.

Another kind of sensitivity analysis is concerned with the impact of the statistical methods used on the conclusions drawn from the analysis. For example one might ask whether the conclusions would have been different if a different effect size measure had been used (e.g. a risk ratio versus an odds ratio or an effect size using covariate adjusted means versus raw means). Alternatively, one might ask whether the conclusions would be the same if fixed-effect versus random-effects methods had been used. We might also ask whether conclusions would be different if the analysis had adjusted for the effects of unreliability or restriction of range within individual studies.

Yet another kind of sensitivity analysis is concerned with how we addressed missing data. One situation is missing data on study characteristics that might be used formally (as in a moderator analysis) or informally (as a basis for grouping or describing studies). A very important form of missing data is the missing data on effect sizes that may result from incomplete reporting or selective reporting of statistical results within studies. When data are selectively reported in a way that is related to the magnitude of the effect size (e.g., when results are only reported when they are statistically significant), such missing data can have biasing effects similar to publication bias on entire studies. In either case, we need to ask how the results would have changed if we had dealt with missing data in another way.

Missing data are not limited just to study characteristics that are potential moderators nor to effect sizes. In some cases information needed to compute effect size estimates or their variances may not be reported and will be imputed in the meta-analysis (such as pretest-posttest correlations used to compute effect sizes). In this context, sensitivity analyses can be used to investigate whether the conclusions would differ substantially across a range of plausible imputed values.

In the next chapter we discuss cumulative analyses, which show how the summary effect and variance shift as studies are added to the analysis. This approach can also be used as part of a sensitivity analysis, for example by showing how our conclusions would (or would not) shift as new studies (perhaps representing a broader range of populations) are added.

SUMMARY POINTS

- The questions being asked by the analysis, as well as the empirical findings, will help to shape the structure of the report, and this will vary from one analysis to the next. If the effect size is consistent across all studies in the analysis we are likely to focus on this effect and the fact that it is consistent. If the effect size varies somewhat we will want to estimate the amount of dispersion in true effects and consider the implications of this dispersion. If the effect size varies substantially, or if a goal of the analysis had been to explore expected variation in effect size, then the report would likely focus on the dispersion itself.
- The report of a meta-analysis should generally include a forest plot. This provides an intuitive sense of the data, and helps to ensure that the statistics will be interpreted in context.
- A sensitivity analysis is important to determine how robust the findings are. It would be important to know how the findings would shift if we changed the criteria for including studies, of if we changed some of the assumptions that we made when performing the analysis.

Further Reading

Lewis, S. & Clarke, M. (2001). Forest plots: trying to see the wood and the trees. *BMJ* 322: 1479–1480.

Light, R.J. & Pillemer, D.B. (1984). *Summing Up: The Science of Reviewing Research.* Cambridge, MA: Harvard University Press.

Light, R.J. & Pillemer, D.B. (1994). The visual presentation and interpretation of meta-analyses. In Cooper, H.M. & Hedges, L.V. (eds), *The Handbook of Research Synthesis.* New York: Russell Sage Foundation.

CHAPTER 42

Cumulative Meta-Analysis

Introduction
Why perform a cumulative meta-analysis?

INTRODUCTION

A cumulative meta-analysis is a meta-analysis that is performed first with one study, then with two studies, and so on, until all relevant studies have been included in the analysis. As such, a cumulative analysis *is not a different analytic method* than a standard analysis, but simply *a mechanism for displaying a series of separate analyses* in one table or plot. When the series are sorted into a sequence based on some factor, the display shows how our estimate of the effect size (and its precision) shifts as a function of this factor. When the studies are sorted chronologically, the display shows how the evidence accumulated, and how the conclusions may have shifted, over a period of time.

For example, consider the systematic review published by Lau *et al.* (1992) that looked at the impact of streptokinase in preventing death following a myocardial infarction. Streptokinase is a drug that has the potential to dissolve the blood clot that is causing a heart attack, and thus reduce the damage to heart muscle.

The systematic review synthesizes data from 33 studies that had been published over a period of 29 years. All the studies followed the same basic format, with patients who had suffered a myocardial infarction being assigned to either strepto-kinase or a placebo, and physicians recording the mortality rates in each group.

The standard meta-analysis is shown in Figure 42.1. Fletcher appears on the first row, with a risk ratio of 0.229, 95% confidence interval of 0.030 to 1.750. The *p*-value is 0.155, the sample size is 23, and the year is 1959. Dewar appears on the next row, with a risk ratio of 0.571, 95% confidence interval from 0.196 to 1.665. The *p*-value is 0.305, the sample size is 42, and the year is 1963. And so on for the remaining 31 studies.

Introduction to Meta-Analysis   M. Borenstein, L. V. Hedges, J. P. T. Higgins, H. R. Rothstein
© 2009, John Wiley & Sons, Ltd

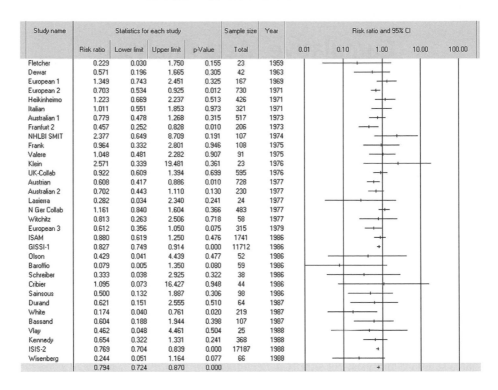

Figure 42.1 Impact of streptokinase on mortality – forest plot.

The studies varied substantially in size, with five having fewer than 40 patients while one (GISSI-1 in 1986) enrolled 11,712 patients and one (ISIS-2 in 1988) enrolled 17,187 patients. Across all studies a total of 18,532 patients were assigned to treatment and 18,442 to control. The number of deaths in the two groups was 1892 versus 2375. The summary effect (using the random-effects model) is shown as a risk ratio of 0.794 with a 95% confidence interval from 0.724 to 0.870 and a *p*-value of 0.0000008.

The cumulative meta-analysis is shown in Figure 42.2. Here, we have the same 33 studies but the values on each row are not the statistics for that study. Rather, they are the summary values for a meta-analysis based on all studies up to and including that row. The line marked *Fletcher* is based only on Fletcher, and so is identical to the first line on the previous figure. The line marked *Dewar* shows the results of a meta-analysis based on Fletcher and Dewar. And so on. (Note that the scale of the forest plot has been changed.)

As one would expect, as we move down the plot the effect size tends to stabilize (as the volume of data accumulates, any new study is less likely to produce a sudden shift) and the confidence intervals tend to narrow (since the amount of data increases). The last study on the plot is Wisenberg. Since the analysis on this row includes data from all 33 studies, the statistics on this row are identical to

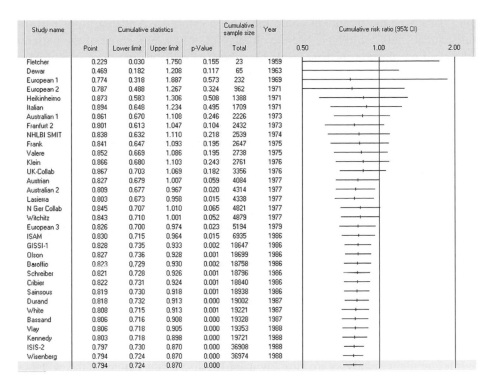

Study name	Cumulative statistics				Cumulative sample size	Year	Cumulative risk ratio (95% CI)		
	Point	Lower limit	Upper limit	p-Value	Total		0.50	1.00	2.00
Fletcher	0.229	0.030	1.750	0.155	23	1959			
Dewar	0.469	0.182	1.208	0.117	65	1963			
European 1	0.774	0.318	1.887	0.573	232	1969			
European 2	0.787	0.488	1.267	0.324	962	1971			
Heikinheimo	0.873	0.583	1.306	0.508	1388	1971			
Italian	0.894	0.648	1.234	0.495	1709	1971			
Australian 1	0.861	0.670	1.108	0.246	2226	1973			
Franfurt 2	0.801	0.613	1.047	0.104	2432	1973			
NHLBI SMIT	0.838	0.632	1.110	0.218	2539	1974			
Frank	0.841	0.647	1.093	0.195	2647	1975			
Valere	0.852	0.669	1.086	0.195	2738	1975			
Klein	0.866	0.680	1.103	0.243	2761	1976			
UK-Collab	0.867	0.703	1.069	0.182	3356	1976			
Austrian	0.827	0.679	1.007	0.059	4084	1977			
Australian 2	0.809	0.677	0.967	0.020	4314	1977			
Lasierra	0.803	0.673	0.958	0.015	4338	1977			
N Ger Collab	0.845	0.707	1.010	0.065	4821	1977			
Witchitz	0.843	0.710	1.001	0.052	4879	1977			
European 3	0.826	0.700	0.974	0.023	5194	1979			
ISAM	0.830	0.715	0.964	0.015	6935	1986			
GISSI-1	0.828	0.735	0.933	0.002	18647	1986			
Olson	0.827	0.736	0.928	0.001	18699	1986			
Darolfio	0.823	0.729	0.930	0.002	18758	1986			
Schreiber	0.821	0.728	0.926	0.001	18796	1986			
Cribier	0.822	0.731	0.924	0.001	18840	1986			
Sainsous	0.819	0.730	0.918	0.001	18938	1986			
Durand	0.818	0.732	0.913	0.000	19002	1987			
White	0.808	0.715	0.913	0.001	19221	1987			
Bassand	0.806	0.716	0.908	0.000	19328	1987			
Vlay	0.806	0.718	0.905	0.000	19353	1988			
Kennedy	0.803	0.718	0.898	0.000	19721	1988			
ISIS-2	0.797	0.730	0.870	0.000	36908	1988			
Wisenberg	0.794	0.724	0.870	0.000	36974	1988			
	0.794	0.724	0.870	0.000					

Figure 42.2 Impact of streptokinase on mortality – cumulative forest plot.

those shown on the summary line. This also matches the summary line in Figure 42.1.

WHY PERFORM A CUMULATIVE META-ANALYSIS?

Cumulative meta-analysis as an educational tool

Lau *et al.* used the streptokinase analysis to show the potential impact of meta-analysis as part of the research process. They argued that if meta-analysis had been available to researchers several decades earlier, then the benefits of streptokinase could have been established as early as 1977. Had researchers performed a meta-analysis in 1977 using the studies prior to and including the Australian-2 study, they would have found that the risk ratio was 0.81, with a *p*-value of 0.020. Since meta-analysis was not yet recognized as a useful tool, researchers continued to perform additional studies (Lau *et al.*, 1992; Lau & Chalmers, 1995; Lau, Schmid, & Chalmers, 1995).

The studies published subsequent to the Australian-2 study enrolled a total of 32,660 patients, with approximately 50% assigned to placebo. In these studies there were 414 more deaths among the placebo patients than among the treated patients. Lau *et al.* argued that if meta-analysis had been conducted in 1977, then the efficacy of the treatment could have been established at that point and the subsequent trials could have been avoided. Not only would some of the patients who died on placebo in these trials have been saved, but the drug would have become the standard of care and countless premature deaths worldwide could have been avoided.

One can argue with the specific numbers. In particular, when we repeatedly look at the cumulative data we may need to use a more conservative criterion for significance than 0.05 before deciding that the treatment is effective (see *Using a cumulative analysis prospectively* on page 375). Additionally, some trials that were published subsequent to the Australian-2 study were already under-way when the Australian-2 study was published. Nevertheless, the basic argument is compelling, and captured the attention of the medical community. This cumulative analysis played an important role in gaining acceptance for meta-analysis as a useful mechanism for decision making.

The above should not be taken as a criticism of the people who performed the later studies. Meta-analysis was not widely accepted in the 1970s and 1980s (indeed it is not universally accepted even now) and so was simply not an option at the time.

To identify patterns in the data

While cumulative analyses are most often used to display the pattern of the evidence over time, the same technique can be used for other purposes as well. Rather than sort the data chronologically, we can sort it by any variable, and then display the pattern of effect sizes.

For example, assume that we have 100 studies that looked at the impact of homeopathic medicines, and we think that the effect is related to the quality of the blinding process. We anticipate that studies with complete blinding will show no effect, those with lower quality blinding will show a minor effect, those that blind only some people will show a larger effect, and so on. We could sort the studies based on the quality of the blinding (from high to low), and then perform a cumulative analysis. If our expectations were correct, the cumulative effect would initially be near zero, would increase as we moved to the next (lower) level of quality, and would increase some more at the next level.

Similarly, we could use cumulative analyses to display the possible impact of publication bias. The details will not be repeated here (this is covered in Chapter 30), but the problem being addressed is that the large studies are assumed to be unbiased, but the smaller studies may tend to over-estimate the effect size. We could perform a cumulative analysis, entering the larger studies at the top and adding the smaller studies at the bottom. If the effect was initially small when the large (nonbiased) studies were included, and then increased as the smaller studies were added, we would indeed be concerned that the effect size was related to sample size. A benefit of the cumulative analysis is that it displays not only *if* there is a shift in effect size, but also *the magnitude* of the shift.

Display, not analysis

It is important to recognize that cumulative meta-analysis is a mechanism for display, rather than analysis. If we sort studies chronologically, we can see how the weight of the evidence has shifted over time. If we sort studies by the effectiveness of blinding, we can see how the effect size shifts with the addition of poor-quality studies. If we sort studies by sample size, we can display the potential impact of publication bias.

These kinds of displays are compelling and can serve an important function. However, if our goal is actually to examine the relationship between a factor and effect size, then the appropriate analysis is a meta-regression, which looks at the relationship between each the study's effect size and the study's covariates (whether year of publication, or sample size, or something else).

Using a cumulative analysis prospectively

As noted, the primary function of a cumulative analysis is to provide a mechanism for display. For example, when we sort the studies by year of publication and perform cumulative meta-analysis retrospectively, the analysis serves to provide us with historical context.

A very different situation emerges when the concept is applied prospectively (a process sometimes called *prospective* cumulative meta-analysis). In this case, a researcher performs a meta-analysis at time X using all the available data. If the cumulative effect is not definitive, then the analysis is repeated at time X+1 with the addition of the next study (when that study becomes available). The process is repeated until such time as the results become definitive, at which time the process is stopped.

There is a serious problem with this use of cumulative analysis if the criterion for stopping is based on the analysis reaching a level of statistical significance. The problem is that the 0.05 (or any other) criterion only works as advertised when the data are subjected to a single statistical test. If the test is applied repeatedly, then (assuming that the null is true) the likelihood of a false positive is 0.05 *for any given test*, but exceeds 0.05 when accumulated over all tests. This is analogous to a problem that arises in longitudinal studies where researchers follow a cohort of patients over time, look at the data periodically, and will stop the study if the *p*-value at any time crosses a given threshold.

There is an entire body of research on the best ways to allocate this risk and much of this can be applied to cumulative meta-analysis as well (Devereaux *et al.*, 2005; Pogue & Yusuf, 1998; Whitehead, 1997). For example, one solution used in longitudinal trials is to work with a more stringent criterion for stopping the trial, such as 0.01 rather than 0.05 (if 5 peeks are planned) so that the overall risk of a type I error is kept at an acceptable level.

At the same time, we need to recognize that researchers, clinicians and patients do not always have the luxury of waiting until enough studies have been completed before they make a decision. People who need to make a decision at a given point may need to base that decision on the evidence available at that point, and for this purpose a cumulative analysis of all available studies may be the best option. However, we can still continue to perform new studies and add to the cumulative evidence until the relevant questions have been fully addressed.

SUMMARY POINTS

- Cumulative meta-analysis is a mechanism for displaying results from a series of separate analyses in one table or plot. The studies are typically sorted chronologically, which shows how the evidence has accumulated (and possibly how the results have shifted) over time. However, the studies may also be sorted by other variables, to show how the results shift as a function of some other factor (such as study quality).
- Cumulative analysis is a mechanism for display, not for analysis. If our goal is to test the hypothesis that the effect size has shifted over time, the correct approach would be to use subgroup analysis or meta-regression.
- A variant of cumulative analyses calls for study results to be added to a meta-analysis as each study is completed, with the analysis repeated every time the list of studies is updated. While this approach may provide the most up-to-date data for someone needing to make a decision about the utility of a treatment, if the plan is to stop adding studies when the analysis becomes definitive, then we need to adjust for the fact that we are having multiple looks at the data.

Criticisms of Meta-Analysis

INTRODUCTION

While meta-analysis has been widely embraced by large segments of the research community, this point of view is not universal and people have voiced numerous criticisms of meta-analysis.

Some of these criticisms are worth mentioning for their creative use of metaphor. The first set of Cochrane reviews dealt with studies in neonatology, and one especially creative critic, cited by Mann (1990), called the reviewers *an obstetrical Baader Meinhof gang* (*obstetrical* being a reference to the field of research, and *Baader Meinhof gang* a reference to the terrorist group that operated in Europe during the 1970s and 1980s).

Others were more circumspect in their comments. Eysenck (1978) criticized a meta-analysis as *an exercise in mega-silliness*. Shapiro (1994) published a paper entitled *Meta-Analysis / Shmeta Analysis*. Feinstein (1995) wrote an editorial in which he referred to meta-analysis as 'statistical alchemy for the 21st century'.

Introduction to Meta-Analysis   M. Borenstein, L. V. Hedges, J. P. T. Higgins, H. R. Rothstein
© 2009, John Wiley & Sons, Ltd

These critics share not only an affinity for allegory and alliteration but also a common set of concerns about meta-analysis. In this chapter we address the following criticisms that have been leveled at meta-analysis, as follows.

- One number cannot summarize a research field
- The file drawer problem invalidates meta-analysis
- Mixing apples and oranges
- Garbage in, garbage out
- Important studies are ignored
- Meta-analysis can disagree with randomized trials
- Meta-analyses are performed poorly

After considering each of these questions in turn, we ask whether a traditional narrative review fares any better than a systematic review on these criticisms. And, we summarize the legitimate criticisms of meta-analysis that need to be considered whenever meta-analysis is applied.

ONE NUMBER CANNOT SUMMARIZE A RESEARCH FIELD

Criticism

A common criticism of meta-analysis is that the analysis focuses on the summary effect, and ignores the fact that the treatment effect may vary from study to study. Bailar (1997), for example, writes, 'Any attempt to reduce results to a single value, with confidence bounds, is likely to lead to conclusions that are wrong, perhaps seriously so.'

Response

In fact, the goal of a meta-analysis should be to *synthesize* the effect sizes, and not simply (or necessarily) to report a summary effect. If the effects are consistent, then the analysis shows that the effect is robust across the range of included studies. If there is modest dispersion, then this dispersion should serve to place the mean effect in context. If there is substantial dispersion, then the focus should shift from the summary effect to the dispersion itself. Researchers who report a summary effect and ignore heterogeneity are indeed missing the point of the synthesis.

THE FILE DRAWER PROBLEM INVALIDATES META-ANALYSIS

Criticism

While the meta-analysis will yield a mathematically sound synthesis of the studies included in the analysis, if these studies are a biased sample of all possible studies, then the mean effect reported by the meta-analysis will reflect this bias. Several lines of evidence show that studies finding relatively high treatment effects are more likely to be published than studies finding lower treatment effects. The latter, unpublished, research lies dormant in the researchers' filing cabinets, and has led to the use of the term *file drawer problem* for meta-analysis.

Response

Since published studies are more likely to be included in a meta-analysis than their unpublished counterparts, there is a legitimate concern that a meta-analysis may overestimate the true effect size.

Chapter 30 (entitled *Publication Bias*) explores this question in some detail. In that chapter we discuss methods to assess the likely amount of bias in any given meta-analysis, and to distinguish between analyses that can be considered robust to the impact of publication bias from those where the results should be considered suspect.

We must remember that publication bias is a problem for any kind of literature search. The problem exists for the clinician who searches a database to locate primary studies about the utility of a treatment. It exists for persons performing a narrative review. And, it exists for persons performing a meta-analysis. Publication bias has come to be identified with meta-analysis because meta-analysis has the goal of providing a more accurate synthesis than other methods, and so we are concerned with biases that will interfere with this goal. However, it would be a mistake to conclude that this bias is not a problem for the narrative review. There, it is simply easier to ignore.

MIXING APPLES AND ORANGES

Criticism

A common criticism of meta-analysis is that researchers combine different kinds of studies (*apples and oranges*) in the same analysis. The argument is that the summary effect will ignore possibly important differences across studies.

Response

The studies that are brought together in a meta-analysis will inevitably differ in their characteristics, and the difficulty is deciding just how similar they need to be. The decision as to which studies should be included is always a judgment, and people will have different opinions on the appropriateness of combining results across studies. Some meta-analysts may make questionable judgments, and some critics may make unreasonable demands on similarity.

We need to remember that meta-analyses almost always, by their very nature, address broader questions than individual studies. Hence a meta-analysis may be thought of as asking a question about fruit, for which both apples and oranges (and indeed pears and melons) contribute valuable information. One of the strengths of meta-analysis is that the consistency, and hence generalizability, of findings from one type of study to the next can be assessed formally.

Of course, we always need to remember that we are dealing with different kinds of fruit, and to anticipate that effects may vary from one kind to the other. It is a further strength of meta-analysis that these differences, if identified, can be investigated formally. Assume, for example, that a treatment is very effective for patients with acute symptoms but has no effect for patients with chronic symptoms. If we were to combine data from studies that used both types of patients, and conclude that the treatment was modestly effective (on average), this conclusion would not be accurate for either kind of patient. If we were to restrict our attention to studies in only patients with acute symptoms, or only patients with chronic symptoms, we could report how the treatment worked with one type of patient, but could only speculate about how it would have worked with the other type. By contrast, a meta-analysis that includes data for both types of patients may allow us to address this question empirically.

GARBAGE IN, GARBAGE OUT

Criticism

The often-heard metaphor *garbage in, garbage out* refers to the notion that if a meta-analysis includes many low-quality studies, then fundamental errors in the primary studies will be carried over to the meta-analysis, where the errors may be harder to identify.

Response

Rather than thinking of meta-analysis as a process of *garbage in, garbage out* we can think of it as a process of waste management. A systematic review or meta-analysis will always have a set of inclusion criteria and these should include criteria based on the quality of the study. For trials, we may decide to limit the studies to those that use random assignment, or a placebo control. For observational studies we may decide to limit the studies to those where confounders were adequately addressed in the design or analysis. And so on. In fact, it is common in a systematic review to start with a large pool of studies and end with a much smaller set of studies after all inclusion/exclusion criteria are applied.

Nevertheless, the studies that do make it as far as a meta-analysis are unlikely to be perfect, and close attention should be paid to the possibility of bias due to study limitations. A meta-analysis of a collection of studies that is each biased in the same direction will suffer from the same bias and have higher precision. In this case, performing a meta-analysis can indeed be more dangerous than not performing one.

However, as noted in the response to the previous criticism about *apples and oranges*, a strength of meta-analysis is the ability to investigate whether variation in characteristics of studies is related to the size of the effect. Suppose that ten studies used an acceptable method to randomize patients while another ten used a questionable method. In the analysis we can compare the effect size in these two subgroups, and determine whether or not the effect size actually differs between the two. Note that such analyses (those comparing effects in different subgroups) can have very low power so need to be interpreted carefully, especially when there are not many studies within subgroups.

IMPORTANT STUDIES ARE IGNORED

Criticism

Whereas the *garbage in, garbage out* problem relates to the inclusion of studies that perhaps should not be included, a common complementary criticism is that important studies were left out. The criticism is often leveled by people who are uncomfortable with the findings of a meta-analysis. For example, a meta-analysis to assess the effects of antioxidant supplements (beta-carotene, vitamin A, vitamin C, vitamin E, and selenium) on overall mortality was met with accusations on the web site of the Linus Pauling Institute (Oregon State University) that in this 'flawed analysis of flawed data' the authors looked at 815 human clinical trials of antioxidant supplements, but only 68 were included in the meta-analysis.

Response

We have explained that systematic reviews and meta-analyses require explicit mechanisms for deciding which studies to include and which ones to exclude. These eligibility criteria are determined by a combination of considerations of relevance and considerations of bias, and are typically decided before the search for studies is implemented. Studies should be sufficiently similar to yield results that can be interpreted, and sufficiently free of bias to yield results that can be believed. For both purposes, judgments are required, and not all meta-analysts or readers would reach the same judgments on each occasion. Importantly, in meta-analysis the criteria are transparent and are described as part of the report.

META-ANALYSIS CAN DISAGREE WITH RANDOMIZED TRIALS

Criticism

LeLorier *et al.* (1997) published a paper in which they pointed out that meta-analyses sometimes yield different results than large scale randomized trials. Specifically, they located cases in the medical literature where someone had performed a meta-analysis, and someone else subsequently performed a large scale randomized trial that addressed the same question (e.g. *Does the treatment work?*). The authors reported that the results of the meta-analysis and the randomized trial *matched* (both were statistically significant, or neither was statistically significant) in about 66% of cases, but did not match (one was statistically significant but the other was not) in the remaining 34%. Since randomized trials are generally accepted as the gold standard they conclude that some 34% of these meta-analyses were wrong, and that meta-analyses in general cannot be trusted.

Response

There are both technical and conceptual flaws in this criticism. The technical flaws relate to the question of what we mean by *matching*, and the authors' decision to define *matching* as both studies being (or not being) statistically significant. The discussion that follows draws in part on comments by Ioannidis *et al.* (1998), Lelorier *et al.* (1997, 536–543) and others (see further readings at the end of this chapter).

Consider Figure 43.1, which shows a meta-analysis of five randomized controlled trials (RCTs) at the top, and a subsequent large-scale randomized trial at the bottom.

In this fictional example the five studies in the meta-analysis each showed precisely the same effect, an odds ratio of 0.80. The summary effect in the meta-analysis is (it follows) an odds ratio of 0.80. And, the subsequent study showed the same effect, an odds ratio of 0.80.

The only difference between the summary effect in the meta-analysis and the effect in the subsequent study is that the former is reported with greater precision (since it is based on more data) and therefore yields a *p*-value under 0.05. By the LeLorier criterion these two conclusions would be seen as conflicting, when in fact they have the identical effect size.

Additionally, LeLorier concludes that in the face of this conflict the single randomized trial is correct and the meta-analysis is wrong. In fact, though, it is the meta-analysis, which incorporates data from five randomized trials rather than one, that has the more powerful position. (What would happen if we performed a new meta-analysis which incorporated the most recent randomized trial? Would

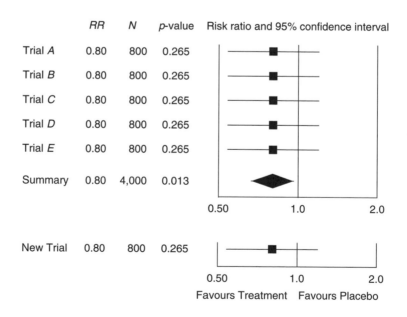

Figure 43.1 Forest plot of five fictional studies and a new trail (consistent effects).

LeLorier now see this new meta-analysis as flawed?) In fact, the real issue is not that a meta-analysis disagrees with a randomized trial, but that randomized trials disagree with each other.

At a meeting of The Cochrane Collaboration in Baltimore (1996), a plenary speaker made the same argument being made by LeLorier *et al.* (that meta-analyses sometimes yield different results than randomized trials) and, like the paper, cited the statistic that roughly a third of meta-analyses fail to match the *comparable* randomized trial. A distinguished member of the audience, Harris Cooper, asked the speaker if he knew what percentage of randomized trials fail to match the next randomized trial on the same topic. It turns out that the percentage is roughly a third.

However, to move on to a more interesting question, let's assume that the results from a meta-analysis and a randomized trial really do differ. Suppose that the meta-analysis yields a risk ratio of 0.67 (with a 95% confidence interval of 0.84 to 0.77) while the new trial yields a risk ratio of 0.91 (0.82 to 1.0). According to the meta-analysis the treatment reduces the risk by at least 23%, while the new trial says that its impact is no more than 18%.

In this case the effect *is different* in the two analyses, but that does not mean that one is wrong and the other is right. Rather, it behooves us to ask why the two results should differ, much as we would if we had two large scale randomized trials with significantly different results. Often, it will turn out that the different analyses either were asking different questions or differed in some important way. A careful examination of the differences in method, patient population, and so on, may help to uncover the source of the difference.

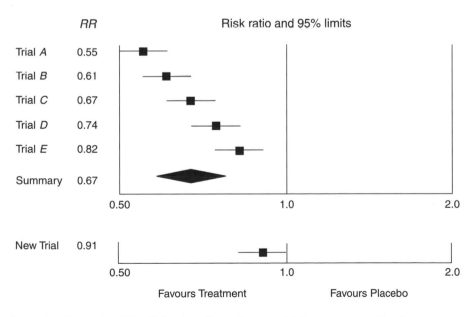

Figure 43.2 Forest plot of five fictional studies and a new trial (heterogeneous effects).

Consider the following scenario, depicted in Figure 43.2. A new compound is introduced, which is meant to minimize neurological damage in stroke patients. In 1990, the compound is tested in a randomized trial involving patients with a very poor prognosis, and yields a risk ratio of 0.55. Based on these encouraging results, in 1994 it is tested in patients with a somewhat better prognosis. Since the patients in this group are more likely to recover without treatment, the impact of the drug is less pronounced, and the risk ratio is 0.61. By 1998 the drug is being tested with all patients, and the risk ratio is 0.82. These are the studies included in the meta-analysis. The new trial is performed using a relatively healthy population and (following the trend seen in the meta-analysis) yields a risk ratio of 0.91.

If one were to report a mean effect of 0.67 for the meta-analysis versus 0.91 for the new trial there would indeed be a problem. But, as we have emphasized throughout this volume, the meta-analysis should focus on the dispersion in effects and try to identify the reason for the dispersion. In this example, using either health status or study year as a covariate we can explain the pattern of the effects, and would have predicted that the effect size in the new study would fall where it did.

META-ANALYSES ARE PERFORMED POORLY

Criticism

John C. Bailar, in an editorial for the *New England Journal of Medicine* (Bailar, 1997), writes that mistakes such as those outlined in the prior criticisms are common in meta-analysis. He argues that a meta-analysis is inherently so complicated that mistakes by the persons performing the analysis are all but inevitable. He also argues that journal editors are unlikely to uncover all of these mistakes.

Response

The specific points made by Bailar about problems with meta-analysis are entirely reasonable. He is correct that many meta-analyses contain errors, some of them important ones. His list of potential (and common) problems can serve as a bullet list of mistakes to avoid when performing a meta-analysis.

However, the mistakes cited by Bailar are flaws in the application of the method, rather than problems with the method itself. Many primary studies suffer from flaws in the design, analyses, and conclusions. In fact, some serious kinds of problems are endemic in the literature. The response of the research community is to locate these flaws, consider their impact for the study in question, and (hopefully) take steps to avoid similar mistakes in the future. In the case of meta-analysis, as in the case of primary studies, we cannot condemn a method because some people have used that method improperly. As Bob Abelson once remarked in a related context, 'Think of all the things that people abuse. There are college educations. And oboes.'

IS A NARRATIVE REVIEW BETTER?

In his editorial Bailar concludes that, until such time as the quality of meta-analyses is improved, he would prefer to work with the traditional narrative reviews: 'I still prefer conventional narrative reviews of the literature, a type of summary familiar to readers of the countless review articles on important medical issues.'

We disagree with the conclusion that narrative reviews are preferable to systematic reviews, and that meta-analyses should be avoided. The narrative review suffers from every one of the problems cited for the systematic review. The only difference is that, in the narrative review, these problems are less obvious. For example:

- The process of determining which studies to include in the systematic review or meta-analysis is difficult and prone to error. But at least there is a set of criteria for determining which studies to include. If the narrative review also has such criteria, then it is subject to the same kinds of error. If not, then we have no way of knowing how studies are being selected, which only compounds the problem.
- Meta-analyses can be affected by publication bias. But the same biases exist in the material upon which narrative reviews are based. Meta-analysis offers a means to investigate the likelihood of these biases and their potential impact on the results.
- Meta-analyses may be based on low quality primary research. But a good systematic review includes a careful assessment of the included studies with regard to their quality or risk of bias, and meta-analytic methods enable formal examination of the potential impact of these biases. A narrative reviewer may discount a study because of a belief that the results are suspect for some reason. However, a limitation can be found for virtually any study, so in the absence of a systematic quality assessment of every study, a narrative reviewer is free to be suspect about any study's results and to lay the blame on one or more of its limitations.
- The weighting scheme in a meta-analysis may give a lot (or little) weight to specific studies in ways that may appear inappropriate. But in a meta-analysis the weights reflect specific goals (to minimize the variance, or to reflect the range of effects) and the weighting scheme is detailed as part of the report, so a reader is able to agree or disagree with it. By contrast, in the case of a narrative review, the reviewer assigns *weights* to studies based on criteria that he or she does not communicate, and may not even be able to fully articulate. Here, the problem involves not only the relative weights assigned to small or large studies. It extends also to the propensity of one reviewer to focus on effect sizes, and of another to focus on (and possibly be misled by) significance tests.
- Some meta-analyses focus on the summary effect and ignore the pattern of dispersion in the results. To ignore the dispersion is clearly a mistake both in a narrative review and in a meta-analysis. However, meta-analysis provides a full complement of tools to assess the pattern of dispersion, and possibly to explain it as a function of study-level covariates. By contrast, it would be an almost

impossible task for a narrative reviewer to accurately assess the pattern of dispersion, or to understand its relationship to other variables.

- In support of the narrative review, Bailer cites the role of the expert with substantive knowledge of the field, who can identify flaws in specific studies, or the presence of potentially important moderator variables. However, this is not an advantage of the narrative review, since the expert is expected to play the same role in a meta-analysis. Steve Goodman (1991) wrote, 'The best meta-analyses knit clinical insight with quantitative results in a way that enhances both. They should combine the careful thought and synthesis of a good review with the scientific rigor of a good experiment.'

CONCLUDING REMARKS

Most of the criticisms raised in this chapter point to problems with meta-analysis, and make the implicit argument that the problem would go away if we dispensed with the meta-analysis and performed a narrative review. We have argued that these problems exist also for the narrative review, and that the key advantage of the systematic approach of a meta-analysis is that all steps are clearly described so that the process is transparent.

Is meta-analysis so difficult that the method should be abandoned, as some have suggested? Our answer is obviously that it is not. Most of the criticisms raised deal with the application of the method, rather than with the method itself. What we should do is take the valid criticisms seriously and protect against them in planned analyses and by thoughtful interpretation of results.

Steven Goodman, in his editorial for *Annals of Internal Medicine* (1991) writes,

> Regardless of the summary number, meta-analysis should shed light on why trial results differ; raise research and editorial standards by calling attention to the strengths and weaknesses of the body of research in an area; and give the practitioner an objective view of the research literature, unaffected by the sometimes distorting lens of individual experience and personal preference that can affect a less structured review.

SUMMARY POINTS

- Meta-analyses are sometimes criticized for a number of flaws, and critics have argued that narrative reviews provide a better solution.
- Some of these flaws, such as the idea that we cannot summarize a body of data in a single number, are based on misunderstandings of meta-analysis.
- Many of the flaws (such as ignoring dispersion in effect sizes) reflect problems in the way that meta-analysis is used, rather than problems in the method itself.

- Other flaws (such as publication bias) are a problem for meta-analysis. However, the suggestion that these problems do not exist in narrative reviews is wrong. These problems exist for narrative reviews as well, but are simply easier to ignore since those reviews lack a clear structure.

Further Reading

Bailar, J.C. (1995). The practice of meta-analysis. *J Clin Epidemiol* 48: 149–157.

Bailar, J.C. (1997). The promise and problems of meta-analysis. *New Engl J Med* 337: 559–561.

Boden, W.E. (1992). Meta-analysis in clinical trials reporting: has a tool become a weapon? *Am J Cardiol* 69: 681–686.

Egger, M, & Davey Smith, G. (1998). Bias in location and selection of studies. *BMJ* 316: 61–66.

Eysenck, H.J. (1978). An exercise in mega-silliness. *Am Psychol* 33: 517.

Lau, J., Ioannidis, J.P., Terrin, N., Schmid, C.H., & Olkin, I. (2006). The case of the misleading funnel plot. *BMJ* 333: 597–600.

LeLorier, J., Gregoire, G., Benhaddad, A., Lapierre, J., & Derderian, F. (1997). Discrepancies between meta-analyses and subsequent large randomized, controlled trials. *N Engl J Med* 337: 536–543.

Responses to Lelorier *et al.*

- Bent, S., Kerlikowske, K., & Grady, D. (1998). *NEJM*, 338(1), 60.
- Imperiale, T.F. (1998). *NEJM*, 338(1), 61.
- Ioannidis, J.P., Cappelleri, J.C., & Lau, J. (1998). *NEJM*, 338(1), 59.
- Khan, S., Williamson, P., & Sutton, R. (1998). *NEJM*, 338(1), 60–61.
- LeLorier, J., & Gregoire, G. (1998). *NEJM*, 338(1), 61–62.
- Song, F. J., & Sheldon, T. A. (1998). *NEJM*, 338(1), 60.
- Stewart, L. A., Parmar, M. K., & Tierney, J. F. (1998). *NEJM*, 338(1), 61

Sharpe, D. (1997) Of apples and oranges, file drawers and garbage: why validity issues in meta-analysis will not go away. *Clin Psychol Rev* 17: 881–901.

Thompson, S.G & Pocock, S. J. (1991). Can meta-analysis be trusted? *Lancet* 338: 1127–1130.

Resources and Software

CHAPTER 44

Software

Introduction
The software
Three examples of meta-analysis software
Comprehensive Meta-Analysis (CMA) 2.0
RevMan 5.0
Stata macros with Stata 10.0

Full disclosure

The authors of this volume are the developers of Comprehensive Meta-Analysis. One of us (*JH*) also contributed to the development of algorithms for RevMan and the Stata macros for meta-analysis. These are the three programs discussed in most detail in this chapter.

The book's web site, www.Meta-Analysis.com offers the following

- Step-by-step instructions for performing a meta-analysis using Excel, CMA, Stata macros, or RevMan
- The datasets used in this book as Excel, CMA, Stata, and RevMan files
- Updated links to the other web sites mentioned in this chapter.

INTRODUCTION

Our goal in this section is to provide an overview of computer programs for meta-analysis.

Three types of software can be used to perform a meta-analysis. One option is to use a spreadsheet such as Microsoft Excel. A second is to use a general purpose statistical package such as SPSS, SAS, R or Stata. A third option is to use a program developed specifically for meta-analysis.

Performing a meta-analysis using a spreadsheet such as Excel is an excellent mechanism for learning (or teaching) meta-analysis since it allows the researcher to

Introduction to Meta-Analysis M. Borenstein, L. V. Hedges, J. P. T. Higgins, H. R. Rothstein
© 2009, John Wiley & Sons, Ltd

develop an appreciation for the formulas, and spreadsheets for this purpose can be downloaded from the book's web site. However, spreadsheets should not generally be used for real analyses as this approach will limit the use of important options (such as forest plots) and is prone to error.

General purpose statistical packages such as SPSS, SAS, R and Stata have no inherent support for meta-analysis. These packages are intended primarily for analysis of primary studies, and do not offer an easy option for assigning weights as required for a meta-analysis (especially for random-effects analyses). Additionally, in the case of subgroup analysis (analysis of variance) or meta-regression, the rules for assigning degrees of freedom are different for meta-analysis than for primary studies, and so using these procedures will yield incorrect p-values.

While the basic routines in these packages should not be used for meta-analysis, it is possible to write code (macros) that can be integrated into the programs and used to perform a meta-analysis. For most major packages, meta-analysis algorithms have been programmed and the code made available for others to use.

- For SPSS, macros have been developed by David Wilson (http://mason.gmu.edu/~dwilsonb/ma.html).
- For SAS, macros have been developed by David Wilson (http://mason.gmu.edu/~dwilsonb/ma.html). Additionally, code is available in tutorials presented by Normand (1999), van Houwelingen (2002), and also in books by Wang and Bushman (1999), and by Arthur, Bennett and Huffcutt (2001).
- For R, packages have been developed by Thomas Lumley (rmeta) and Guido Schwarzer (meta).
- For Stata, numerous authors have developed macros, some of which are discussed below.

The third option is to use software developed specifically for meta-analysis, such as

- Comprehensive Meta-Analysis (CMA), developed by the authors of this volume (see www.Meta-Analysis.com)
- RevMan, developed by the The Cochrane Collaboration (see www.cc-ims.net/RevMan)
- Metawin Version 2.0, developed by Rosenberg, Adams and Gurevitch (see www.metawinsoft.com)

THE SOFTWARE

We focus on two programs that are relatively rich in features and also widely used in meta-analysis. These are Comprehensive Meta-Analysis (CMA) and RevMan. We also discuss a set of macros developed for use with Stata (a general purpose statistical package).

THREE EXAMPLES OF META-ANALYSIS SOFTWARE

Useful functions

We start by outlining the kinds of features that a researcher might need in a program, and discuss which of these features are supported by Comprehensive Meta-Analysis (CMA), RevMan, and the macros available for Stata.

Compute an effect size and variance for each study

The first step in performing a meta-analysis is to compute an effect size and variance from the summary data for each study. In some systematic reviews all studies use a common design and report data in the same way. For example, all studies may report data as a 2×2 table (events and non-events) for independent groups. Or, all studies may report data as means, standard deviations, and sample size for two independent groups. All of the programs can accept data in these formats.

In other cases, however, the meta-analysis will include studies that used different designs (some used independent groups while others used matched groups). Or, it will include studies that reported data in different formats. For example, some studies might report the mean, standard deviation and sample size for each group while others report only a p-value and sample size. CMA is able to accept data in more than 100 formats and allows the user to mix and match formats in the same analysis. RevMan and the Stata macros accept data in the more common formats only, and require that data for all studies be entered in the same format.

Perform the meta-analysis

All of the programs are able to perform fixed-effect and random-effects analyses. They all report the key statistics, such as the summary effect and confidence intervals, measures of heterogeneity (T^2, Q, I^2) and provide enough information so that the researcher can compute additional statistics (such as prediction intervals) on their own, if needed. For binary data all programs offer the option of using inverse variance models, Mantel-Haenszel weights or (for the odds ratio) the one-step (Peto) method.

Sensitivity analysis

It is often useful to see how the results would change if one study (or a set of studies) was removed from the analysis. All of the programs allow the researcher to exclude one study at a time (or to exclude sets of studies) and see how this affects the results. Two of the programs (CMA and the Stata macros) allow the researcher to automate the process, performing the analysis repeatedly and removing a different study on each pass.

Create a forest plot

The forest plot is an important part of any analysis, providing a context for the statistics and also a mechanism for communicating results to others. All of the programs are able to produce a forest plot, but they differ widely in how much control the user has over the forest plot's format. Examples are provided below.

Complex data structures

If some (or all) studies include data from more than one subgroup, outcome, time-point, or comparison, then there needs to be a mechanism to work with this in the analysis. CMA allows the user to define a hierarchical structure (for example, multiple outcomes within studies) and then offers the user a set of options including the option to create a synthetic variable based on some (or all) the outcomes, or to work with each outcome separately. RevMan allows the user to work with each outcome separately. The Stata macros do not include a provision for complex data structures but the user could write code to address this situation.

Subgroup analyses and meta-regression

In some cases the researcher will want to classify studies on the basis of a moderator variable and compare the effect size in two or more groups of studies. All three programs can do this. In other cases, the researcher will want to code each study for one or more continuous moderators, and perform a meta-regression to assess the relationship between effect size and the covariate(s). Two of the programs (CMA and the Stata macros) support these kinds of analyses.

Publication bias

Often, it is important to perform one or more analyses to assess the possible impact of publication bias. Two of the programs (CMA and the Stata macros) offer a full set of tools to assess publication bias. RevMan will produce a funnel plot but will not perform any statistical analyses for publication bias.

Look and feel

We also try to give a sense for the look and feel of each program. For example, some programs offer a point-and-click interface while others allow the researcher to write code.

COMPREHENSIVE META-ANALYSIS (CMA) 2.0

In Comprehensive Meta-Analysis (CMA) the researcher enters summary data into a spreadsheet, and then clicks 'Run' to display the results of the meta-analysis. The program's strengths are its flexibility in working with many different kinds of data, its ease of use, its ability to customize and export forest plots, and its Windows look and feel. The program also incorporates a number of features for educational purposes, such as the option to display the formulas that are used to compute effect sizes, and the option to display a spreadsheet that shows how the summary effects were computed.

The program is available in several versions. The entry-level version includes some 50 formats for data entry, all of the basic computational options, and high-resolution forest plots. Advanced versions add 50 additional formats for data entry, and advanced computational options such as subgroup analysis, meta-regression, and procedures to assess publication bias, as well as additional forest plot options.

Data entry

The data entry sheet looks similar to Excel. The user enters the data into the white columns. The program computes the effect size and variance, and displays these in the shaded columns. In Figure 44.1 the user has entered the events and total n for each study, and the program has computed the odds ratio, log odds ratio, risk ratio, log risk ratio, and risk difference.

In this example the data were events and sample size, but this is only one of more than 100 formats available. For example, if the user wanted to enter means, standard deviations, and sample size for each study, the program would display the corresponding set of columns for data entry. The screenshot has been cropped for clarity (additional columns are normally displayed as well).

The program will accept data for different study designs, such as independent groups, matched groups, and cross-over designs. The program will accept data in various formats and allows the user to mix and match formats within the same analysis. For example, the user can provide means, standard deviations, and sample size for some studies, and the p-value and sample size for others. Or, the user can

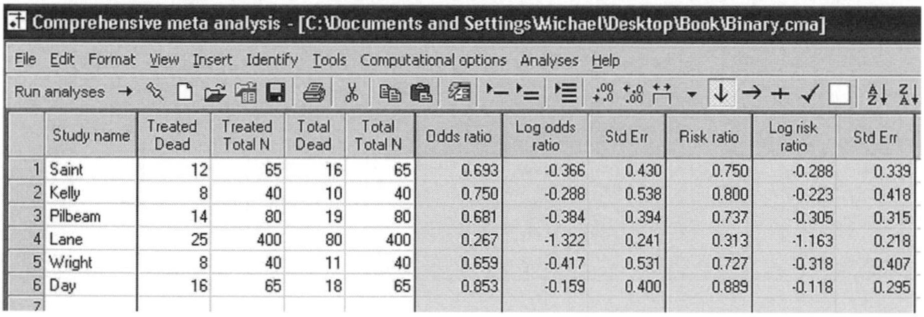

	Study name	Treated Dead	Treated Total N	Total Dead	Total Total N	Odds ratio	Log odds ratio	Std Err	Risk ratio	Log risk ratio	Std Err
1	Saint	12	65	16	65	0.693	-0.366	0.430	0.750	-0.288	0.339
2	Kelly	8	40	10	40	0.750	-0.288	0.538	0.800	-0.223	0.418
3	Pilbeam	14	80	19	80	0.681	-0.384	0.394	0.737	-0.305	0.315
4	Lane	25	400	80	400	0.267	-1.322	0.241	0.313	-1.163	0.218
5	Wright	8	40	11	40	0.659	-0.417	0.531	0.727	-0.318	0.407
6	Day	16	65	18	65	0.853	-0.159	0.400	0.889	-0.118	0.295
7											

Figure 44.1 CMA – data entry screen for 2 × 2 tables.

provide the number of events and non-events for some studies, the odds ratio and its confidence interval for others, and the log odds ratio and its standard error for others. The program also displays the formula used to compute the effect size and variance.

The program will work with the following effect sizes: raw mean difference, standardized mean difference (*d* and *g*), odds ratio (and log odds ratio) risk ratio (and log risk ratio) risk difference, correlation (and Fisher's *z*), rate ratio, and hazard ratio. It will also work with point estimates in single group designs such as the mean, proportion, or rate in a single group. Finally, the program will work with a generic effect size.

Analysis

To perform an analysis, the user clicks the 'Run' button to display a screen similar to the one shown here (see Figure 44.2). Menus and toolbars are used to customize many elements of the computational model and display, including the following.

- Display results for fixed and/or random-effects models.
- Display weights for the two models simultaneously.
- Display a table of statistics including effect size, variance, standard error, confidence limits, Q, T^2, T, and I^2.

Create a forest plot

The main analysis is displayed as a forest plot (Figure 44.2). Additionally, the program allows the user to create a high-resolution plot, customize the plot by specifying what columns to display, what symbols to use, and so on (Figure 44.3). The program features a one-click export to Word and PowerPoint, and the plots can also be inserted into any other program.

Sensitivity analysis

The program can run the analysis repeatedly, removing a different study on each pass, to show the impact of that study on the results. The user can also define sets of studies and include or remove these as a block by using a checkbox.

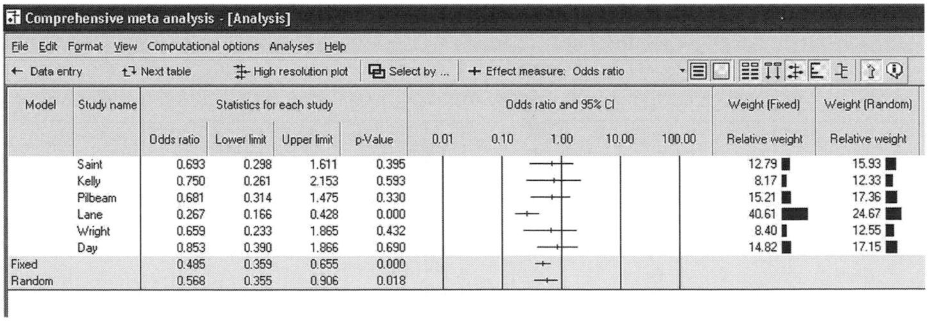

Figure 44.2 CMA – analysis screen.

Impact of Intervention

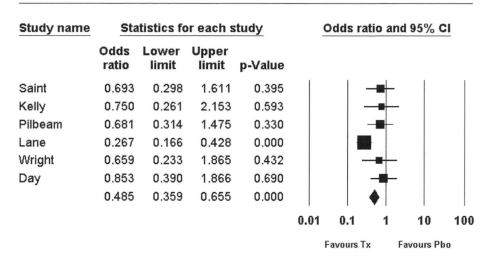

Study name	Statistics for each study				Odds ratio and 95% CI
	Odds ratio	Lower limit	Upper limit	p-Value	
Saint	0.693	0.298	1.611	0.395	
Kelly	0.750	0.261	2.153	0.593	
Pilbeam	0.681	0.314	1.475	0.330	
Lane	0.267	0.166	0.428	0.000	
Wright	0.659	0.233	1.865	0.432	
Day	0.853	0.390	1.866	0.690	
	0.485	0.359	0.655	0.000	

Fixed-effect model

Figure 44.3 CMA – high resolution forest plot.

Work with subgroups within studies and with multiple outcomes

The program is able to work with complex data structures. On the data entry sheet the user can specify that some (or all) studies include more than one subgroup, outcome, time-point, and/or comparison. In this case the program will provide room for additional rows of data within each study.

In the analysis, the program will offer any relevant options. For example, if some studies include several independent subgroups, the user will be able to limit an analysis to one or more subgroups while excluding others, or to merge data across subgroups within studies. Or, if some studies include more than one outcome, the user will be able to limit the analysis to one or more outcomes, and/or create synthetic effects, and/or compare the effect in different outcomes.

Perform subgroup analysis and meta-regression

When entering data the user can create categorical variables and enter a value (for example, acute or chronic) for each study. In the analysis, the program will allow the user to group by the categorical variables and perform a subgroups analysis (analysis of variance). Similarly, when entering data the user can create continuous variables, and then perform a meta-regression.

Perform analyses for publication bias

The program will create a funnel plot, will perform the Begg and Mazumdar and the Egger tests for bias, and will report Rosenthal's and Orwin's Fail-safe N. It will also perform the Trim and Fill analysis, and a cumulative analysis sorted by sample size or precision.

Interface with other programs

Users can copy and paste summary data from any Windows-based spreadsheet into CMA. They can also copy any computed values from CMA to the clipboard, and from there into other programs.

Contact information

Web site www.Meta-Analysis.com
e-mail info@Meta-Analysis.com

REVMAN 5.0

RevMan (Review Manager) is the software developed by The Cochrane Collaboration for use with Cochrane reviews, though the program may be used outside the organization as well (see the web site for details). Whereas CMA and the Stata macros provide a mechanism solely for the meta-analysis, RevMan provides a mechanism for all facets of the systematic review, of which the meta-analysis is but one part. This is an advantage for people who want a mechanism for managing all parts of the review, and a critical advantage for researchers who want to upload the completed review to *The Cochrane Library*, as this is the only mechanism for doing so. However, it can be a disadvantage for others as the user needs to go through multiple steps before getting to the analysis itself.

Data entry

The data entry sheet is shown in Figure 44.4. The user enters the data into the white cells. The program computes various statistics and displays these in the shaded cells.

In this example the user has entered the events and total n for each study, and the program has computed the odds ratio. The screenshot has been cropped for clarity (a forest plot is normally displayed as well).

Study or Subgroup	Treated Events	Treated Total	Control Events	Control Total	Weight	Odds Ratio IV, Fixed, 95% CI
☑ Saint	12	65	16	65	12.8%	0.69 [0.30, 1.61]
☑ Kelly	8	40	10	40	8.2%	0.75 [0.26, 2.15]
☑ Pibeam	14	80	19	80	15.2%	0.68 [0.31, 1.48]
☑ Lane	25	400	80	400	40.6%	0.27 [0.17, 0.43]
☑ Wright	8	40	11	40	8.4%	0.66 [0.23, 1.86]
☑ Day	16	65	18	65	14.8%	0.85 [0.39, 1.87]
Total (95% CI)		690		690	100.0%	0.48 [0.36, 0.66]
Total events	83		154			
Heterogeneity: Chi² = 10.55, df = 5 (P = 0.06); I² = 53%						
Test for overall effect: Z = 4.71 (P < 0.00001)						

Figure 44.4 RevMan – data entry screen for 2 x 2 tables.

RevMan will accept data in four formats, which are: events and sample size, means, standard deviations and sample size, O minus E and V, and a generic effect size. All studies in the analysis must be in the same format. A researcher whose data had been provided in multiple formats would need to compute effect sizes and variance for each study externally (for example, using Excel) and then copy the computed effect size and variance into the program.

The program will work with the following effect sizes: Raw mean difference, standardized mean difference (g), odds ratio, risk ratio, and risk difference. The program will also work with a generic effect size.

Analysis

The program displays a screen similar to the one shown here (Figure 44.5). Menus are used to customize many elements of the computational model and display, including the following.

- Display results for fixed or random-effects models.
- Display weights for either model.
- Display a table of statistics including effect size, variance, standard error, confidence limits, Q, T^2, and I^2.

Create a forest plot

The analysis engine can generate a separate forest plot image. While there is limited flexibility in the plot, the design is well thought out and is appropriate for most analyses.

Sensitivity analysis

The user can manually exclude one or more studies from the analysis.

Perform subgroup analysis and meta-regression

Within each study comparison, the program allows the user to enter data by subgroup. The program produces an analysis for each comparison, and, when subgroup variables are entered, groups the results by subgroup. The program will

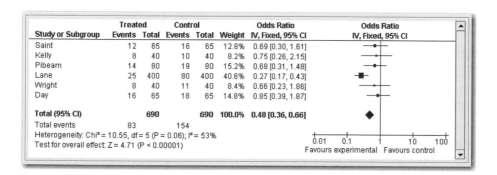

Figure 44.5 RevMan – analysis screen.

perform a separate analysis for each subgroup and will compare the effect across subgroups, but cannot perform a meta-regression.

Perform analyses for publication bias
RevMan will display a funnel plot option but does not offer any tests or procedures for publication bias.

Interface with other programs
Users can copy and paste summary data from any Windows-based spreadsheet into RevMan.

Contact information
Web site www.cc-ims.net/RevMan

STATA MACROS WITH STATA 10.0

Stata is a general purpose statistical package for primary studies, and there are no meta-analysis routines included in the program itself. However, Stata encourages users to develop special-purpose macros (blocks of code) which can then be posted to the Stata web site, and a full set of such macros has been developed for meta-analysis.

Stata is a command-driven program, which means that the user types in a command (for example 'metan TreatedDead TreatedAlive ControlDead ControlAlive, fixed rr') rather than clicking a button to perform an analysis. However, it is generally possible to use a dialog box to generate the command, which simplifies the process.

Someone not familiar with Stata would need to acquire and learn the program before turning to the meta-analysis procedures. However, for researchers who are already using this program, the macros are certainly worth a look. For these people the advantages of this program are the number of available macros, which can perform most of the procedures discussed in this volume, and the number of options available for many of these procedures. The only real disadvantage to using the Stata macros is the rather limited number of data entry formats these macros will accept.

Data entry
The data entry sheet is a spreadsheet. In Figure 44.6 the user has entered the events and non-events for each study.

The standard meta-analysis macro *metan* will accept data in two formats, which are events and non-events, means, standard deviations and sample size, and also in a generic format of effect size and variance. All studies in the analysis must be in the same format. To use the generic format the user would either compute these values for each study outside of Stata, or compute them inside Stata using a series of 'generate' commands prior to calling the meta-analysis macros.

Preserve | Restore | Sort | << | >> | Hide | Delete...

TreatedDead[12] =

	Study	TreatedDead	TreatedAlive	ControlDead	ControlAlive
1	Saint	12	53	16	49
2	Kelly	8	32	10	30
3	Pibeam	14	66	19	61
4	Lane	25	375	80	320
5	Wright	8	32	11	29
6	Day	16	49	18	47

Figure 44.6 Stata macros – data entry screen for 2 × 2 data.

The program will work with the following effect sizes: Raw mean difference, standardized mean difference (Cohen's *d*, Hedges' *g* and Glass' *g*), odds ratio (and log odds ratio), risk ratio (and log risk ratio), and risk difference. Finally, the program will work with a generic effect size.

Analysis

To perform an analysis, the user types a command with the names of the variables and the desired options. The program displays a screen similar to the one shown in Figure 44.7, and will

- Display results for fixed or random-effects models
- Display weights for either model
- Display a table of statistics including effect size, variance, standard error, confidence limits, Q, T^2, and I^2.

```
. db metan

. metan TreatedDead TreatedAlive ControlDead ControlAlive, label(namevar=Study)
> fixedi or

           Study     |     OR     [95% Conf. Interval]     % Weight
---------------------+-----------------------------------------------
Saint                |  0.693       0.298     1.611        12.79
Kelly                |  0.750       0.261     2.153         8.17
Pibeam               |  0.681       0.314     1.475        15.21
Lane                 |  0.267       0.166     0.428        40.61
Wright               |  0.659       0.233     1.865         8.40
Day                  |  0.853       0.390     1.866        14.82
---------------------+-----------------------------------------------
I-V pooled OR        |  0.485       0.359     0.655       100.00
---------------------+-----------------------------------------------

  Heterogeneity chi-squared =  10.55 (d.f. = 5) p = 0.061
  I-squared (variation in OR attributable to heterogeneity) =  52.6%

  Test of OR=1 : z=   4.71 p = 0.000
```

Figure 44.7 Stata macros – analysis screen.

Create a forest plot

The Stata macros will create a forest plot as shown in Figure 44.8. The program allows the user a few options for customizing the plot.

Sensitivity analysis

Macros are available to run the analysis repeatedly, removing a different study on each pass, to show the impact of that study on the results. The user can also define sets of studies and include or remove these as a block by writing the appropriate code.

Perform subgroup analysis and meta-regression

When entering data the user can create categorical variables and enter a value (for example, acute or chronic) for each study. In the analysis, the user can group by the categorical variables and perform a subgroups analysis (analysis of variance). Similarly, when entering data the user can create continuous variables, and then perform a meta-regression.

Perform analyses for publication bias

Macros can create a funnel plot, and perform the Begg and Mazumdar and the Egger tests for bias. They can also perform the Trim and Fill analysis, and a cumulative analysis sorted by sample size or precision.

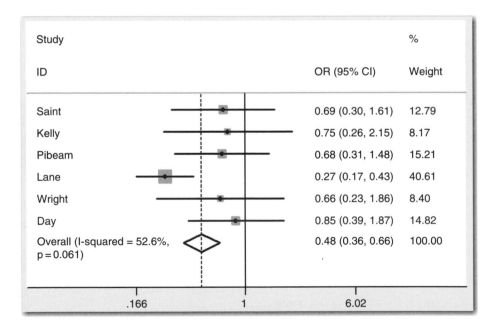

Figure 44.8 Stata macros – high resolution forest plot.

Interface with other programs

Users can copy and paste summary data from any Windows-based spreadsheet into Stata. They can also copy any computed values from Stata to the clipboard, and from there into other programs.

Programs to compute effect sizes only

Some programs are available to assist the effect size calculation alone. For example

- Effect Size Version 2, developed by Will Shadish (http://faculty.ucmerced.edu/wshadish/es.htm)
- An Excel spreadsheet by David Wilson incorporates formulas for many common conversions. (es_calculator.zip, available from http://mason.gmu.edu/~dwilsonb/ma.html)

Microsoft Excel, SPSS, SAS, Stata, Comprehensive Meta Analysis, Metawin, are trademarks of their respective publishers.

SUMMARY POINTS

- We provide an overview of several meta-analysis programs.
- Detailed instructions for using these programs are available at www.Meta-Analysis.com

CHAPTER 45

Books, Web Sites and Professional Organizations

BOOKS ON SYSTEMATIC REVIEW METHODS

Cooper, H., Hedges, L.V., Valentine, J. (eds) (2009) *The Handbook of Research Synthesis*. New York, NY: Russell Sage.

Cooper, H. (2009). *Research Synthesis and Meta-Analysis: A Step-by-Step Approach*. Thousand Oaks, CA: Sage.

Cooper, H. (1998). *Synthesizing Research: A Guide for Literature Reviews*. (3rd edn). Thousand Oaks, CA: Sage.

Egger, M., Smith, G.W. & Altman, D.G. (2001). *Systematic Reviews in Health Care: Meta-analysis in Context* (2nd edn). London, UK: BMJ Books.

Glasziou, P., Irwig, L., Bain, C., Colditz, G. (2001). *Systematic Reviews in Health Care: A Practical Guide*. Cambridge, (UK): Cambridge University Press.

Higgins, J.P.T. & Green, S. (2008). *Cochrane Handbook for Systematic Reviews of Interventions*. Chichester, (UK): John Wiley & Sons, Ltd.

Littell, J.H., Corcoran, J., & Pillai, V. (eds) (2008). *Systematic Reviews and Meta-analysis*. New York, NY: Oxford University Press.

Khan, K.S., Kunz, R., Kleijnen, J., & Antes, G. (2003). *Systematic Reviews to Support Evidence-Based Medicine: How to Apply Findings of Healthcare Research*. London, UK: Royal Society of Medical Press Ltd.

Petticrew, M. & Roberts, H. (2006). *Systematic Reviews in the Social Sciences: A Practical Guide*. Malden, MA: Blackwell.

Sutton, A.J., Abrams, K.R., Ades, A.S., Cooper, N.J., Welton, N. J. (2009) *Evidence Synthesis for Decision Making in Healthcare*. Chichester, UK: John Wiley & Sons, Ltd.

BOOKS ON META-ANALYSIS

Hartung, J., Knapp, G. & Sinha, B.K. (2008). *Statistical Meta-Analysis with Applications*. Hoboken, NJ: John Wiley & Sons, Inc.

Hedges, L.V. & Olkin, I. (1985). *Statistical Methods for Meta-analysis*. San Diego, CA: Academic Press.

Hunter, J.E. & Schmidt, F.L. (2004). *Methods of Meta-analysis: Correcting Error and Bias in Research Findings* (2nd edn). Newbury Park, CA: Sage.

Lipsey, M.W. & Wison, D.B. (2001). *Practical Meta-analysis*. Thousand Oaks, CA: Sage.

Rothstein, H.R., Sutton, A.J., Borenstein, M. *Publication Bias in Meta-analysis: Prevention, Assessment and Adjustments* (2005). Chichester, UK: John Wiley & Sons, Ltd.

Stangl, D.K. & Berry, D.A. (2000). *Meta-analysis inn Medicine and Health Policy*. New York, NY: Marcel Dekker.

Sutton, A.J., Abrams, K.R., Jones, D.R, Song, F. (2000). *Methods for Meta-Analysis in Medical Research*. Chichester, UK: John Wiley & Sons, Ltd.

Whitehead, A. (2002). *Meta-Analysis of Controlled Clinical Trials*. Chichester, UK: John Wiley & Sons, Ltd.

Journals, special issues dedicated to meta-analysis

- *Statistics in Medicine* 1987, vol. 6, no. 3: themed issue on meta-analysis
- *Journal of Educational and Behavioral Statistics* 1992, vol. 17, no. 4: special issue on meta-analysis
- *Statistical Methods in Medical Research* 1993, vol. 2, no. 2: themed issue on meta-analysis
- *International Journal of Epidemiology* 2002, vol. 11, no. 1: themed issue on Systematic reviews and meta-analysis
- *Statistics in Medicine* 2002 vol 21, no 11: proceedings from the 3rd Symposium on Systematic Review Methodology
- *Statistical Methods in Medical Research* 2001, vol. 10, no. 4: themed issue on meta-analysis, overviews and publication bias

WEB SITES

The James Lind Library

www.jameslindlibrary.org

This web site is dedicated to 'Explaining and illustrating the development of fair tests of treatments in health care'. As such, it provides a history of the field, from the earliest randomized trials to the most recent developments. Iain Chalmers and his colleagues have gathered key historical documents that help to put all current work in fascinating perspective.

Comprehensive Meta-Analysis

www.Meta-Analysis.com

This is the site for this book and for the program Comprehensive Meta-Analysis. The site includes the following

- Free trial of Comprehensive Meta-Analysis
- Worked examples for this book and for other books on meta-analysis
- Papers on meta-analysis
- Links to web sites on meta-analysis and systematic reviews
- Links to courses and workshops on meta-analysis and systematic reviews
- Links to relevant conferences

The Cochrane Collaboration

www.Cochrane.org

The Cochrane Collaboration is composed of thousands of persons who work in various fields related to health-care and volunteer some part of their time to collaborate on systematic reviews.

The organization publishes (through Wiley) a database with results of systematic reviews (currently more than 3700) on the utility of healthcare interventions. The organization sponsors an annual international colloquium.

The Campbell Collaboration

www.campbellcollaboration.org

The Campbell Collaboration has a similar set of goals to Cochrane's, but focuses on the social sciences with working groups in such areas as crime and justice, education, and social welfare. The organization sponsors an annual international colloquium.

The Human Genome Epidemiology Network

www.cdc.gov/genomics/hugenet

The Human Genome Epidemiology Network (HuGENet) is a global collaboration committed to the assessment of the impact of human genome variation on population health. Their web site includes numerous systematic reviews (HuGE reviews) and other resources to support meta-analyses of genetic association studies.

References

Abelson, R.P. (1997). A retrospective on the significance test ban of 1999 (If there were no significance tests, they would be invented). In L.L. Harlow, S.A. Mulaik & J.H. Steiger (eds), *What if There Were No Significance Tests? Mahwah*, NJ: Lawrence Erlbaum Associates.

Arthur Jr., W., Bennett Jr., W. & Huffcutt, A. I. (2001). *Conducting Meta-Analysis Using SAS*. Mahwah, NJ: Lawrence Erlbaum Associates.

Bailar, J.C., 3rd. (1997). The promise and problems of meta-analysis. *New England Journal of Medicine*, 337, 559–561.

Becker, B.J. (2005). Failsafe N or file-drawer number. In H.R. Rothstein, A.J. Sutton & M. Borenstein (eds), *Publication Bias in Meta-Analysis: Prevention, Assessment and Adjustments*. Chichester, UK: John Wiley & Sons, Ltd.

Begg, C.B., & Mazumdar, M. (1994). Operating characteristics of a rank correlation test for publication bias. *Biometrics*, 50, 1088–1101.

Berkey, C.S., Hoaglin, D.C., Mosteller, F., & Colditz, G.A. (1995). A random-effects regression model for meta-analysis. *Statistics in Medicine*, 14, 395–411.

Birge, R.T. (1941). The general physical constants. *Reports on Progress in Physics*, 8, 90–101.

Boccia, S., Hung, R., Ricciardi, G., *et al*. (2008). Meta- and pooled analyses of the methylenetetrahydrofolate reductase C677T and A1298C polymorphisms and gastric cancer risk: a huge-GSEC review. *American Journal of Epidemiology*, 167, 505–516.

Borenstein, M. (1994). The case for confidence intervals in controlled clinical trials. *Controlled Clinical Trials*, 15, 411–428.

Borenstein, M. (2000). The shift from significance testing to effect size estimation. In A.S. Bellack & M. Hersen (eds), *Comprehensive Clinical Psychology* (Volume 3, pp. 313–349) Oxford, UK: Pergamon.

Borenstein, M., Hedges, L., Higgins, J., & Rothstein, H. R. (2009). *Computing Effect Sizes for Meta-analysis*. Chichester: John Wiley & Sons, Ltd.

Butler, T.L. (1988). The relationship of passive smoking to various health outcomes among Seventh-Day Adventists in California. University of California: Los Angeles (Dissertation).

Cannon, C.P., Steinberg, B.A., Murphy, S.A., Mega, J.L., & Braunwald, E. (2006). Meta-analysis of cardiovascular outcomes trials comparing intensive versus moderate statin therapy. *Journal of the American College Cardiology*, 48, 438–445.

Chalmers, I. (2006). The scandalous failure of scientists to cumulate scientifically. Abstract to paper presented at: Ninth World Congress on Health Information and Libraries; 2005 Sep 20–23; Salvador, Brazil. (Available online: http://www.icml9.org/program/activity.php?lang=pt&id=21. Accessed on February 3, 2009.

Chalmers, I. (2007). The lethal consequences of failing to make use of all relevant evidence about the effects of medical treatments: the need for systematic reviews. In P. Rothwell (ed.), *Treating Individuals*: *From Randomized Trials to Personalised Medicine* (pp. 37–58). London, UK: Elsevier.

Chan, A.W., Hróbjartsson, A., Haahr, M.T., Gøtzsche, P.C., & Altman, D.G. (2004). Empirical evidence for selective reporting of outcomes in randomized trials: comparison of protocols to published articles. *Journal of the American Medical Association,* 291, 2457–2465.

Chan, W.C., & Fung, S.C. (1982). Lung cancer in non-smokers in Hong Kong. In: E. Grundmann (ed.), *Cancer Campaign.* (Vol 6. Cancer Epidemiology, pp. 199–202). New York, NY: Gustav Fischer.

Clarke, M., & Chalmers, I. (1998). Discussion sections in reports of controlled trials published in general medical journals: islands in search of continents? *Journal of the American Medical Association*, 280, 280–282.

Clarke, M., & Clarke, T. (2000). A study of the references used in Cochrane protocols and reviews. Three bibles, three dictionaries, and nearly 25,000 other things. *International Journal of Technology Assessment in Health Care,* 16, 907–909.

Cohen, J. (1962). The statistical power of abnormal-social psychological research: a review. *Journal of Abnormal and Social Psychology*, 65, 145–153.

Cohen, J. (1969). *Statistical Power Analysis for the Behavioral Sciences.* New York, NY: Academic Press.

Cohen, J. (1987). *Statistical Power Analysis for the Behavioral Sciences.* Hillside, NJ: Lawrence Erlbaum Associates.

Colditz, G.A., Brewer, T.F., Berkey, C.S., *et al.* (1994). Efficacy of BCG vaccine in the prevention of tuberculosis. Meta-analysis of the published literature. *Journal of the American Medical Association*, 271, 698–702.

Crocker, L., & Algina, J. (1986). *Introduction to Classical and Modern Test Theory.* New York, NY: Holt, Rinehart, & Winston.

Devereaux, P.J., Beattie, W.S., Choi, P.T., *et al.* (2005). How strong is the evidence for the use of perioperative beta blockers in non-cardiac surgery? Systematic review and meta-analysis of randomised controlled trials. *BMJ*, 331, 313–321.

Dickersin, K., & Min, Y.I. (1993a). NIH clinical trials and publication bias. *Online Journal of Current Clinical Trials, Doc No 50.*

Dickersin, K., & Min, Y. I. (1993b). Publication bias: the problem that won't go away. *Annals of the New York Academy of Sciences*, 703, 135–146; discussion 146–148.

Dickersin, K., Min, Y.I., & Meinert, C.L. (1992). Factors influencing publication of research results. Follow-up of applications submitted to two institutional review boards. *Journal of the American Medical Association*, 267, 374–378.

Duval, S., & Tweedie, R. (2000a). A nonparametric 'trim and fill' method of accounting for publication bias in meta-analysis. *Journal of the American Statistical Association*, 95, 89–98.

Duval, S., & Tweedie, R. (2000b). Trim and fill: A simple funnel-plot-based method of testing and adjusting for publication bias in meta-analysis. *Biometrics*, 56, 455–463.

Easterbrook, P.J., Berlin, J.A., Gopalan, R., & Matthews, D.R. (1991). *Publication bias in clinical research. Lancet*, 337, 867–872.

Egger, M., Davey Smith, G., Schneider, M., & Minder, C. (1997). Bias in meta-analysis detected by a simple, graphical test. *BMJ*, 315, 629–634.

Egger, M., Smith, G.W., & Altman, D.G. (2001). Systematic Reviews in Health Care: Meta-analysis in Context (2nd edn). London, UK: BMJ Books.

Eysenck, H.J. (1978). An exercise in mega-silliness. *American Psychologist*, 33, 517–519.

Feinstein, A.R. (1995). Meta-analysis: statistical alchemy for the 21st century. *Journal of Clinical Epidemiology*, 48, 71–79.

Freiman, J.A., Chalmers, T.C., Smith, Jr., H., & Kuebler, R.R. (1978). The importance of beta, the type II error and sample size in the design and interpretation of the randomized control trial. Survey of 71 'negative' trials. *New England Journal of Medicine*, 299, 690–694.

Gilbert, R., Salanti, G., Harden, M., & See, S. (2005). Infant sleeping position and the sudden infant death syndrome: systematic review of observational studies and historical review of recommendations from 1940 to 2002. *International Journal of Epidemiology*, 34, 874–887.

Goodman, S.N. (1991). Have you ever meta-analysis you didn't like? *Annals Internal Medicine*, 114, 244–246.

Gøtzsche, P.C. (1987). Reference bias in reports of drug trials. *BMJ*, 295, 654–656.

Grissom, R.J., & Kim, J.J. (2005). *Effect Sizes for Research: A Broad Practical Approach*. Mahwah, NJ: Lawrence Erlbaum Associates.

Hackshaw, A.K., Law, M.R., & Wald, N.J. (1997). The accumulated evidence on lung cancer and environmental tobacco smoke. *BMJ*, 315, 980–988.

Halpern, S.D., & Berlin, J.A. (2005). Beyond conventional publication bias: other determinants of data suppression. In H.R. Rothstein, A.J. Sutton & M. Borenstein (eds), *Publication Bias in Meta-analysis: Prevention, Assessment and Adjustments*. Chichester, UK: John Wiley & Sons, Ltd.

Hartung, J., Cottrell, J.E., & Giffin, J.P. (1983). Absence of evidence is not evidence of absence. *Anesthesiology*, 58, 298–300.

Hasselblad, V., & Hedges, L.V. (1995). Meta-analysis of screening and diagnostic tests. *Psychological Bulletin*, 117, 167–178.

Hedges, L. (1981). Distribution theory for Glass's estimator of effect size and related estimators. *Journal of Educational Statistics*, 6, 107–128.

Hedges, L. (1984) Estimation of effect size under nonrandom sampling: The effects of censoring studies yielding statistically insignificant mean differences. *Journal of Educational Statistics*, 9, 61–85.

Hedges, L. (1989) Estimating the normal mean and variance under a selection model. In L. Gleser, M.D. Perlman, S.J. Press, A.R. Sampson. *Contributions to Probability and Statistics: Essays in Honor of Ingram Olkin* (pp. 447–458). New York, NY: Springer Verlag.

Hedges, L., & Olkin, I. (1980). Vote-counting methods in research synthesis. *Psychological Bulletin*. 88:359–369.

Hedges, L., & Olkin, I. (1985). *Statistical Methods for Meta-analysis*. San Diego, CA: Academic Press.

Hedges, L. and Pigott, T.D. (2001). The power of statistical tests in meta-analysis, *Psychological Methods*, 6, 203–17.

Hedges, L. & Pigott, T.D. (2004). The power of statistical tests for moderators in meta-analysis. *Psychological Methods*, 9, 426–445.

Hedges, L., Gurevitch, J., & Curtis, P. (1999). The meta-analysis of response ratios in experimental ecology. *Ecology*, 80, 1150–1156.

Higgins, J. P. T. & Green S. (2008). *Cochrane Handbook for Systematic Reviews of Interventions*. Chichester, UK: John Wiley & Sons, Ltd.

Higgins, J., & Thompson, S.G. (2002). Quantifying heterogeneity in a meta-analysis. *Statistics in Medicine*, 21, 1539–1558.

Higgins, J., Thompson, S.G., Deeks, J.J., & Altman, D.G. (2003). Measuring inconsistency in meta-analyses. *BMJ*, 327, 557–560.

Higgins, J., & Thompson, S.G. (2004). Controlling the risk of spurious findings from meta-regression. *Statistics in Medicine*, 23: 1663–1682.

Hopewell, S., Clarke, M., & Mallett, S. (2005). Grey literature and systematic reviews. In H.R. Rothstein, A. J. Sutton & M. Bornstein (Eds). *Publication Bias in Meta-Analysis*: *Prevention, Assessment and Adjustments*. Chichester, UK: John Wiley & Sons, Ltd.

Hunter, J.E., & Schmidt, F.L. (1990). *Methods of Meta-analysis: Correcting Error and Bias in Research Findings*. Newbury Park, CA: Sage Publications.

Hunter, J.E., & Schmidt, F.L. (2004). *Methods of Meta-analysis: Correcting Error and Bias in Research Findings* (2nd edn). Newbury Park, CA: Sage Publications.

Jüni, P., Holenstein, F., Sterne, J., Bartlett, C., & Egger, M. (2002). Direction and impact of language bias in meta-analyses of controlled trials: empirical study. *International Journal of Epidemiology*, 31, 115–123.

Kane, J.M., & Borenstein, M. (1985). Compliance in the long-term treatment of schizophrenia. *Psychopharmacology Bulletin*, 21, 23–27.

Knapp, G. & Hartung, J. (2003). Improved tests for a random effects meta-regression with a single covariate. *Statistics in Medicine*, 22, 2693–2710.

Lacasaña-Navarro, M., Galvan-Portillo, M., Chen, J., Lopez-Cervantes, M., & Lopez-Carrillo, L. (2006). Methylenetetrahydrofolate reductase 677C > T polymorphism and gastric cancer susceptibility in Mexico. *European Journal of Cancer*, 42, 528–533.

Lau, J., Antman, E. M., Jimenez-Silva, J., Kupelnick, B., Mosteller, F., & Chalmers, T. C. (1992). Cumulative meta-analysis of therapeutic trials for myocardial infarction. *New England Journal of Medicine*, 327, 248–254.

Lau, J., & Chalmers, T. C. (1995). The rational use of therapeutic drugs in the 21st century. Important lessons from cumulative meta-analyses of randomized control trials. *International Journal of Technology Assessment in Health Care*, 11, 509–522.

Lau, J., Schmid, C.H., & Chalmers, T.C. (1995). Cumulative meta-analysis of clinical trials builds evidence for exemplary medical care. *Journal of Clinical Epidemiology*, 48, 45–57; discussion 59–60.

LeLorier, J., Gregoire, G., Benhaddad, A., Lapierre, J., & Derderian, F. (1997). Discrepancies between meta-analyses and subsequent large randomized, controlled trials. *New England Journal of Medicine*, 337, 536–542.

Lewis, S., & Clarke, M. (2001). Forest plots: trying to see the wood and the trees. *BMJ*, 322(7300), 1479–1480.

Light, R.J., & Pillemer, D.B. (1984). *Summing up: The Science of Reviewing Research*. Cambridge, MA: Harvard University Press.

Light, R.J., Singer, J.D., & Willett, J.B. (1994). The visual presentation and interpretation of meta-analyses. In M. Cooper & L.V. Hedges (eds), *The Handbook of Research Synthesis*. New York, NY: Russell Sage Foundation.

Lord, F.M., & Novick, M.R. (1968). *Statistical Theories of Mental Test Scores*. Reading, MA: Addison-Wesley.

Mallet, S., Hopewell, S., & Clarke, M. (2002). The use of grey literature in the first 1000 Cochrane reviews. Paper presented at the Fourth Symposium on Systematic Reviews: Pushing the Boundaries; 2002 Jul 2-4; Oxford, UK.

Mann, C. (1990). Meta-analysis in the breech, *Science,* 249, 476–480.

Meehl, P.E. (1978). Theoretical risks and tabular asterisks: Sir Karl, Sir Ronald, and the slow progress of soft psycholoy. *Journal of Consulting and Clinical Psychology*, 46, 806–834.

Meehl, P.E. (1990). Why summaries of research on psychological theories are often uninterpretable. *Psychological Reports*, 66, 195–244.

Normand, S. L. (1999). Meta-analysis: formulating, evaluating, combining, and reporting. *Statistics in Medicine*, 18: 321–59.

O'Farrell, N., & Egger, M. (2000). Circumcision in men and the prevention of HIV infection: a 'meta-analysis' revisited. *International Journal of STD and AIDS*, 11, 137–142.

Orwin, R.G., & Boruch, R.F. (1983). RRT meets RDD: statistical strategies for assuring response privacy in telephone surveys. *Public Opinion Quarterly,* 46, 560–571.

Phillips, W.C., Scott, J.A., & Blasczcynski, G. (1983). Statistics for diagnostic procedures. II. The significance of 'no significance': what a negative statistical test really means. *American Journal of Roentgenology*, 141, 203–206.

Pogue, J., & Yusuf, S. (1998). Overcoming the limitations of current meta-analysis of randomised controlled trials. *Lancet*, 351, 47–52.

Ravnskov, U. (1992). Frequency of citation and outcome of cholesterol lowering trials. *BMJ*, 305, 717.

Reed, J.F., 3rd, & Slaichert, W. (1981). Statistical proof in inconclusive 'negative' trials. *Archives of Internal Medicine*, 141, 1307–1310.

Reed, J.G., & Baxter, P.M. (2009). Using reference databases. In H. Cooper, L.V. Hedges & J. Valentine (eds), *The Handbook of Research Synthesis* (2nd edn). New York, NY: Sage Publications.

Reynolds, T.B. (1980). Type II error in clinical trials (editor's reply to letter). *Gastroenterology*, 79, 180.

Rona, R.J., Keil, T., Summers, C., *et al.* (2007). The prevalence of food allergy: a meta-analysis. *Journal of Allergy and Clinical Immunology*, 120, 638–646.

Rosenthal, R. (1979). The File drawer problem and tolerance for null results. *Psychological Bulletin*, 86, 638–641.

Rossi, J. (1997). A case study in the failure of psychology as a cumulative science: The spontaneous recovery of verbal learning. In L.L. Harlow, S.A. Mulaik & J.H. Steiger (eds), *What if There Were No Significance Tests?* (pp. 175–198). Mahwah, NJ: Laurence Erlbaum Associates.

Rossi, J.S. (1990). Statistical power of psychological research: what have we gained in 20 years? *Journal of Consulting and Clinical Psychology*, 58, 646–656.

Rothstein, H.R. (2006). Use of unpublished data in systematic reviews in the *Psychological Bulletin* 1995–2005. Unpublished manuscript.

Rothstein, H.R., & Hopewell, S. (2009). The Grey literature. In H. Cooper, L. V. Hedges & J. Valentine (eds), *The Handbook of Research Synthesis* (2nd edn). New York, NY: Sage Publications.

Sanchez-Meca, J., Marin-Martinez, F., & Chacon-Moscoso, S. (2003). Effect-size indices for dichotomized outcomes in meta-analysis. *Psychological Methods*, 8, 448–467.

Schmidt, F.L. (1996). Statistical significance testing and cumulative knowledge in psychology: Implications for training of researchers. *Psychological Methods*, 1, 115–129.

Sedlmeier, P., & Gigerenzer, G. (1989). Do studies of statistical power have an effect on the power of studies? *Psychological Bulletin*, 105, 309–316.

Shapiro, S. (1994). Meta-analysis/shmeta-analysis. *American Journal of Epidemiology*, 140, 771–778.

Sirmans, G.S., Macdonald, L., Macpherson, D.A., & Zietz, E.N. (2006). The value of housing characteristics: a meta analysis. *Journal of Real Estate Finance and Economics*, 33, 215–240.

Sterne, J.A., & Egger, M. (2001). Funnel plots for detecting bias in meta-analysis: guidelines on choice of axis. *Journal of Clinical Epidemiology*, 54, 1046–1055.

Sterne, J.A., Egger, M., & Smith, G.D. (2001). Systematic reviews in health care: Investigating and dealing with publication and other biases in meta-analysis. *BMJ*, 323, 101–105.

Sterne, J.A., Gavaghan, D., & Egger, M. (2000). Publication and related bias in meta-analysis: power of statistical tests and prevalence in the literature. *Journal of Clinical Epidemiology*, 53, 1119–1129.

Stewart, L.A., & Tierney, J.F. (2002). To IPD or not to IPD? Advantages and disadvantages of systematic reviews using individual patient data. *Evaluation and the Health Professions*, 25, 76–97.

Sutton, A.J., Abrams, K.R., Jones, D.R., & Song, F. (2000). *Methods for Meta-analysis in Medical Research*. Chichester, UK: John Wiley & Sons, Ltd.

Tramer, M.R., Reynolds, D.J., Moore, R.A., & McQuay, H.J. (1997). Impact of covert duplicate publication on meta-analysis: a case study. *BMJ*, 315, 635–640.

van Houwelingen, H. C., Arends, L.R., Stijnen, T. (2002). Advanced methods in meta-analysis: multivariate approach and meta-regression. *Statistics in Medicine*, 21: 589–624.

Van Howe, R.S. (1999). Circumcision and HIV infection: review of the literature and meta-analysis. *International Journal of STD and AIDS*, 10, 8–16.

Wade, A., Turner, H.M., Rothstein, H.R., & Lavenberg, J. (2006). Information retrieval and the role of the information specialist in producing high quality systematic reviews in the social, behavioral, and education sciences. *Evidence and Policy*, 2, 89–108.

Wang, M.C. and Bushman, B.J. (1999). *Integrating results through Meta-Analytic Review Using SAS Software*. Cart, NC: SAS Institute.

Weisz, J.R., Weiss, B., Han, S.S., Granger, D.A., & Morton, T. (1995). Effects of psychotherapy with children and adolescents revisited: a meta-analysis of treatment outcome studies. *Psychological Bulletin*, 117, 450–468.

Whitehead, A. (2002). *Meta-analysis of Controlled Clinical Trials*. Chichester, UK: John Wiley & Sons, Ltd.

Whitehead, J. (1997). *The Design and Analysis of Sequential Clinical Trials* (*rev.* 2nd edn). NY: Chichester, UK: John Wiley & Sons, Inc.

Williams, J., Brayne, C., & Higgins, J.P.T. (2006). Systematic review of prevalence studies of autism spectrum disorders. *Archives of Disease in Childhood*, 91, 8–15.

Wilson, S.J., Lipsey, M.W., & Derzon, J. H. (2003a). The effects of school-based intervention programs on aggressive behavior: A meta-analysis. *Journal of Consulting and Clinical Psychology*, 71, 136–149.

Wilson, S. J., Lipsey, M. W., & Soydan, H. (2003b). Are mainstream programs for juvenile delinquency less effective with minority youth than majority youth? A meta-analysis of outcomes research. *Research on Social Work Practice*, 13, 3–26.

Index

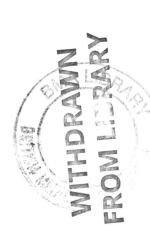